AF389395

10th Anniversary of JCM—Recent Diagnostic and Therapeutic Advance in Gastroenterology and Hepatopancreatobiliary Medicine

10th Anniversary of JCM—Recent Diagnostic and Therapeutic Advance in Gastroenterology and Hepatopancreatobiliary Medicine

Editor

Hidekazu Suzuki

MDPI • Basel • Beijing • Wuhan • Barcelona • Belgrade • Manchester • Tokyo • Cluj • Tianjin

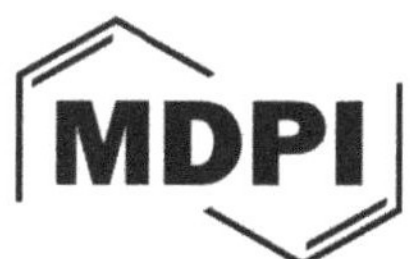

Editor
Hidekazu Suzuki
Tokai University School of
Medicine
Isehara, Japan

Editorial Office
MDPI
St. Alban-Anlage 66
4052 Basel, Switzerland

This is a reprint of articles from the Special Issue published online in the open access journal *Journal of Clinical Medicine* (ISSN 2077-0383) (available at: https://www.mdpi.com/journal/jcm/special_issues/Gastroenterology_Hepatopancreatobiliary).

For citation purposes, cite each article independently as indicated on the article page online and as indicated below:

LastName, A.A.; LastName, B.B.; LastName, C.C. Article Title. *Journal Name* **Year**, *Volume Number*, Page Range.

ISBN 978-3-0365-8392-1 (Hbk)
ISBN 978-3-0365-8393-8 (PDF)

Contents

Journal of
Clinical Medicine

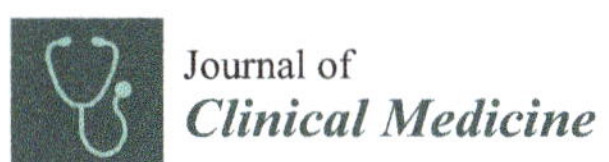

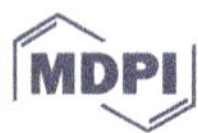

Editorial

Special Issue: "10th Anniversary of JCM—Recent Diagnostic and Therapeutic Advances in Gastroenterology and Hepatopancreatobiliary Medicine"

Takashi Ueda and Hidekazu Suzuki *

Division of Gastroenterology and Hepatology, Department of Internal Medicine, Tokai University School of Medicine, 143 Shimokasuya, Isehara, Kanagawa 259-1193, Japan
* Correspondence: hsuzuki@tokai.ac.jp

Citation: Ueda, T.; Suzuki, H. Special Issue: "10th Anniversary of JCM—Recent Diagnostic and Therapeutic Advances in Gastroenterology and Hepatopancreatobiliary Medicine". *J. Clin. Med.* **2022**, *11*, 6008. https://doi.org/10.3390/jcm11206008

Received: 29 September 2022
Accepted: 10 October 2022
Published: 12 October 2022

Publisher's Note: MDPI stays neutral with regard to jurisdictional claims in published maps and institutional affiliations.

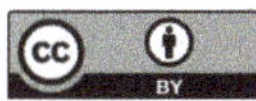

This Special Issue, "10th Anniversary of JCM—Recent Diagnostic and Therapeutic Advances in Gastroenterology and Hepatopancreatobiliary Medicine", presents five original articles and two review articles.

In this issue, three original articles from Japan are related to the evaluation of the latest endoscopic technology, from which we can see that advanced innovations are being made that are constantly evolving. Among them, the progress of new endoscopic diagnoses using image enhancement technology is remarkable. Nishizawa et al. in our team investigated the effectiveness of texture- and color-enhancement imaging (TXI, Olympus Co. Ltd. Tokyo, Japan) in the imaging of serrated colorectal polyps, including sessile serrated lesions (SSLs) [1]. In their investigation, SSLs were observed using white-light imaging (WLI), TXI, narrow-band imaging (NBI), and chromoendoscopy with and without magnification. We concluded that TXI was significantly superior to WLI but inferior to chromoendoscopy in the imaging of serrated polyps and the sub-analysis of SSLs [1]. In addition to TXI, each endoscope manufacturer introduced new technologies one after another.

Remarkable advances have also been made in treatment instruments for endoscopic submucosal dissection. Fujinami et al. evaluated the utility of the S-O clip during colorectal endoscopic submucosal dissection (ESD) [2]. They compared the time required for endoscopic treatment, the dissection speed, the en bloc resection rate, and the complication rate between the groups. The S-O clip group had a significantly shorter surgery duration, a significantly higher dissection speed, a significantly higher en bloc resection rate (98.8% vs. 80.9%; $p \leq 0.001$), and a significantly lower perforation rate (1.3% vs. 4.3%) than the non-S-O clip group, especially in cases of lesions in the right colon [2].

On the other hand, insufflation during endoscopy may cause gastrointestinal symptoms. Therefore, the amount of insufflation should be as small as possible. Furthermore, it is thought that these symptoms can be alleviated by replacing ordinary air with CO_2. Fujisawa et al. reported the effectiveness of CO_2 insufflation in patients undergoing nasal endoscopy without sedation [3]. According to their study, visual analog scale (VAS) scores for abdominal distension (15.4 vs. 25.5; $p < 0.001$) and distress from flatus (16.0 vs. 28.8; $p < 0.001$) 2 h postprocedure were significantly reduced in the CO_2 group [3].

Gastric cancer screening programs are a major problem, especially in East Asian countries where gastric cancer deaths are high. In Japan, while endoscopic gastric cancer screening has been initiated nationwide, the incidence of *Helicobacter pylori* infection has decreased, and the number of cases following *H. pylori* eradication has increased. Moreover, the importance of ABC classification (combination of anti-*H. pylori* IgG antibody test with serum pepsinogen test), which reflects *H. pylori* infection status and gastric atrophy before endoscopic screening, is increasingly recognized. Yashima et al. emphasized that considering its cost effectiveness, disseminating the use of endoscopic screening would be advantageous in establishing a new medical examination provision system that conducts examinations at appropriate screening intervals according to the individual's background and gastric cancer risks [4].

Gastrointestinal bleeding is a disease with a poor prognosis, especially in older adults and in patients with comorbidities; not only might hemostasis affect prognosis, but so might early drug intervention. In this Special Issue, Ting et al. examined whether early tranexamic acid (TXA) administration reduced the risk of mortality in Taiwanese patients with gastrointestinal bleeding [5]. The incidence of mortality significantly decreased during the first and fourth weeks (adjusted HR (aHR): 0.65, 95% CI: 0.56–0.75). A Kaplan–Meier curve revealed a significant decrease in the cumulative incidence of mortality in the early TXA treatment group (log-rank test, $p < 0.0001$). Conversely, thromboembolic events were not significantly associated with early or late TXA treatment (aHR: 1.03, 95% CI: 0.94–1.12). The Kaplan–Meier curve also revealed no significant difference in either venous or arterial events (log-rank test: $p = 0.3654$ and 0.0975, respectively). They concluded that early TXA treatment was associated with a reduced risk of mortality in patients with gastrointestinal bleedig, without an increase in thromboembolic events [5].

For the treatment of ulcerative colitis and Crohn's disease, many therapeutic options, including biological agents, have been introduced in recent years. Such new therapeutic interventions are expected to have positive effects on the long-term prognosis and quality of life of patients. As you all know, Crohn's disease (CD) is known to lead to a poor health-related quality of life (HRQoL). Presented in this Special Issue is a systematic review by Aladraj et al., who evaluated the effects of biological agents and small-molecule drugs in improving the HRQoL of patients with moderate-to-severe CD [6]. Among the 16 multicenter, multinational RCTs, 13 studies showed a significant ($p < 0.05$) improvement in the HRQoL of patients with CD, and finally, revealed a substantial improvement in the HRQoL of patients with CD using biological agents and small-molecule drugs [6].

Furthermore, from the field of liver surgery, Katou et al. also presented new findings regarding surgery for liver metastases [7]. They evaluated the outcomes of patients who underwent liver surgery for liver metastasis of non-colorectal and non-neuroendocrine tumors (NCRNNELMs) and colorectal liver metastases (CRLMs) [7]; they analyzed the prognostic factors of overall and recurrence-free survival, and compared survival between the two groups. The 5-year overall survival rates were 38% for NCRNNELM and 55% for CRLM, suggesting that resection for NCRNNELM showed comparable results to resection for CRLM [7].

In this Special Issue, we assemble these seven outstanding articles showing advances in endoscopic technology, the current state of gastric cancer screening programs in Japan, drug interventions for gastrointestinal bleeding, quality of life in patients with Crohn's disease with recent new biological treatment options, and liver metastasis surgery. We believe that this special feature will bring further progress in the field of Gastroenterology and Hepatopancreatobiliary Medicine.

Funding: This research received no external funding.

Conflicts of Interest: The authors declare no conflict of interest.

References

1. Nishizawa, T.; Toyoshima, O.; Yoshida, S.; Uekura, C.; Kurokawa, K.; Munkhjargal, M.; Obata, M.; Yamada, T.; Fujishiro, M.; Ebinuma, H.; et al. TXI (Texture and Color Enhancement Imaging) for Serrated Colorectal Lesions. *J. Clin. Med.* **2021**, *11*, 119. [CrossRef] [PubMed]
2. Fujinami, H.; Teramoto, A.; Takahashi, S.; Ando, T.; Kajiura, S.; Yasuda, I. Effectiveness of S-O Clip-Assisted Colorectal Endoscopic Submucosal Dissection. *J. Clin. Med.* **2021**, *11*, 141. [CrossRef]
3. Fujisawa, T.; Fukuda, H.; Sakamoto, N.; Hojo, M.; Tomishima, K.; Ishii, S.; Yokokawa, H.; Saita, M.; Naito, T.; Nagahara, A.; et al. Relief Effect of Carbon Dioxide Insufflation in Transnasal Endoscopy for Health Checks—A Prospective, Double-Blind, Case-Control Trial. *J. Clin. Med.* **2022**, *11*, 1231. [CrossRef]
4. Yashima, K.; Shabana, M.; Kurumi, H.; Kawaguchi, K.; Isomoto, H. Gastric Cancer Screening in Japan: A Narrative Review. *J. Clin. Med.* **2022**, *11*, 4337. [CrossRef] [PubMed]

5. Ting, K.H.; Shiu, B.H.; Yang, S.F.; Liao, P.L.; Huang, J.Y.; Chen, Y.Y.; Yeh, C.B. Risk of Mortality among Patients with Gastrointestinal Bleeding with Early and Late Treatment with Tranexamic Acid: A Population-Based Cohort Study. *J. Clin. Med.* **2022**, *11*, 1741. [CrossRef]
6. Aladraj, H.; Abdulla, M.; Guraya, S.Y.; Guraya, S.S. Health-Related Quality of Life of Patients Treated with Biological Agents and New Small-Molecule Drugs for Moderate to Severe Crohn's Disease: A Systematic Review. *J. Clin. Med.* **2022**, *11*, 3743. [CrossRef]
7. Katou, S.; Schmid, F.; Silveira, C.; Schafer, L.; Naim, T.; Becker, F.; Radunz, S.; Juratli, M.A.; Seifert, L.L.; Heinzow, H.; et al. Surgery for Liver Metastasis of Non-Colorectal and Non-Neuroendocrine Tumors. *J. Clin. Med.* **2022**, *11*, 1906. [CrossRef] [PubMed]

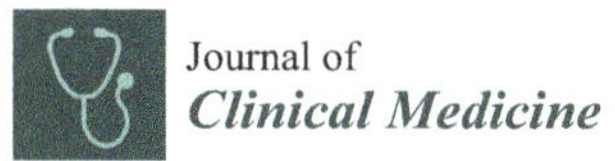

Journal of
Clinical Medicine

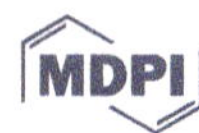

Article

TXI (Texture and Color Enhancement Imaging) for Serrated Colorectal Lesions

Toshihiro Nishizawa [1,2], Osamu Toyoshima [1], Shuntaro Yoshida [1], Chie Uekura [1,3], Ken Kurokawa [1,3], Munkhbayar Munkhjargal [2], Miho Obata [1,3], Tomoharu Yamada [1,3], Mitsuhiro Fujishiro [3], Hirotoshi Ebinuma [2] and Hidekazu Suzuki [4,*]

1   Gastroenterology, Toyoshima Endoscopy Clinic, Tokyo 157-0066, Japan; nisizawa@kf7.so-net.ne.jp (T.N.); t@ichou.com (O.T.); shungtang@hotmail.com (S.Y.); kouchiei@gmail.com (C.U.); kurokawak-int@h.u-tokyo.ac.jp (K.K.); miho.littlefield@hotmail.com (M.O.); tyism123@gmail.com (T.Y.)
2   Department of Gastroenterology and Hepatology, International University of Health and Welfare, Narita Hospital, Narita 286-8520, Japan; mb99md@gmail.com (M.M.); ebinuma@me.com (H.E.)
3   Department of Gastroenterology, Graduate School of Medicine, The University of Tokyo, Tokyo 113-8655, Japan; mtfujish@gmail.com
4   Division of Gastroenterology and Hepatology, Department of Internal Medicine, Tokai University School of Medicine, Isehara 259-1193, Japan
*   Correspondence: hsuzuki@tokai.ac.jp; Tel.: +81-463-93-1121

Abstract: Background and aim: Olympus Corporation released the texture and color enhancement imaging (TXI) technology as a novel image-enhancing endoscopic technique. We investigated the effectiveness of TXI in the imaging of serrated colorectal polyps, including sessile serrated lesions (SSLs). Methods: Serrated colorectal polyps were observed using white light imaging (WLI), TXI, narrow-band imaging (NBI), and chromoendoscopy with and without magnification. Serrated polyps were histologically confirmed. TXI was compared with WLI, NBI, and chromoendoscopy for the visibility of the lesions without magnification and for that of the vessel and surface patterns with magnification. Three expert endoscopists evaluated the visibility scores, which were classified from 1 to 4. Results: Twenty-nine consecutive serrated polyps were evaluated. In the visibility score without magnification, TXI was significantly superior to WLI but inferior to chromoendoscopy in the imaging of serrated polyps and the sub-analysis of SSLs. In the visibility score for vessel patterns with magnification, TXI was significantly superior to WLI and chromoendoscopy in the imaging of serrated polyps and the sub-analysis of SSLs. In the visibility score for surface patterns with magnification, TXI was significantly superior to WLI but inferior to NBI in serrated polyps and in the sub-analysis of SSLs and hyperplastic polyps. Conclusions: TXI provided higher visibility than did WLI for serrated, colorectal polyps, including SSLs.

Keywords: TXI; sessile serrated lesion; hyperplastic polyp; colonoscopy

Citation: Nishizawa, T.; Toyoshima, O.; Yoshida, S.; Uekura, C.; Kurokawa, K.; Munkhjargal, M.; Obata, M.; Yamada, T.; Fujishiro, M.; Ebinuma, H.; et al. TXI (Texture and Color Enhancement Imaging) for Serrated Colorectal Lesions. *J. Clin. Med.* **2022**, *11*, 119. https://doi.org/10.3390/jcm11010119

Academic Editors: Hiroyuki Yoshida and Hajime Isomoto

Received: 3 December 2021
Accepted: 24 December 2021
Published: 27 December 2021

Publisher's Note: MDPI stays neutral with regard to jurisdictional claims in published maps and institutional affiliations.

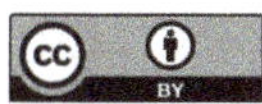

1. Introduction

Globally, colorectal cancer is the third most diagnosed malignancy [1]. The endoscopic resection of colorectal polyps could reduce colorectal cancer mortality by over 50%, providing evidence for the importance of endoscopic resection [2,3].

Recently, the serrated polyp–cancer sequence has received considerable attention, and it is responsible for up to 20% of all sporadic colorectal cancers. Serrated polyps are classified into three categories: hyperplastic polyps (HPs), sessile serrated lesions (SSLs), and traditional serrated adenomas [4]. Of these, SSL and traditional serrated adenoma are both precursors of cancer [5]. SSL predominantly occurs in the right side of the colon and is associated with B-RAF mutation and high microsatellite instability [6]. SSL is often difficult to detect because it typically has indistinct borders, and the color is similar to the background mucosa or is slightly faded [7]. SSL is often overlooked, though it accounts for a significant proportion of interval cancers [8]. Thus, it is desirable to improve the detection sensitivity for SSL.

Recently, Olympus Corporation released texture and color enhancement imaging (TXI) as an image-enhanced endoscopy technology in the new endoscopy system EVIS X1. Briefly, TXI enhances texture and color and adjusts brightness. TXI consists of six consecutive processes: (i) The input image is split into a base layer and detail layer. (ii) The brightness in the dark regions of the base layer is adjusted. (iii) Tone-mapping is applied to the corrected base layer. (iv) Texture enhancement is applied to the detail layer to enhance the subtle contrast. (v) The base layer after tone-mapping and the detail layer after texture enhancement are recombined. A TXI image produced in the fifth step is TXI mode 2 (texture and brightness enhancement). (vi) Color enhancement is applied to the output of TXI mode 1 to more clearly define the slight color contrast. The color enhancement algorithm of TXI was designed to expand the color difference between red and white hues in the image. TXI more greatly improves the visibility for colorectal adenoma than does white light imaging (WLI). In this study, we investigate the effectiveness of TXI for colorectal serrated polyps, especially SSLs.

2. Methods

2.1. Patients

We enrolled patients who underwent endoscopic resection for serrated colorectal lesions at Toyoshima Endoscopy Clinic from March to June 2021. When colorectal lesions were endoscopically diagnosed or were suspected to be SSLs, they were removed. When patients had multiple polyps, the polyps were treated individually. All of the resected specimens were examined histologically under hematoxylin and eosin staining. Indications for colonoscopy included the evaluation for symptoms, examination for a positive fecal occult blood test, polyp surveillance, and a medical check-up [9].

2.2. Ethics

This study was conducted in accordance with the ethical guidelines of the Declaration of Helsinki. This study was approved by the Certificated Review Board of Yoyogi Mental Clinic on 16 July 2021 (approval no. RKK227).

2.3. Endoscopy

We used the EVIS X1 video system center (CV-1500), a 4K resolution ultra-high-definition liquid crystal display monitor (OEV321UH), and a CF-HQ290Z colonoscope (Olympus Corp., Tokyo, Japan). For chromoendoscopy, we used 0.05% indigo carmine [10].

One expert endoscopist performed the colonoscopy and observation using the WLI, TXI, narrow band imaging (NBI), and chromoendoscopy modalities [11]. Lesions were first washed carefully with water to remove the mucus. Images were then obtained through WL, TXI, and NBI with distanced observation, followed by magnified observation. The lesions were subsequently stained for chromoendoscopy with indigo carmine, and images were obtained with and without magnification. TXI has mode 1 and mode 2. Mode 2 involves texture enhancement and brightness adjustment, and mode 1 adds color enhancement to mode 2. Mode 1 was used in this study.

2.4. Visibility Scoring

We investigated the visibility of the lesions, the vessel patterns, and surface patterns.

The visibility of the lesions was defined as the detectability of the lesions without magnification. The visibility of the vessel patterns was defined as the visibility of microvessels and varicose microvascular vessels using magnification. The visibility of the surface patterns was defined as the visibility of the mucosal structure, including the white zone, pit, and expanded crypt opening, using magnification. An expanded crypt opening is a feature of SSLs.

As in previous reports, the visibility score was defined as follows: 4, excellent (easily detectable); 3, good (detectable with careful observation); 2, fair (hardly detectable without careful examination); and 1, poor (not detectable without repeated careful examination) [12,13]. Representative images of each score are shown in Figures 1 and 2. Three expert endoscopists evaluated the visibility scores.

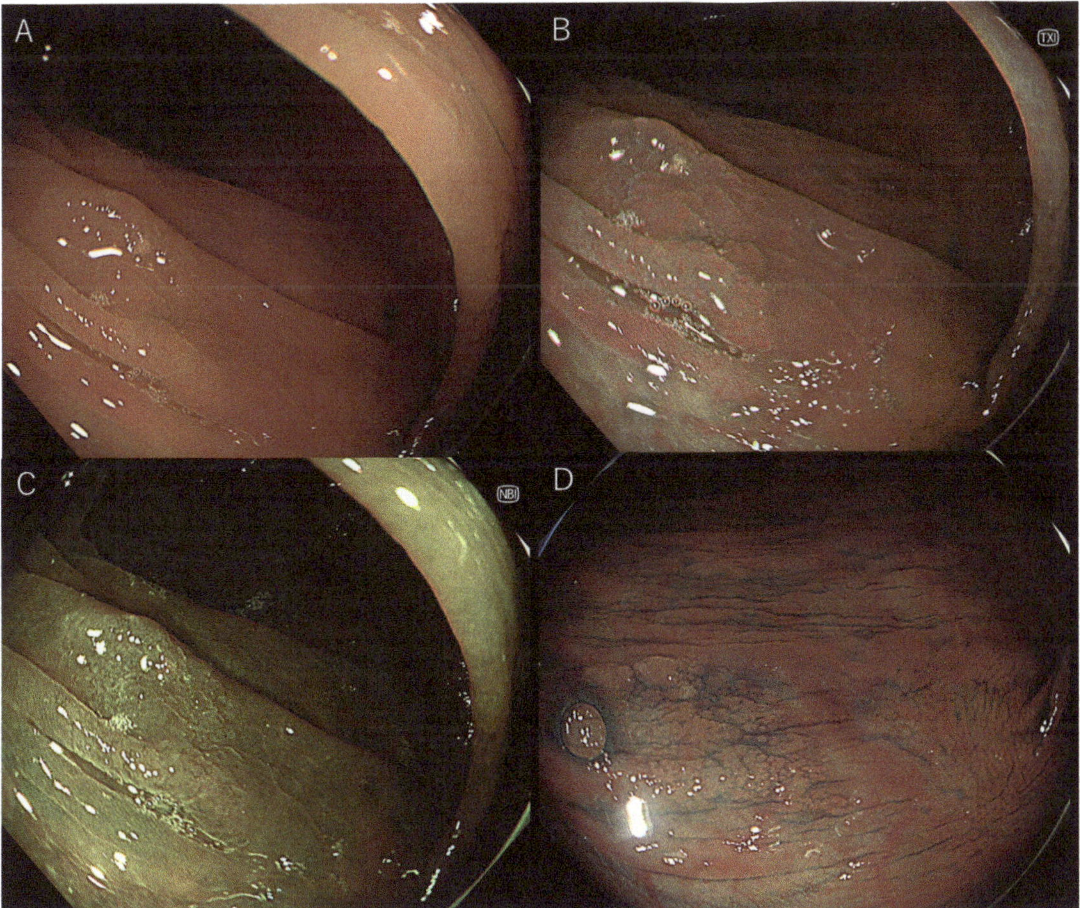

Figure 1. Representative images of a sessile serrated lesion without magnification. (**A**) white-light imaging, (**B**) texture and color enhancement imaging, (**C**) narrow-band imaging, (**D**) chromoendoscopy.

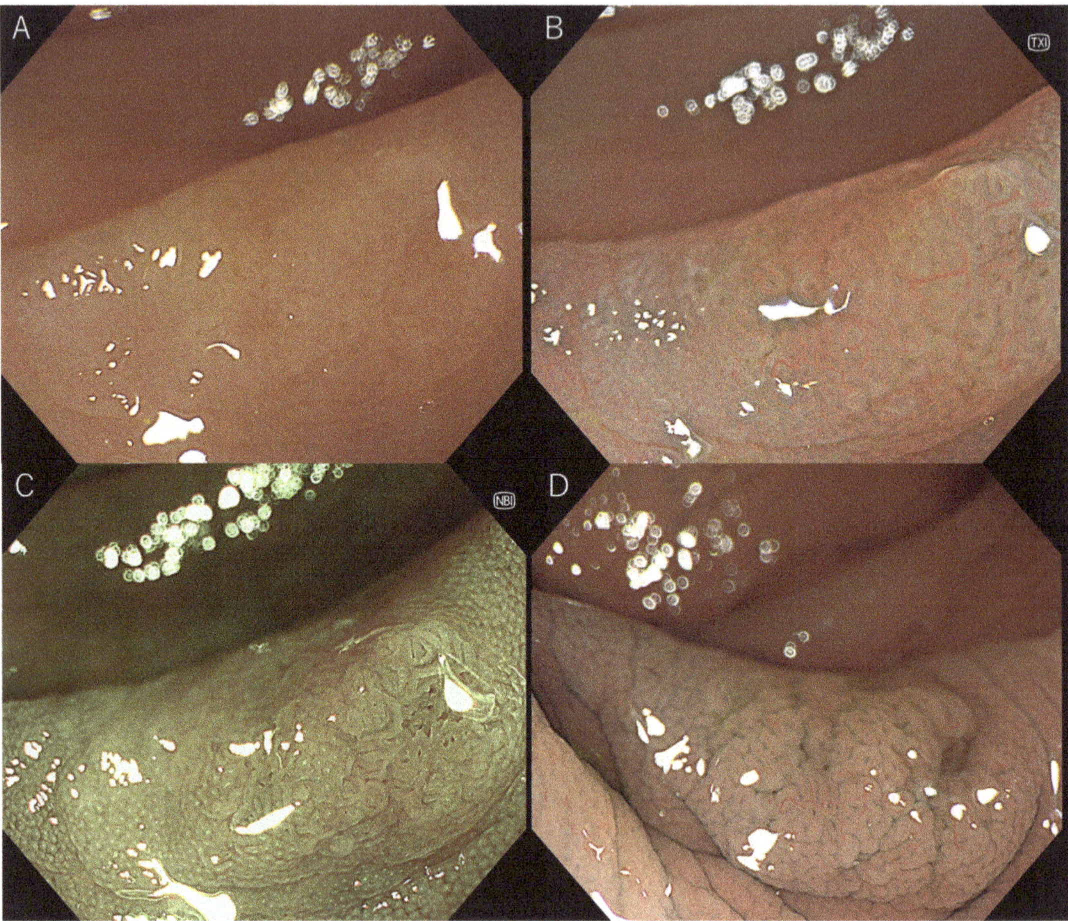

Figure 2. Representative images of sessile serrated lesion with magnification. (**A**) white-light imaging, (**B**) texture and color enhancement imaging, (**C**) narrow-band imaging, (**D**) chromoendoscopy.

2.5. Statistical Analysis

The continuous variables are expressed as mean ± standard deviation (SD). Continuous data between the four groups were compared using Dunn's test with the Kruskal–Wallis test. Continuous data between the two groups were compared using the signed-rank test. Calculations were performed using Stat Mate IV software (version 4.01, ATOMS, Tokyo, Japan). Statistical significance was defined as a $p < 0.05$.

3. Results

3.1. Patients

Table 1 shows the clinicopathological characteristics of the 27 consecutive patients with 29 serrated polyps evaluated in this study. Histologically, there were 18 SSLs and 11 microvesicular mucin-rich type hyperplastic polyps.

Table 1. Clinicopathological characteristics of patients and adenomas.

Serrated Polyps, *n.*	29
Histological subtype; *n.*	
Sessile serrated lesion	18
Microvesicular mucin-rich type hyperplastic polyp	11
Goblet cell-rich type hyperplastic polyp	0
Location; *n.*, cecum, ascending, transverse, descending, sigmoid, rectum	4, 12, 10, 0, 3, 0
Size, mean (standard deviation, range); mm	9.0 (4.29, 3–18)
Morphology; *n.*, Ip, Is, IIa, IIb	0, 0, 29, 0

3.2. Visibility Score for the Lesion without Magnification

The lesion visibility score of TXI was significantly higher than that of WLI but lower than that of chromoendoscopy in serrated polyps and the sub-analysis of SSLs (Table 2).

Table 2. Visibility scores without magnification for WLI, TXI, NBI, and chromoendoscopy.

	WLI	TXI	NBI	Chromoendoscopy
All serrated polyps				
Mean visibility score (SD)	2.27 (0.75)	2.93 (0.76) ***	2.74 (0.79) **	3.45 (0.68) ***, †††, ‡‡‡
SSLs				
Mean visibility score (SD)	2.25 (0.76)	2.90 (0.77) ***	2.65 (0.79)	3.45 (0.64) ***, ††, ‡‡‡
Hyperplastic polyps				
Mean visibility score (SD)	2.30 (0.72)	2.97 (0.67) **	2.88 (0.77) *	3.45 (0.74) ***, ‡

The visibility score was defined as follows: 4, excellent (easily detectable); 3, good (detectable with careful observation; 2, fair (hardly detectable without careful examination); and 1 poor (not detectable without repeated careful examination). WLI, white light imaging; TXI, texture and color enhancement imaging; NBI, narrow-band imaging; SD, standard deviation. ***: *p* value < 0.001 compared with WLI, **: *p* value < 0.01 compared with WLI, *: *p* value < 0.05 compared with WLI, †††: *p* value < 0.001 compared with TXI, ††: *p* value < 0.01 compared with TXI, ‡‡‡: *p* value < 0.001 compared with NBI, ‡: *p* value < 0.05 compared with NBI.

3.3. Visibility Score for Vessel Pattern with Magnification

The visibility score of TXI for the vessel pattern with magnification was significantly higher than that of WLI and chromoendoscopy in serrated polyps and the sub-analysis of SSLs (Table 3).

Table 3. Visibility scores of vessel pattern and surface pattern with magnification for WLI, TXI, NBI, and chromoendoscopy.

	WLI	TXI	NBI	Chromoendoscopy
All serrated polyps				
Vessel pattern (SD)	2.30 (0.74)	2.91 (0.80) ***, †††	3.23 (0.84) ***, †††	2.21 (0.83)
Surface pattern (SD)	1.86 (0.64)	2.75 (0.68) ***	3.46 (0.70) ***, ‡‡‡, †††	2.79 (0.75) ***
SSLs				
Vessel pattern (SD)	2.24 (0.74)	2.89 (0.81) ***, ††	3.19 (0.86) ***, †††	2.30 (0.87)
Surface pattern (SD)	1.80 (0.62)	2.70 (0.66) ***	3.39 (0.78) ***, ‡‡‡, ††	2.83 (0.76) ***
Hyperplastic polyps				
Vessel pattern (SD)	2.41 (0.73)	2.96 (0.79) †††	3.33 (0.77) ***, †††	2.04 (0.69)
Surface pattern (SD)	2.00 (0.67)	2.85 (0.70) **	3.59 (0.49) ***, ‡‡, †††	2.70 (0.71) *

WLI, white light imaging; TXI, texture and color enhancement imaging; NBI, narrow-band imaging; SD, standard deviation. ***: *p* value < 0.001 compared with WLI, **: *p* value < 0.01 compared with WLI, *: *p* value < 0.05 compared with WLI, †††: *p* value < 0.001 compared with chromoendoscopy, ††: *p* value < 0.01 compared with chromoendoscopy, ‡‡‡: *p* value < 0.001 compared with TXI, ‡‡: *p* value < 0.01 compared with TXI.

3.4. Visibility Score for Surface Pattern with Magnification

The visibility score of TXI for the surface pattern with magnification was significantly higher than that of WLI but lower than that of NBI in serrated polyps and the sub-analysis of SSLs and hyperplastic polyps (Table 3).

3.5. Visibility Scores for WLI and TXI by Each Expert Endoscopist

The visibility scores of TXI with and without magnification were significantly higher than those of WLI (Table 4). The visibility improvement in TXI was consistent among the three expert endoscopists.

Table 4. Visibility scores for WLI and TXI assigned by each expert endoscopist.

	WLI	TXI
Mean visibility scores without magnification (SD)		
Expert endoscopist 1	2.29 (0.71)	2.75 (0.75) ***
Expert endoscopist 2	2.46 (0.83)	3.00 (0.77) ***
Expert endoscopist 3	2.07 (0.66)	3.04 (0.69) ***
Visibility scores of vessel pattern with magnification		
Expert endoscopist 1	1.85 (0.60)	2.37 (0.74) ***
Expert endoscopist 2	2.52 (0.85)	2.89 (0.70) **
Expert endoscopist 3	2.52 (0.58)	3.48 (0.58) ***
Visibility scores of surface pattern with magnification		
Expert endoscopist 1	1.62 (0.88)	2.48 (0.80) ***
Expert endoscopist 2	1.89 (0.51)	2.74 (0.59) ***
Expert endoscopist 3	2.07 (0.38)	3.04 (0.52) ***

WLI, white light imaging; TXI, texture and color enhancement imaging; SD, standard deviation. ***: p value < 0.001 compared with WLI, **: p value < 0.01 compared with WLI.

4. Discussion

This study showed that TXI with and without magnification provided higher visibility than WLI did for serrated colorectal polyps, including SSL. However, non-magnified TXI was inferior to chromoendoscopy, and magnified TXI for surface patterns was inferior to magnified NBI. This is the first report on the efficacy of TXI for serrated colorectal polyps, including SSL.

Olympus Corp. first developed the NBI as an innovative image-enhanced endoscopy technology in 2007 [14]. Fujifilm Corp. developed blue light imaging (BLI) as a similar product. NBI and BLI are mainly used for magnified endoscopy and the detection of esophageal cancer [15,16]. Fujifilm Corp. also developed the linked color imaging (LCI) method, which is mainly used to detect lesions without magnification [17]. A randomized controlled trial (RCT) showed that LCI was significantly superior to standard WLI for polyp detection [18]. Currently, LCI-based observations are becoming standard instead of WLI. However, Olympus did not have a mode corresponding to that of LCI until recently. Olympus released TXI as a mode similar to that of LCI. Although LCI and TXI have similar concepts, there are several differences in their principles. LCI uses ambient light with wavelengths of 410 nm and 450 nm, the images are converted to resemble those of WLI, and color is enhanced such that red is changed to vivid red and white is changed to clear white. On the other hand, TXI uses white light, texture and color are enhanced, and brightness is adjusted. There is no study that directly compares TXI and LCI. The comparison between TXI and LCI is a future issue. The global share of Olympus Corp. is 70% for gastrointestinal endoscopy, so the spread of TXI may exceed that of LCI.

TXI provides higher visibility than does WLI for colorectal adenomas. In the present study, we found that TXI provided higher visibility than did WLI for serrated colorectal polyps. Taken together, this might imply that TXI can replace WLI in the detection of premalignant polyps in colonoscopy.

It is controversial whether LCI allows for better SSL detection. Fujimoto et al. showed that LCI was the most sensitive mode for SSL detection among WLI, BLI, and LCI in still-image examinations. Furthermore, their RCT of tandem colonoscopy with WLI and LCI suggested that LCI is superior to WLI in SSL detection [19]. An RCT by Dos Santos showed that LCI enables better adenoma detection, with a borderline significance for a higher detection of sessile serrated adenomas ($p = 0.05$) [20]. Conversely, an RCT by Paggi et al. showed that LCI allowed for better adenoma detection, but not for SSL detection [21]. Our study showed that TXI was significantly superior to WLI for SSL detection in still-image examinations. With regard to the SSL detection rate during colonoscopy, prospective RCTs are required in the future.

In this study, TXI was inferior to chromoendoscopy in SSL detection. Furthermore, the magnified TXI was inferior to the magnified NBI in terms of the visibility of surface patterns. On the other hand, Kitagawa et al. found that magnified LCI with indigo carmine was superior to magnified BLI [22]. Sakamoto et al. also reported that magnified LCI with crystal violet staining provided more diagnostic information than magnified blue light imaging (BLI) and WLI [23]. TXI with chromoendoscopy might be also promising, and needs to be further investigated in future studies.

Texture plays an important role in the identification of regions of interest in an image; hence, texture enhancement is a meaningful component in digital image processing [24,25]. There are several reports on the quantitative analysis of TXI. Sato et al. performed a quantitative analysis using endoscopic images of the gastrointestinal tract from an in vivo porcine study [26]. Their quantitative analysis included edge-based contrast measurements, the standard deviation of the averaged illumination, and the color difference. In the analysis of edge-based contrast measure, TXI had higher value than WLI, showing that TXI can enhance image contrast, arising from texture enhancement. This study also revealed that TXI can reduced the standard deviation of the illumination nonuniformity compared with white light imaging (WLI). This improvement was achieved by selectively enhancing the brightness in dark areas. In the analysis of color difference, TXI had a higher color difference than WLI due to color enhancement. Ishikawa et al. also analyzed the color difference between neoplastic and peripheral areas of twelve gastric neoplasms in WLI and TXI [27]. The color difference was significantly higher in TXI than in WLI.

The present study had some limitations. The sample size was small, although statistically significant differences were observed. Larger prospective studies are required in the future. Even though this was a single-center, retrospective study, because our institution specializes in endoscopy, the endoscopic environment was well managed.

5. Conclusions

The visibility provided by non-magnified TXI was higher than that provided by WLI and lower than that provided by chromoendoscopy for serrated polyps, including SSLs. The visibility provided by magnified TXI was higher than that provided by WLI but lower than that provided by NBI. TXI could be a suitable modality for the detection of premalignant colorectal polyps.

Author Contributions: T.N.: conception of article, writing of article, statistical analysis, review of endoscopic images; O.T.: conception of article, taking endoscopic images, review of endoscopic images, and final manuscript approval; S.Y., C.U., K.K., M.M., M.O. and T.Y.: review of endoscopic images, critical review; M.F., H.E. and H.S.: critical review and final manuscript approval. All authors have read and agreed to the published version of the manuscript.

Funding: This research received no external funding.

Institutional Review Board Statement: This study was reviewed and approved by the Certificated Review Board, Yoyogi Mental Clinic on 16 July 2021 (approval no. RKK227).

Informed Consent Statement: Informed consent was obtained from all subjects involved in the study.

Data Availability Statement: No additional data are available.

Conflicts of Interest: MF received a research grant and honoraria from Olympus Corporation.

References

1. Goyal, H.; Mann, R.; Gandhi, Z.; Perisetti, A.; Ali, A.; Aman Ali, K.; Sharma, N.; Saligram, S.; Tharian, B.; Inamdar, S. Scope of Artificial Intelligence in Screening and Diagnosis of Colorectal Cancer. *J Clin. Med.* **2020**, *9*, 3313. [CrossRef] [PubMed]
2. Zauber, A.G.; Winawer, S.J.; O'Brien, M.J.; Lansdorp-Vogelaar, I.; van Ballegooijen, M.; Hankey, B.F.; Shi, W.; Bond, J.H.; Schapiro, M.; Panish, J.F.; et al. Colonoscopic polypectomy and long-term prevention of colorectal-cancer deaths. *N. Engl. J. Med.* **2012**, *366*, 687–696. [CrossRef] [PubMed]
3. Albeniz, E.; Pellise, M.; Gimeno Garcia, A.Z.; Lucendo, A.J.; Alonso Aguirre, P.A.; Herreros de Tejada, A.; Alvarez, M.A.; Fraile, M.; Herraiz Bayod, M.; Lopez Roses, L.; et al. Clinical guidelines for endoscopic mucosal resection of non-pedunculated colorectal lesions. *Gastroenterol. Hepatol.* **2018**, *41*, 175–190. [CrossRef] [PubMed]
4. Nishizawa, T.; Yoshida, S.; Toyoshima, A.; Yamada, T.; Sakaguchi, Y.; Irako, T.; Ebinuma, H.; Kanai, T.; Koike, K.; Toyoshima, O. Endoscopic diagnosis for colorectal sessile serrated lesions. *World J. Gastroenterol.* **2021**, *27*, 1321–1329. [CrossRef]
5. Kinoshita, S.; Nishizawa, T.; Uraoka, T. Progression to invasive cancer from sessile serrated adenoma/polyp. *Dig. Endosc.* **2018**, *30*, 266. [CrossRef]
6. Dhillon, A.S.; Ibraheim, H.; Green, S.; Suzuki, N.; Thomas-Gibson, S.; Wilson, A. Curriculum review: Serrated lesions of the colorectum. *Frontline Gastroenterol.* **2020**, *11*, 243–248. [CrossRef]
7. Riu Pons, F.; Andreu, M.; Naranjo, D.; Alvarez-Gonzalez, M.A.; Seoane, A.; Dedeu, J.M.; Barranco, L.; Bessa, X. Narrow-band imaging and high-definition white-light endoscopy in patients with serrated lesions not fulfilling criteria for serrated polyposis syndrome: A randomized controlled trial with tandem colonoscopy. *BMC Gastroenterol.* **2020**, *20*, 111. [CrossRef]
8. JE, I.J.; van Doorn, S.C.; van der Brug, Y.M.; Bastiaansen, B.A.; Fockens, P.; Dekker, E. The proximal serrated polyp detection rate is an easy-to-measure proxy for the detection rate of clinically relevant serrated polyps. *Gastrointest. Endosc.* **2015**, *82*, 870–877. [CrossRef]
9. Nishizawa, T.; Yoshida, S.; Toyoshima, O.; Matsuno, T.; Irokawa, M.; Arano, T.; Ebinuma, H.; Suzuki, H.; Kanai, T.; Koike, K. Risk Factors for Prolonged Hospital Stay after Endoscopy. *Clin. Endosc.* **2021**, *54*, 851–856. [CrossRef]
10. Toyoshima, O.; Yoshida, S.; Nishizawa, T.; Yamakawa, T.; Sakitani, K.; Hata, K.; Takahashi, Y.; Fujishiro, M.; Watanabe, H.; Koike, K. CF290 for pancolonic chromoendoscopy improved sessile serrated polyp detection and procedure time: A propensity score-matching study. *Endosc. Int. Open* **2019**, *7*, E987–E993. [CrossRef]
11. Toyoshima, O.; Nishizawa, T.; Yoshida, S.; Sekiba, K.; Kataoka, Y.; Hata, K.; Watanabe, H.; Tsuji, Y.; Koike, K. Expert endoscopists with high adenoma detection rates frequently detect diminutive adenomas in proximal colon. *Endosc. Int. Open* **2020**, *8*, E775–E782. [CrossRef]
12. Yoshida, N.; Hisabe, T.; Hirose, R.; Ogiso, K.; Inada, Y.; Konishi, H.; Yagi, N.; Naito, Y.; Aomi, Y.; Ninomiya, K.; et al. Improvement in the visibility of colorectal polyps by using blue laser imaging (with video). *Gastrointest. Endosc.* **2015**, *82*, 542–549. [CrossRef] [PubMed]
13. Suzuki, T.; Hara, T.; Kitagawa, Y.; Takashiro, H.; Nankinzan, R.; Sugita, O.; Yamaguchi, T. Linked-color imaging improves endoscopic visibility of colorectal nongranular flat lesions. *Gastrointest. Endosc.* **2017**, *86*, 692–697. [CrossRef] [PubMed]
14. Kurumi, H.; Nonaka, K.; Ikebuchi, Y.; Yoshida, A.; Kawaguchi, K.; Yashima, K.; Isomoto, H. Fundamentals, Diagnostic Capabilities and Perspective of Narrow Band Imaging for Early Gastric Cancer. *J. Clin. Med.* **2021**, *10*, 2918. [CrossRef] [PubMed]
15. Wagner, A.; Zandanell, S.; Kiesslich, T.; Neureiter, D.; Klieser, E.; Holzinger, J.; Berr, F. Systematic Review on Optical Diagnosis of Early Gastrointestinal Neoplasia. *J. Clin. Med.* **2021**, *10*, 2794. [CrossRef]
16. Okumura, K.; Hojo, Y.; Tomita, T.; Kumamoto, T.; Nakamura, T.; Kurahashi, Y.; Ishida, Y.; Hirota, S.; Miwa, H.; Shinohara, H. Accuracy of Preoperative Endoscopy in Determining Tumor Location Required for Surgical Planning for Esophagogastric Junction Cancer. *J. Clin. Med.* **2021**, *10*, 3371. [CrossRef] [PubMed]
17. Matsumura, S.; Dohi, O.; Yamada, N.; Harusato, A.; Yasuda, T.; Yoshida, T.; Ishida, T.; Azuma, Y.; Kitae, H.; Doi, T.; et al. Improved Visibility of Early Gastric Cancer after Successful Helicobacter pylori Eradication with Image-Enhanced Endoscopy: A Multi-Institutional Study Using Video Clips. *J. Clin. Med.* **2021**, *10*, 3649. [CrossRef]
18. Min, M.; Deng, P.; Zhang, W.; Sun, X.; Liu, Y.; Nong, B. Comparison of linked color imaging and white-light colonoscopy for detection of colorectal polyps: A multicenter, randomized, crossover trial. *Gastrointest. Endosc.* **2017**, *86*, 724–730. [CrossRef]
19. Fujimoto, D.; Muguruma, N.; Okamoto, K.; Fujino, Y.; Kagemoto, K.; Okada, Y.; Takaoka, Y.; Mitsui, Y.; Kitamura, S.; Kimura, T.; et al. Linked color imaging enhances endoscopic detection of sessile serrated adenoma/polyps. *Endosc. Int. Open* **2018**, *6*, E322–E334. [CrossRef]
20. Oliveira Dos Santos, C.E.; Malaman, D.; Pereira-Lima, J.C.; de Quadros Onofrio, F.; Ribas Filho, J.M. Impact of linked-color imaging on colorectal adenoma detection. *Gastrointest. Endosc.* **2019**, *90*, 826–834. [CrossRef]
21. Paggi, S.; Radaelli, F.; Senore, C.; Maselli, R.; Amato, A.; Andrisani, G.; Di Matteo, F.; Cecinato, P.; Grillo, S.; Sereni, G.; et al. Linked-color imaging versus white-light colonoscopy in an organized colorectal cancer screening program. *Gastrointest. Endosc.* **2020**, *92*, 723–730. [CrossRef] [PubMed]
22. Kitagawa, Y.; Hara, T.; Ikebe, D.; Nankinzan, R.; Takashiro, H.; Kobayashi, R.; Nakamura, K.; Yamaguchi, T.; Suzuki, T. Magnified endoscopic observation of small depressed gastric lesions using linked color imaging with indigo carmine dye. *Endoscopy* **2018**, *50*, 142–147. [CrossRef] [PubMed]

23. Sakamoto, T.; Inoki, K.; Takamaru, H.; Sekiguchi, M.; Yamada, M.; Nakajima, T.; Matsuda, T.; Saito, Y. Efficacy of linked colour imaging in magnifying chromoendoscopy with crystal violet staining: A pilot study. *Int. J. Colorectal Dis.* **2019**, *34*, 1341–1344. [CrossRef] [PubMed]
24. Haralick, R.; Shanmugam, K.; Dinstein, I. Textural features for image classification. *IEEE Trans. Syst. Man Cybern.* **1973**, *3*, 610–621. [CrossRef]
25. Yu, Q.; Vegh, V.; Liu, F.; Turner, I. A Variable Order Fractional Differential-Based Texture Enhancement Algorithm with Application in Medical Imaging. *PLoS ONE* **2015**, *10*, e0132952. [CrossRef]
26. Sato, T. TXI: Texture and Color Enhancement Imaging for Endoscopic Image Enhancement. *J. Healthc. Eng.* **2021**, *2021*, 5518948. [CrossRef]
27. Ishikawa, T.; Matsumura, T.; Okimoto, K.; Nagashima, A.; Shiratori, W.; Kaneko, T.; Oura, H.; Tokunaga, M.; Akizue, N.; Ohta, Y.; et al. Efficacy of Texture and Color Enhancement Imaging in visualizing gastric mucosal atrophy and gastric neoplasms. *Sci. Rep.* **2021**, *11*, 6910. [CrossRef]

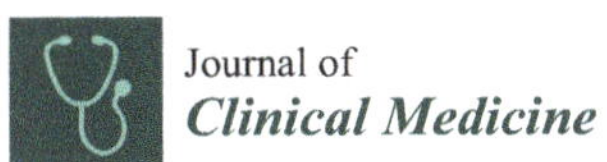

Journal of
Clinical Medicine

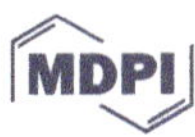

Article

Effectiveness of S-O Clip-Assisted Colorectal Endoscopic Submucosal Dissection

Haruka Fujinami [1,*], Akira Teramoto [2], Saeko Takahashi [2], Takayuki Ando [2], Shinya Kajiura [3] and Ichiro Yasuda [2]

[1]   Department of Endoscopy, Toyama University Hospital, Toyama 930-0194, Japan
[2]   Third Department of Internal Medicine, University of Toyama, Toyama 930-0194, Japan;
      akira_teramoto@hotmail.com (A.T.); aec56260@hotmail.co.jp (S.T.); taando33@gmail.com (T.A.);
      yasudaich@gmail.com (I.Y.)
[3]   Department of Clinical Oncology, University of Toyama, Toyama 930-0194, Japan; shin-ya@nsknet.or.jp
*   Correspondence: haruka52@med.u-toyama.ac.jp; Tel.: +81-76-4347301

Abstract: This study aimed to assess the utility of the S-O clip during colorectal endoscopic submucosal dissection (ESD). We conducted a retrospective study on 185 patients who underwent colorectal ESD from January 2015 to January 2020. The patients were divided into two groups: before and after the introduction of the S-O clip. Forty-two patients underwent conventional ESD (CO group) and 29 patients underwent ESD using the S-O clip (SO group). We compared the surgery duration, dissection speed, en bloc resection rate, and complication rate between both groups. Compared with the CO group, the SO group had a significantly shorter surgery duration (70.7 ± 37.9 min vs. 51.2 ± 18.6 min; $p = 0.017$), a significantly higher dissection speed (15.1 ± 9.0 min vs. 26.3 ± 13.8 min; $p < 0.001$), a significantly higher en bloc resection rate (80.9% vs. 98.8%; $p \leq 0.001$), and a significantly lower perforation rate (4.3% vs. 1.3%). In the right colon, the surgery duration was significantly shorter and the dissection speed was significantly higher in the SO group than in the CO group. Moreover, the rate of en bloc resection improved significantly in the right colon. S-O clip-assisted ESD reduces the procedure time and improves the treatment effects, especially in the right colon.

Keywords: endoscopic submucosal dissection; colorectal tumor; traction method

Citation: Fujinami, H.; Teramoto, A.; Takahashi, S.; Ando, T.; Kajiura, S.; Yasuda, I. Effectiveness of S-O Clip-Assisted Colorectal Endoscopic Submucosal Dissection. *J. Clin. Med.* **2022**, *11*, 141. https://doi.org/10.3390/jcm11010141

Academic Editor: Hidekazu Suzuki

Received: 18 November 2021
Accepted: 24 December 2021
Published: 27 December 2021

Publisher's Note: MDPI stays neutral with regard to jurisdictional claims in published maps and institutional affiliations.

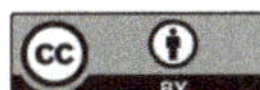

1. Introduction

Endoscopic submucosal dissection (ESD) is an established treatment for intramucosal tumors of the gastrointestinal tract, including the colon and rectum. This method, compared to conventional endoscopic mucosal resection (EMR), enables en bloc resection of larger lesions and has a low recurrence rate of 0.4–1.0% [1,2]. Colorectal ESD has several limitations, including an anatomically difficult procedure, a longer procedure compared to that of endoscopic mucosal resection, and a high risk of perforation and bleeding [2–5]. Moreover, some studies have reported life-threatening complications, such as perforation, the incidence of which was 4.1–5.3% [6,7].

Performing traction-assisted ESD will be easier if the submucosal layer can be directly visualized after the mucosal cut. Several traction techniques on lesions have been reported to be effective during ESD for large early gastric and colorectal cancers [8]. In particular, the S-O clip (TC1H05; Zeon Medical Co., Ltd., Tokyo, Japan) has been reported to be safe to use and to hasten colorectal ESD [9,10]. This study aimed to assess the utility of colorectal ESD using the S-O clip.

2. Materials and Methods

2.1. Patients

In this retrospective study, medical record of all patients who underwent colorectal ESD at the Toyama University Hospital were reviewed. Patients were divided into two groups according to the date of ESD procedure as S-O clip (Figure 1) were introduced in

May 2017: the CO group underwent conventional ESD from September 2015 to April 2017, and the SO group underwent S-O clip-assisted ESD from May 2017 to January 2020. The indications for ESD included (1) a colonic neoplasm (adenoma and carcinoma) measuring >20 mm that was difficult to resect en bloc by conventional EMR, (2) a suspicion of an intramucosal lesion, and (3) the absence of submucosal invasion on magnifying endoscopy. Patients were excluded if they (1) had a rectal lesion, (2) showed a non-lifting sign or had residual lesions after endoscopic resection, or (3) had a lesion measuring >50 mm. All procedures were performed by five endoscopists who had performed more than 20 gastric ESD procedures.

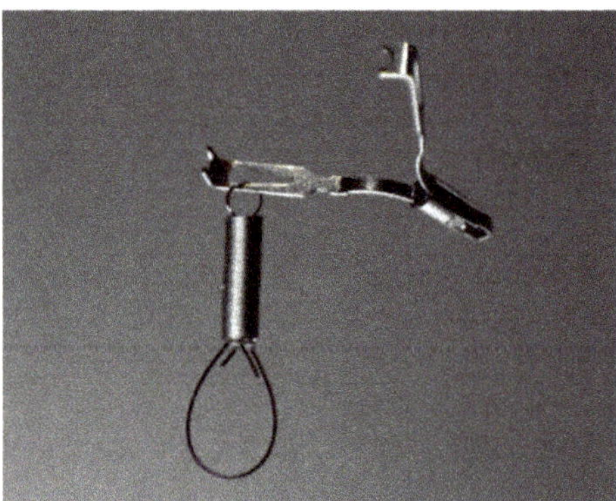

Figure 1. The external appearance of an S-O clip. The S-O clip comprised a metal clip (ZEOCLIP; Zeon Medical Co., Ltd.) and a 5 mm long spring. A nylon loop is attached to the other side of the spring and fixed to the colon wall using a second clip. The S-O clip can be passed through the channel of a conventional endoscope.

2.2. ESD Preparation

A single-channel endoscope with a water-jet function (PCF-Q260AZI or PCF-H290ZI; Olympus Optical Co., Ltd., Tokyo, Japan) was prepared for the ESD. A transparent hood was attached to the endoscope to provide sufficient space and facilitate submucosal dissection. A solution containing sodium hyaluronate (MucoUp; Boston Scientific Co., Tokyo, Japan), saline, and a small quantity of indigo carmine were injected into the submucosal layer. As the border of the colonic neoplasm was generally clearly visible, no marking was carried out. Carbon dioxide (CO_2) was used in all cases for insufflation.

Using the Jet-B knife (BSJB15B; Zeon Medical Co., Ltd.) and the SB Knife Jr (MD-47703; Sumitomo Bakelite, Tokyo, Japan), a circumferential mucosal incision was made and submucosal dissection was performed. Hemostasis was performed using Coagrasper (FD-411QR; Olympus Optical Co., Ltd.) with an electric surgical unit (VIO 300D; ERBE, Tübingen, Germany). The electrical power setting for the Jet-B knife was as follows: (1) dry-cut mode, effect 2, 50 W for the mucosal incision; and (2) forced-coagulation mode, effect 2, 50 W for the submucosal dissection. The setting for the SB Knife Jr was endo-cut Q-mode, effect 1, duration 1, interval 1, and that for the soft-coagulation mode was effect 4, 40 W for hemostasis. The setting for the Coagrasper was the soft-coagulation mode, effect 2, 40 W. All procedures were recorded on DVDs.

2.3. Conventional Colonic ESD

Using the Jet-B knife, an initial mucosal incision was made on the anal side of the lesion, followed by submucosal dissection. Next, the mucosal incision was extended to the right and to the left, and the submucosal layer under the extended area was dissected. When hemorrhage occurred during surgery, hemostasis was achieved using the Jet-B knife in the forced-coagulation mode or by using the Coagrasper [11]. In technically difficult situations, the SB Knife Jr was used thanks to its safety and usefulness [12,13]. Mucosal incisions and submucosal dissections were repeated; then, circumferential mucosal incisions and submucosal dissections were performed.

2.4. S-O Clip-Assisted ESD

First, a circumferential incision on the mucosal layer was performed using the Jet-B knife or the SB Knife Jr. Then, the S-O clip was attached to the proximal edge of the lesion (Figure 2A,B). Another clip was used to grasp the nylon loop attached to the tip of the spring and then pulled one in front and was fixed to the colon wall opposite the lesion (Figure 2C,D). This traction force allowed for adequate visualization of the submucosal cutting line, which resulted in a fast and safe dissection (Figure 2E). After the dissection, the S-O clip was detached from the colon wall and the specimen was collected (Figure 2F).

2.5. Evaluation of Therapeutic Efficacy and Complications

The surgery duration, dissection speed, complete resection rate, perforation rate, and bleeding rate were compared between the two groups and assessed separately for the right colon (i.e., transverse colon, ascending colon, and cecum) and the left colon (i.e., descending colon and sigmoid colon). The surgery duration was calculated from the initial mucosal incision to the end of submucosal dissection. The dissection time was defined as the time-lapse from the end of the circumferential mucosal cut to the end of submucosal dissection. The lesion area, which was approximated as an ellipse, was determined by measuring the major axis (A) and the minor axis (B). The resected area was calculated as $\pi AB/4$. The dissection speed was calculated by dividing the resected area by the duration of the dissection. Perforation was confirmed endoscopically during ESD, and free air was confirmed on abdominal computed tomography. Hemorrhage was defined as massive intraoperative bleeding that required blood transfusion or as postoperative bleeding that required hemostatic treatment such as endoscopic clipping or coagulation.

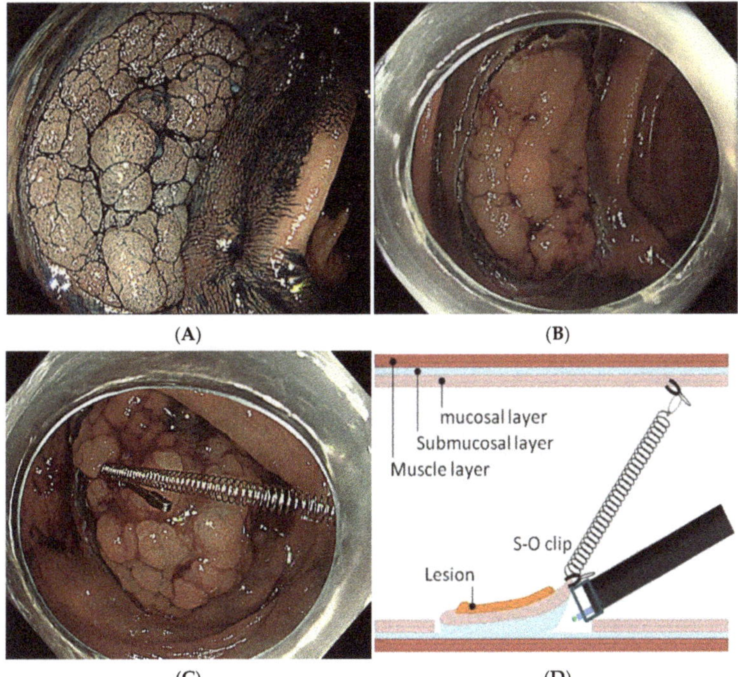

Figure 2. *Cont.*

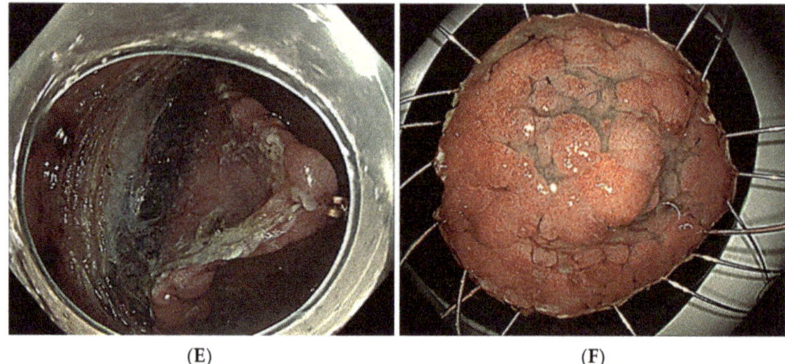

(E)   (F)

Figure 2. Method of S-O clip-assisted ESD. (**A**) An endoscopic examination with narrow-band imaging and 0.4% indigo carmine is conducted before ESD; (**B**) A circumferential incision of the mucosal layer is performed; (**C,D**) The S-O clip is attached to the proximal edge of the lesion, and another clip is used to grasp the nylon loop and pull one in front to fix to the colon wall opposite the lesion; (**E**) A counter-traction force allows good visualization of the submucosal cutting line; (**F**) Resected specimen.

2.6. Statistical Analysis

The chi-squared test was used for comparisons between categorical data, whereas the Mann–Whitney U test was used for comparing continuous data. A p-value of < 0.05 was considered statistically significant. StatView 5.0 (Abacus Concepts Inc., Berkeley, CA, USA) was used to perform all statistical analyses.

3. Results

From September 2015 to January 2020, 185 colorectal tumors underwent ESD at our hospital. We divided the patients into two groups according to the timing of ESD; Conventional ESD group (CO group, $n = 66$) or S-O clip-assisted group (SO group, $n = 119$). In CO group, 19 patients were excluded from enrollment because they had rectal lesion ($n = 15$), non-lifting sign ($n = 2$), and a lesion measuring over 50 mm ($n = 2$). In SO group, 39 patients were excluded from enrollment. Finally, analysis was performed on 47 and 80 patients in the CO and SO groups, respectively (Figure 3).

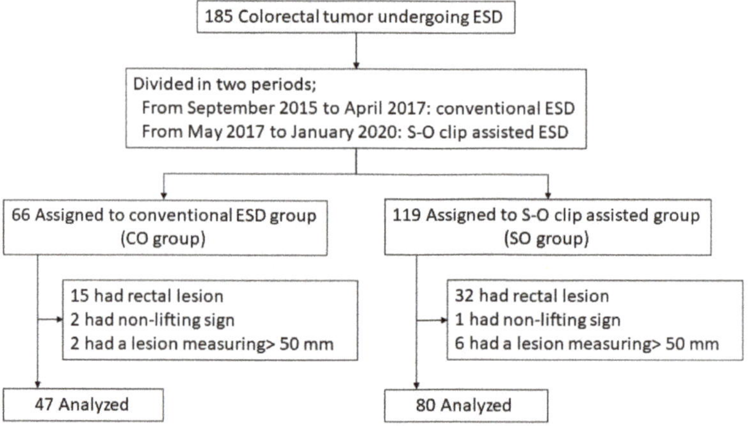

Figure 3. Flow diagram of the study patients.

As shown in Table 1, the demographics and clinicopathologic features of the cases did not differ between the two groups. The overall outcomes are shown in Table 2. Compared with the CO group, the SO group had a significantly shorter surgery duration (73.9 ± 43.5 min vs. 52.3 ± 21.8 min; p = 0.0006), a significantly greater dissection speed (14.8 ± 8.7 min vs. 24.4 ± 12.9 min; p = 0.0014), and a significantly higher en bloc resection rate (80.9% vs. 98.8%; $p \leq$ 0.001). Overall, S-O clip-assisted ESD was able to reduce the procedure time of conventional ESD. No statistical significance in either group experienced massive hemorrhage or postoperative bleeding that required blood transfusion.

The results were analyzed separately for the right and left colon (Table 3). In the right colon, both surgery duration was significantly shorter and the dissection speed was significantly higher in the SO group than in the CO group; however, there was no significant difference in the lesion area between the two groups. Furthermore, the en bloc resection rate was significantly improved in the right colon. On the other hand, there was no such trend in the left colon as in the right colon.

Table 1. Patient demographics and clinicopathologic features.

	CO Group (n = 47)	SO Group (n = 80)	p-Value
Male/Female, n	32/15	47/33	0.345
Mean age (range), years	65.5 (38–80)	69.7 (39–89)	0.531
Lesion size, mean ± SD (range), mm	29.4 ± 9.1 (20–48)	30.6 ± 7.5 (20–50)	0.272
Lesion location			0.685
Right colon, n	35	56	
Left colon, n	12	24	

Table 2. Overall outcomes.

	CO Group (n = 47)	SO Group (n = 80)	p-Value
Surgery duration, mean ± SD (range), min	73.9 ± 43.5 (31–226)	52.3 ± 21.8 (16–113)	0.0006 *
Lesion area, mean ± SD (range), mm^2	616.8 ± 576.8 (235.6–1507.9)	660.6 ± 333.6 (259.2–1696.4)	0.227
Dissection time, mean ± SD (range), min	49.7 ± 37.1 (17–189)	31.9 ± 16.4 (7–82)	<0.001 *
Dissection speed, mean ± SD (range), mm^2/min	14.8 ± 8.7 (4.1–50.1)	24.4 ± 12.9 (5.5–70.6)	0.0014 *
En bloc resection rate, % (n)	80.9 (38/47)	98.8 (79/80)	<0.001 *
Perforation rate, % (n)	4.3 (2/47)	1.3 (1/80)	0.554
Hemorrhage rate, % (n)	0 (0/47)	2.5 (2/80)	0.530

* A p value of < 0.05 was considered statistically significant.

Table 3. Separate analysis for the left colon and the right colon.

	CO Group	SO Group	p-Value
Right colon, n	35	56	
Surgery duration, mean ± SD (range), min	78.1 ± 48.0 (33–226)	52.2 ± 21.3 (16–113)	0.0054 *
Lesion area, mean ± SD (range), mm^2	648.4 ± 660.4 (235.6–1507.9)	685.5 ± 324.3 (259.1–1445.1)	0.1220
Dissection time, mean ± SD (range), min	51.5 ± 40.9 (17–189)	30.7 ± 15.2 (7–64)	0.0019 *
Dissection speed, mean ± SD (range), mm^2/min	14.9 ± 9.1 (4.0–50.1)	25.4 ± 11.7 (9.5–61.7)	<0.001 *
En bloc resection rate, % (n)	77.1 (27/35)	98.2 (55/56)	0.0018 *
Left colon, n	12	24	
Surgery duration, mean ± SD (range), min	61.5 ± 24.1 (31–121)	51.9± 18.2 (26–112)	0.3139
Lesion area, mean ± SD (range), mm^2	524.6 ± 175.4 (314.1–824.6)	563.0 ± 291.4 (311.0–1696.4)	0.9464
Dissection time, mean ± SD (range), min	44.4 ± 23.4 (20–100)	33.3 ± 18.1 (14–82)	0.1488
Dissection speed, mean ± SD (range), mm^2/min	14.0 ± 8.0 (5.7–32.1)	22.0 ± 15.5 (5.4–70.6)	0.1587
En bloc resection rate, % (n)	91.7 (11/12)	100 (24/24)	0.3333

* A p value of < 0.05 was considered statistically significant.

4. Discussion

The maintenance of tension and good visibility of the submucosal layer is an important prerequisite for a fast and safe submucosal dissection. In surgery, the assistant usually maintains tension using a proper force to allow for easier tissue dissection. However, during ESD, it is not easy to maintain good traction because the endoscope has only one working channel for the electrical surgical knife. Therefore, a so-called "second hand" is necessary during ESD.

To achieve traction force during ESD, several methods have been developed. A distal hood with a transparent tip was the first device used to apply tension to the submucosal layer to enable the endoscope to easily enter the submucosal layer and to stabilize the electric knife during resection or dissection [14]. The use of a transparent hood with a small-caliber tip was reported to provide a clear field during submucosal dissection and for the control of bleeding [15]. A traction force can also be obtained simply by gravity without needing to use additional devices. The direction of the traction force can be controlled by changing the patient's position [16]. However, when the flap is small at the first stage of submucosal dissection, gravity does not work sufficiently, and dissection becomes difficult for small lesions or those accompanied by fibrosis [17].

Several methods have been developed to generate a counter-traction to the lesion. The efficacy of the external forceps method [18,19] was reported for gastric and rectal ESD. In this method, traction is applied to the anal side using grasping vending forceps. This way, dissecting the submucosal layer of the grasped side can push or pull the lesion and make the submucosal layer more visible. However, it is difficult to send the forceps deep into the colon. Therefore, this method is limited for rectal ESD. The use of clips to achieve traction has been attempted by various methods. In the thread-and-clip method (Figure 4A), the clip is attached to the flap of the proximal lesion and the end of the thread is pulled to enable the lifting of the lesion during endoscope manipulation [20,21]. However, this method requires withdrawal and re-insertion of the colonoscope before applying the clip. In the clip-and-rubber-band method, a clip is used with a rubber band for continuous traction between the proximal side of the lesion and the normal mucosa [22,23]. The clip-and-ring-thread method (Figure 4B) can help pull the lesion to the intended direction to set a moderate traction force; the advantage of this method over the thread-and-clip one is its lower cost [24]. Since the thread itself has no contraction force, the traction force decreases as the lesion is dissected. Therefore, it is necessary to add a clip repeatedly to maintain the traction force.

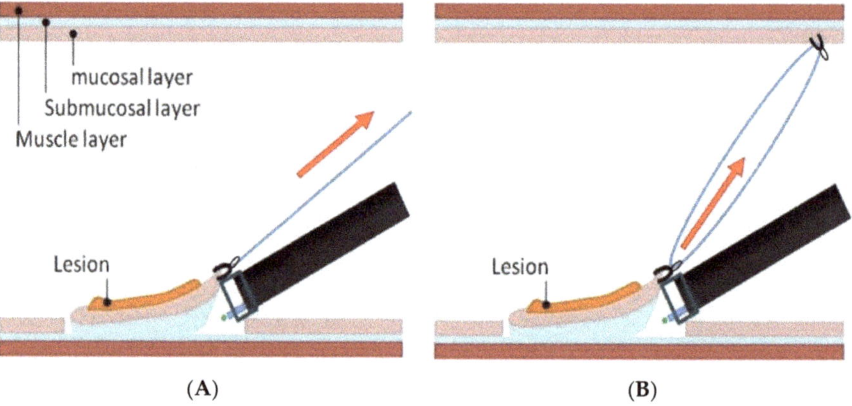

Figure 4. Method of traction-assisted ESD. (**A**) The thread-and-clip method. The clip is attached to the proximal lesion and the end of the thread is pulled to enable the lifting of the lesion; (**B**) The clip-and-ring-thread method. It can help pull the lesion to the intended direction to set a traction force.

The use of the S-O clip can allow for the pulling of the submucosal layer using the spring and can assist in the first phase of dissection during colorectal ESD. Unlike other traction methods, the S-O clip does not require extensive equipment or lengthy preparation and can be used anywhere, regardless of the location of the lesion, including the deep colon. It can be applied through the forceps opening without removing the endoscope, just like a normal clip. Moreover, traction can be applied continuously in the desired direction. The spring of the device has good and constant strength in both extension or contraction and does not cause excessive tension of the muscle layer and is not affected by peristalsis. Stable traction is applied throughout the procedure, and the lesion is automatically pulled. After resection, the lesion is clipped to the intestinal mucosa through a nylon (or silicon) loop, which prevents it from moving to other sites due to peristalsis. Therefore, after ESD, the lesion can be slowly retrieved after hemostasis of the blood vessels of the resected ulcer. In a prospective study, Ritsuno et al. reported that ESD using S-O clip was safe and rapid for en bloc resection of large superficial colorectal tumors [25]. Furthermore, the S-O clip was approved by the pharmaceutical affairs bureau as a medical device for ESD of all gastrointestinal tracts. The efficacy of the S-O clip in gastric ESD has also been reported [26].

Although previous studies on traction methods showed shorter duration of procedure and lower rate of complications, it is unknown which lesions are ideal for this method. Our study is the first to report that lesions located in the right-side colon are strongly associated with shorter treatment time. In general, it has been reported that colorectal ESD is more difficult in the right colon than in the left colon [27]. The reasons are: (1) the longer insertion length of the endoscope and poor operability, (2) the influence of respiratory fluctuation, and (3) the presence of flexure. In the conventional traction method, the traction force decreases as the dissection progresses. However, the major advantage of the S-O clip is that a constant traction force can be maintained throughout procedure, and it can be towed in the intended direction, which provides a stable visual field even in the right colon. In this study, CO group had a longer surgery duration in the right side than in the left side mainly due to difficulty in maintaining visual field and poor maneuverability (Table 3). However, SO group had a significantly faster dissection speed in the right-side colon, which was not observed in the left side colon. Based on these findings, S-O clip is more favorable for right-sided lesions, and application of this method for simple lesions in the left side colon may not be beneficial. Furthermore, we believe that this method can potentially shorten the procedure time and reduce the complication rate effectively when it is performed by less experienced endoscopists, but it may not be necessary for experts to routinely use the S-O clip in all cases. Given that there are cases in which S-O clip-assisted ESD is inapplicable or ineffective, endoscopists should develop their skills based on the conventional method, even in the presence of new technique.

There were several limitations to this study. First, it was a retrospective analysis carried out in a single-center setting, and the experience of the endoscopist and the difficulty of the cases were not uniform. Because it is a regional central hospital, most cases were difficult to treat; therefore, many large lesions of the right colon were treated. However, ESD using S-O clip showed a certain treatment effect to some extent, independent of the surgeon's experience. Secondly, rectal lesions were excluded from this study. The reason for excluding rectal lesions was that the spring part of the S-O clip needed to be pulled to the anal side of the lesion, and the other side of the S-O clip may or may not be able to be fixed to the rectal wall. In general, rectal lesions have relatively large lesion sizes, long ESD procedure times, low perforation rates, and high bleeding rates. Therefore, the exclusion of rectal lesions may have affected the surgery duration and complication rate. Finally, the influence of the learning curve is discussed. Although we compared the learning curves for the entire study, we did not analyze the learning curves separately for experienced and less-experienced endoscopists because the number of cases for less-experienced endoscopists was small. In the future, we will carry out more studies with bigger samples to examine the usefulness of the less experienced and to develop a system for ESD training.

5. Conclusions

The S-O clip-assisted method for ESD shortened the surgery duration and increased the en bloc resection rate and dissection speed, especially in the right colon. Even endoscopists who had less experience in colorectal ESD were able to perform this procedure safely and rapidly. Therefore, S-O clip-assisted ESD can be the most suitable method for introducing colorectal ESD.

Author Contributions: Conceptualization, H.F.; methodology, H.F. and T.A.; software, H.F. and S.K; validation, H.F. and I.Y.; formal analysis, H.F. and S.T.; investigation, H.F.; resources, H.F.; data curation, S.T., A.T., T.A. and S.K.; writing—original draft preparation, H.F.; writing—review and editing, H.F. and A.T.; visualization, H.F.; supervision, I.Y.; project administration, I.Y. All authors have read and agreed to the published version of the manuscript.

Funding: This research received no external funding.

Institutional Review Board Statement: The study was conducted according to the guidelines of the Declaration of Helsinki and approved by Ethics Committee, University of Toyama (30-515).

Informed Consent Statement: Informed consent was obtained from all the participants of the study.

Data Availability Statement: Data sharing is not applicable to this article.

Conflicts of Interest: The authors declare no conflict of interest.

References

1. Shigita, K.; Oka, S.; Tanaka, S.; Sumimoto, K.; Hirano, D.; Tamaru, Y.; Ninomiya, Y.; Asayama, N.; Hayashi, N.; Shimamoto, F.; et al. Long-term outcomes after endoscopic submucosal dissection for superficial colorectal tumors. *Gastrointest. Endosc.* **2017**, *85*, 546–553. [CrossRef]
2. Cao, Y.; Liao, C.; Tan, A.; Gao, Y.; Mo, Z.; Gao, F. Meta-analysis of endoscopic submucosal dissection versus endoscopic mucosal resection for tumors of the gastrointestinal tract. *Endoscopy* **2009**, *41*, 751–757. [CrossRef]
3. Tanaka, S.; Oka, S.; Kaneko, I.; Hirata, M.; Mouri, R.; Kanao, H.; Yoshida, S.; Chayama, K. Endoscopic submucosal dissection for colorectal neoplasia: Possibility of standardization. *Gastrointest. Endosc.* **2007**, *66*, 100–107. [CrossRef]
4. Lee, E.J.; Lee, J.B.; Choi, Y.S.; Lee, S.H.; Lee, D.H.; Kim, D.S.; Youk, E.G. Clinical risk factors for perforation during endoscopic submucosal dissection (ESD) for large-sized, nonpedunculated colorectal tumors. *Surg. Endosc.* **2012**, *26*, 1587–1594. [CrossRef]
5. Mizushima, T.; Kato, M.; Iwanaga, I.; Sato, F.; Kubo, K.; Ehira, N.; Uebayashi, M.; Ono, S.; Nakagawa, M.; Mabe, K.; et al. Technical difficulty according to location, and risk factors for perforation, in endoscopic submucosal dissection of colorectal tumors. *Surg. Endosc.* **2015**, *29*, 133–139. [CrossRef] [PubMed]
6. Lee, E.J.; Lee, J.B.; Lee, S.H.; Kim, D.S.; Lee, D.H.; Lee, D.S.; Youk, E.G. Endoscopic submucosal dissection for colorectal tumors–1000 colorectal ESD cases: One specialized institute's experiences. *Surg. Endosc.* **2013**, *27*, 31–39. [CrossRef] [PubMed]
7. Saito, Y.; Uraoka, T.; Yamaguchi, Y.; Hotta, K.; Sakamoto, N.; Ikematsu, H.; Fukuzawa, M.; Kobayashi, N.; Nasu, J.; Michida, T.; et al. A prospective, multicenter study of 1111 colorectal endoscopic submucosal dissections (with video). *Gastrointest. Endosc.* **2010**, *72*, 1217–1225. [CrossRef] [PubMed]
8. Mizutani, H.; Ono, S.; Ohki, D.; Takeuchi, C.; Yakabi, S.; Kataoka, Y.; Saito, I.; Sakaguchi, Y.; Minatsuki, C.; Tsuji, Y.; et al. Recent development of techniques and devices in colorectal endoscopic submucosal dissection. *Clin. Endosc.* **2017**, *50*, 562–568. [CrossRef]
9. Sakamoto, N.; Osada, T.; Shibuya, T.; Beppu, K.; Matsumoto, K.; Mori, H.; Kawabe, M.; Nagahara, A.; Otaka, M.; Ogihara, T.; et al. Endoscopic submucosal dissection of large colorectal tumors by using a novel spring-action S-O clip for traction (with video). *Gastrointest. Endosc.* **2009**, *69*, 1370–1374. [CrossRef]
10. Sakamoto, N.; Osada, T.; Shibuya, T.; Beppu, K.; Matsumoto, K.; Shimada, Y.; Konno, A.; Kurosawa, A.; Nagahara, A.; Ohkusa, T.; et al. The facilitation of a new traction device (S-O clip) assisting endoscopic submucosal dissection for superficial colorectal neoplasms. *Endoscopy* **2008**, *40* (Suppl. S2), E94–E95. [CrossRef]
11. Yoshida, N.; Naito, Y.; Kugai, M.; Inoue, K.; Wakabayashi, N.; Yagi, N.; Yanagisawa, A.; Yoshikawa, T. Efficient hemostatic method for endoscopic submucosal dissection of colorectal tumors. *World J. Gastroenterol.* **2010**, *16*, 4180–4186. [CrossRef]
12. Yamashina, T.; Takeuchi, Y.; Nagai, K.; Matsuura, N.; Ito, T.; Fujii, M.; Hanaoka, N.; Higashino, K.; Uedo, N.; Ishihara, R.; et al. Scissor-type knife significantly improves self-completion rate of colorectal endoscopic submucosal dissection: Single-center prospective randomized trial. *Dig. Endosc.* **2017**, *29*, 322–329. [CrossRef] [PubMed]
13. Fujinami, H.; Hosokawa, A.; Ogawa, K.; Nishikawa, J.; Kajiura, S.; Ando, T.; Ueda, A.; Yoshita, H.; Sugiyama, T. Endoscopic submucosal dissection for superficial esophageal neoplasms using the stag beetle knife. *Dis. Esophagus* **2014**, *27*, 50–54. [CrossRef] [PubMed]

14. Tanaka, S.; Oka, S.; Chayama, K. Colorectal endoscopic submucosal dissection: Present status and future perspective, including its differentiation from endoscopic mucosal resection. *J. Gastroenterol.* **2008**, *43*, 641–651. [CrossRef] [PubMed]

15. Ishii, N.; Itoh, T.; Horiki, N.; Matsuda, M.; Setoyama, T.; Suzuki, S.; Uemura, M.; Iizuka, Y.; Fukuda, K.; Suzuki, K.; et al. Endoscopic submucosal dissection with a combination of small-caliber-tip transparent hood and flex knife for large superficial colorectal neoplasia including ileocecal lesions. *Surg. Endosc.* **2010**, *24*, 1941–1947. [CrossRef]

16. Lee, B.I. Debates on colorectal endoscopic submucosal dissection—Traction for effective dissection: Gravity is enough. *Clin. Endosc.* **2013**, *46*, 467–471. [CrossRef] [PubMed]

17. Iacopini, F.; Saito, Y.; Bella, A.; Gotoda, T.; Rigato, P.; Elisei, W.; Montagnese, F.; Iacopini, G.; Costamagna, G. Colorectal endoscopic submucosal dissection: Predictors and neoplasm-related gradients of difficulty. *Endosc. Int. Open* **2017**, *5*, 839–846. [CrossRef]

18. Imaeda, H.; Hosoe, N.; Ida, Y.; Kashiwagi, K.; Morohoshi, Y.; Suganuma, K.; Nagakubo, S.; Komatsu, K.; Suzuki, H.; Saito, Y.; et al. Novel technique of endoscopic submucosal dissection using an external grasping forceps for superficial gastric neoplasia. *Dig. Endosc.* **2009**, *21*, 122–127. [CrossRef]

19. Imaeda, H.; Hosoe, N.; Ida, Y.; Nakamizo, H.; Kashiwagi, K.; Kanai, T.; Iwao, Y.; Hibi, T.; Ogata, H. Novel technique of endoscopic submucosal dissection by using external forceps for early rectal cancer (with videos). *Gastrointest. Endosc.* **2012**, *75*, 1253–1257. [CrossRef]

20. Chen, P.J.; Chu, H.C.; Chang, W.K.; Hsieh, T.Y.; Chao, Y.C. Endoscopic submucosal dissection with internal traction for early gastric cancer (with video). *Gastrointest. Endosc.* **2008**, *67*, 128–132. [CrossRef]

21. Okamoto, K.; Muguruma, N.; Kitamura, S.; Kimura, T.; Takayama, T. Endoscopic submucosal dissection for large colorectal tumors using a cross-counter technique and a novel large-diameter balloon overtube. *Dig. Endosc.* **2012**, *24* (Suppl. S1), 96–99. [CrossRef] [PubMed]

22. Matsumoto, K.; Nagahara, A.; Ueyama, H.; Konuma, H.; Morimoto, T.; Sasaki, H.; Hayashi, T.; Shibuya, T.; Sakamoto, N.; Osada, T.; et al. Development and clinical usability of a new traction device "medical ring" for endoscopic submucosal dissection of early gastric cancer. *Surg. Endosc.* **2013**, *27*, 3444–3451. [CrossRef]

23. Parra-Blanco, A.; Nicolas, D.; Arnau, M.R.; Gimeno-Garcia, A.Z.; Rodrigo, L.; Quintero, E. Gastric endoscopic submucosal dissection assisted by a new traction method: The clip-band technique. A feasibility study in a porcine model (with video). *Gastrointest. Endosc.* **2011**, *74*, 1137–1141. [CrossRef]

24. Mori, H.; Kobara, H.; Nishiyama, N.; Fujihara, S.; Matsunaga, T.; Masaki, T. Novel effective and repeatedly available ring-thread counter traction for safer colorectal endoscopic submucosal dissection. *Surg. Endosc.* **2017**, *31*, 3040–3047. [CrossRef]

25. Ritsuno, H.; Sakamoto, N.; Osada, T.; Goto, S.P.; Murakami, T.; Ueyama, H.; Mori, H.; Matsumoto, K.; Beppu, K.; Shibuya, T.; et al. Prospective clinical trial of traction device-assisted endoscopic submucosal dissection of large superficial colorectal tumors using the S-O clip. *Surg. Endosc.* **2014**, *28*, 3143–3149. [CrossRef] [PubMed]

26. Nagata, M. Internal traction method using a spring-and-loop with clip (S-O clip) allows countertraction in gastric endoscopic submucosal dissection. *Surg. Endosc.* **2020**, *34*, 3722–3733. [CrossRef] [PubMed]

27. Isomoto, H.; Nishiyama, H.; Yamaguchi, N.; Fukuda, E.; Ishii, H.; Ikeda, K.; Ohnita, K.; Nakao, S.; Shikuwa, S. Clinicopathological factors associated with clinical outcomes of endoscopic submucosal dissection for colorectal epithelial neoplasms. *Endoscopy* **2009**, *41*, 679–683. [CrossRef]

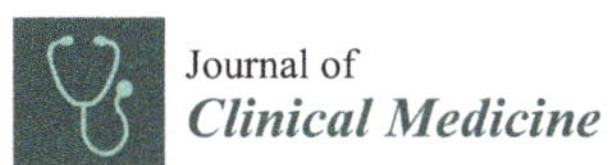

Journal of
Clinical Medicine

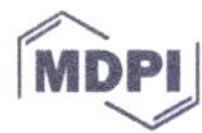

Article

Relief Effect of Carbon Dioxide Insufflation in Transnasal Endoscopy for Health Checks—A Prospective, Double-Blind, Case-Control Trial

Toshio Fujisawa [1], Hiroshi Fukuda [2], Naoto Sakamoto [1], Mariko Hojo [1], Ko Tomishima [1], Shigeto Ishii [1], Hirohide Yokokawa [2], Mizue Saita [2], Toshio Naito [2], Akihito Nagahara [1], Sumio Watanabe [1] and Hiroyuki Isayama [1,*]

[1] Department of Gastroenterology, Graduate School of Medicine, Juntendo University, Tokyo 113-8421, Japan; t-fujisawa@juntendo.ac.jp (T.F.); sakamoto@juntendo.ac.jp (N.S.); mhojo@juntendo.ac.jp (M.H.); tomishim@juntendo.ac.jp (K.T.); sishii@juntendo.ac.jp (S.I.); nagahara@juntendo.ac.jp (A.N.); sumio@juntendo.ac.jp (S.W.)

[2] Department of General Medicine, Graduate School of Medicine, Juntendo University, Tokyo 113-8421, Japan; hiro@juntendo.ac.jp (H.F.); hyokoka@juntendo.ac.jp (H.Y.); msaita@juntendo.ac.jp (M.S.); naito@juntendo.ac.jp (T.N.)

* Correspondence: h-isayama@juntendo.ac.jp; Tel.: +81-3-3813-3111

Citation: Fujisawa, T.; Fukuda, H.; Sakamoto, N.; Hojo, M.; Tomishima, K.; Ishii, S.; Yokokawa, H.; Saita, M.; Naito, T.; Nagahara, A.; et al. Relief Effect of Carbon Dioxide Insufflation in Transnasal Endoscopy for Health Checks—A Prospective, Double-Blind, Case-Control Trial. *J. Clin. Med.* **2022**, *11*, 1231. https://doi.org/10.3390/jcm11051231

Academic Editor: Hidekazu Suzuki

Received: 7 January 2022
Accepted: 22 February 2022
Published: 24 February 2022

Publisher's Note: MDPI stays neutral with regard to jurisdictional claims in published maps and institutional affiliations.

Abstract: CO_2 insufflation has proven effective in reducing patients' pain after colonoscopies but has not been examined in esophagogastroduodenoscopies. Therefore, we examined the effect of CO_2 insufflation in examinees who underwent transnasal endoscopies without sedation. This study is a single-center, prospective, double-blind, case-control trial conducted between March 2017 and August 2018. Subjects were assigned weekly to receive insufflation with either CO_2 or air. The primary outcome was improvement of abdominal pain and distension at 2 h and 1-day postprocedure. In total, 336 and 338 examinees were assigned to the CO_2 and air groups, respectively. Visual analog scale (VAS) scores for abdominal distension (15.4 vs. 25.5; $p < 0.001$) and distress from flatus (16.0 vs. 28.8; $p < 0.001$) at 2 h postprocedure were significantly reduced in the CO_2 group. VAS scores for pain during the procedure (33.5 vs. 37.1; $p = 0.059$) and abdominal pain after the procedure (3.9 vs. 5.7; $p = 0.052$) also tended to be lower at 2 h postprocedure, but all parameters showed no significant difference at 1-day postprocedure. All procedures were safely completed through the planned program, and no apparent adverse events requiring treatment or follow-up occurred. In conclusion, CO_2 insufflation may reduce postprocedural abdominal discomfort from transnasal esophagogastroduodenoscopies. (UMIN000028543).

Keywords: carbon dioxide; CO_2 insufflation; abdominal pain; abdominal distention; transnasal endoscopy; health check

1. Introduction

Carbon dioxide (CO_2) is rapidly absorbed from the gastrointestinal tract and easily eliminated by respiration. It is absorbed approximately 160 times faster than nitrogen, which is the major gaseous ingredient of air [1]. CO_2 insufflation has proven effective in reducing patients' pain after endoscopic procedures. Its effect has been examined mainly in colonoscopies [2–4] and in small numbers, in balloon-assisted endoscopies [5] and endoscopic retrograde cholangiopancreatographies [6–8]. Regarding the upper gastrointestinal tract, the usefulness of CO_2 in therapeutic endoscopies, such as endoscopic submucosal dissections (ESDs) [9,10], has been examined, but it has not been examined in diagnostic endoscopies. The principal source of pain from a colonoscopy is intestinal hyperextension by air insufflation, whereas in an esophagogastroduodenoscopy, pain is largely due to the vomiting reflex. Because the main causes of pain are different, it is difficult for the endoscopist to identify the pain relief effect of CO_2 insufflation. This may be one reason that the effect of CO_2 insufflation has not been studied in esophagogastroduodenoscopies. However, esophagogastroduodenoscopies also require considerable insufflation, similar to colonoscopies, so abdominal pain and distension may occur during and after the procedures in the same way.

Because screening esophagogastroduodenoscopies are performed on healthy examinees during health checks, it should be as painless as possible. Esophagogastroduodenoscopies during health checks are often performed by transnasal endoscopies to reduce patients' discomfort [11], but few institutions perform endoscopies under sedation due to labor shortages and high costs [12]. In addition, patients who receive health check endoscopic examinations have no symptoms, so bias from previous symptoms is low.

Therefore, we examined the effect of CO_2 insufflation on pain relief in examinees who underwent transnasal endoscopies without sedation.

2. Materials and Methods

This study is a prospective, case-control, double-blind trial; its protocol was approved by the institutional review board and the database is open to the public (UMIN000028543).

2.1. Inclusion and Exclusion Criteria

The inclusion criteria consist of subjects who were examinees who underwent esophagogastroduodenoscopies as part of health checks at our hospital from March 2017 to August 2018 and agreed to participate in the present study.

The exclusion criteria consist of the following: 1. examinees under 20 years of age and those unable to understand information about the purpose of the study; 2. examinees with severe chronic obstructive pulmonary disease (COPD) and known CO_2 retention; 3. examinees who were unable to complete questionnaires at 2 h and 1 day after the procedure. If either questionnaire could not be collected, the subject was removed from the analysis.

2.2. Allocation and Blinding

After written agreement to the study procedures was obtained, the subjects were automatically assigned to receive insufflation with either CO_2 (CO_2 group) or air (air group). The selection of CO_2 or air insufflation changed weekly. This method was chosen to eliminate any bias between the groups attributable to the endoscopist because the attending endoscopist was determined by the day of the week. The schedule was established before the study began and was not changed during the study. A weekly gas exchange was chosen to avoid bias from the endoscopist among groups and to avoid unblinding by changing the gas between procedures. All persons directly involved in the endoscopies, including the examinees, the endoscopists, and the nurses, were blinded with a blindfold on the inflation machine regarding which gas was used.

2.3. Endoscopic Procedure

The transnasal endoscopies were performed with video scopes (EG-L580NW; Fujifilm corporation, Tokyo, Japan) with only local anesthetics to the nostrils. Nostril patency was tested using a pretreatment transnasal catheter of comparable scope diameter (N10/18F-W 6.0 mm-6 cm; TOP Corporation, Tokyo, Japan) lubricated with 2% lidocaine gel. If the nostrils were narrow and the endoscope could not be inserted, a nasal endoscope was inserted orally after 50–100 mg of Xylocaine spray (2%) was added to the oral cavity as a local anesthetic. All procedures were performed without any sedative agents because the endoscopy facility did not use sedatives in transnasal endoscopies for health checks. In the endoscopic examination, the pharynx, esophagus, stomach, duodenal bulb, and second portion were observed, and a biopsy was performed when histopathological examination was necessary. Even if a lesion requiring treatment was found, therapeutic endoscopies were performed on another day. In total, 26 endoscopists and 19 nurses oversaw the endoscopic examinations.

2.4. Gas Delivery

CO_2 was delivered using a CO_2 regulator (GW-1; Fujifilm). The gas flow rate was set at 1.8 L/min for both CO_2 and air insufflation. To prevent unblinding, the regulator was placed behind the endoscopy rack and hidden from the endoscopist's view. The gas to be delivered was set by the coordinator before all procedures of the day began.

2.5. Patient Questionnaire

Examinees completed questionnaires at 2 h and at 1-day post-procedure. The 2 h questionnaire was completed at the hospital before leaving for home, and the 1-day questionnaire was filled out at home and returned by mail. Cases in which either questionnaire could not be retrieved were excluded from the analysis. A visual analogue scale (VAS) was used to rate aspects of the procedure from 0 to 100, with 0 being the lowest and 100 being the highest rating for each factor. Patients rated four factors of their procedural experiences on each questionnaire. The questionnaire at 2 h post-procedure asked about pain during the endoscopy, abdominal distension, abdominal pain, and distress from flatus. The questionnaire at 1-day post-procedure asked about the patient's preferences during a future endoscopy instead of pain during this endoscopy. Both questionnaires had space for free-form comments about other discomfort.

2.6. Endoscopist/Nurse Questionnaire

The endoscopists and the attending nurses independently completed questionnaires to objectively assess patient discomfort using a score from 0 to 10, with 0 indicating no discomfort and 10 indicating maximum discomfort. The endoscopist also evaluated the overall procedural aspects of scope handling on a scale from 0 to 10, with 0 indicating the easiest and 10 the most difficult possible procedure. This evaluation was performed immediately after the procedure. In addition to the information provided in the questionnaires, participants' age, sex, length of examination, history of endoscopies, presence of biopsy, and rate of change from a nasal to an oral route were also included in the study.

2.7. Outcomes and Statistical Analysis

The primary outcome was set as improvement of abdominal pain and distension at 2 h and 1-day post-procedure. These data were collected by questionnaire from the patients after the procedure. The secondary outcomes were set as painfulness of endoscopies, procedure times, and rate of adverse events. The results of the questionnaires from the endoscopists and nurses were also analyzed.

We were planning a study of a continuous response variable in control and experimental subjects with one control for each experimental subject. In a previous study [9,10], the responses within each subject group were normally distributed with a standard deviation of 40. If the true difference between the experimental and control means were 10, we would need to study 337 experimental subjects and 337 control subjects to be able to reject the null hypothesis that the population means of the experimental and control groups are equal with a probability (power) of 0.9. The type I error probability associated with this test of the null hypothesis is 0.05. Analyses were performed on a per-protocol basis for patients who underwent the procedure. Characteristics of the study groups were compared with a t-test or Mann–Whitney U test for continuous variables and a chi-squared test (or Fisher's exact test, as appropriate) for categorical variables. A two-sided p-value < 0.05 was considered statistically significant for all tests.

3. Results

3.1. Subject Allocation

From March 2017 to August 2018, 1794 examinees underwent transnasal endoscopies during health checks at our hospital. Twenty-two examinees were excluded from the study due to a history of COPD. The study period was 72 weeks, with 36 weeks each allocated to the CO_2 and air groups. The average number of participants per week was 9.3. Finally,

674 examinees agreed to participate in the present study; 336 and 338 were allocated to the CO_2 group and air group, respectively. The flow chart of subject allocation is shown in Figure 1.

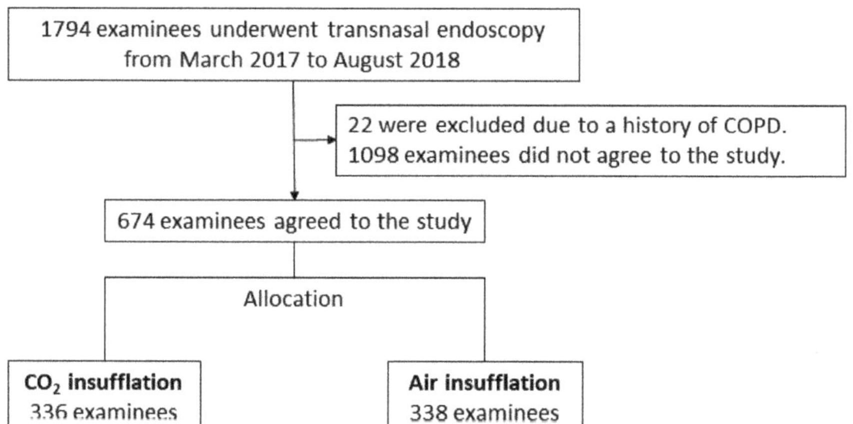

Figure 1. Flow chart of examinee allocation. Of the total 1794 examinees, 674 were finally included in the analysis.

3.2. Participant Characteristics

Participant characteristics and features of endoscopic procedures in the groups receiving CO_2 and air insufflation are shown in Table 1. There were no significant differences between the groups in any parameters, including sex, age, experience of transnasal endoscopy, length of procedure, rate of biopsy, and rate of change to oral endoscopy.

Table 1. Patient characteristics and features of the endoscopic procedures in the groups receiving carbon dioxide (CO_2) and air insufflation.

	CO_2 Group (*n* = 336)	Air Group (*n* = 338)	*p* Value
Sex, M/F	212/124	205/133	0.526
Age (year) *	61.2 ± 11.5	60.1 ± 11.8	0.206
Transnasal endoscopy experienced	167 (49.7%)	178 (52.6%)	0.488
Procedure time (min) *	8.98 ± 2.87	8.95 ± 2.93	0.895
Biopsy performed	33 (9.8%)	43 (12.7%)	0.273
Change to oral	21 (6.2%)	23 (6.8%)	0.876

* expressed as mean ± standard deviation.

3.3. Results of Examinee Questionnaires

The results of examinee questionnaires are summarized in Table 2 and Figure 2A–C. The VAS scores for abdominal distension (15.4 vs. 25.5; $p < 0.001$) and distress from flatus (16.0 vs. 28.8; $p < 0.001$) at 2 h post-procedure were significantly reduced in the CO_2 group compared to the air group, respectively. With regard to pain during the procedure and abdominal pain afterward, the VAS scores of the CO_2 group tended to be lower than those of the air group at 2 h post-procedure, but the difference was not significant (33.5 vs. 37.1, respectively; $p = 0.059$ for pain during the procedure; 3.9 vs. 5.7, respectively; $p = 0.052$ for postprocedure abdominal pain). At 1-day post-procedure, there were no differences between the CO_2 and air groups, respectively, in any parameter including abdominal distension (8.1 vs. 7.0; $p = 0.383$), distress from flatus (11.4 vs. 12.5; $p = 0.490$), abdominal pain (4.1 vs. 3.0; $p = 0.166$), and preference in a future endoscopy (19.1 vs. 18.8; $p = 0.844$). For abdominal distension, distress from flatus, and abdominal pain, the change in VAS score over time from 2 h to the next day is shown in Figure 2A–C.

Table 2. Results of examinees' questionnaires.

Timing	Abdominal Distention			Distress by Flatus			Abdominal Pain		
	CO_2	Air	*p* Value	CO_2	Air	*p* Value	CO_2	Air	*p* Value
2 h	15.4 ± 1.1	25.5 ± 1.4	<0.001 *	16.0 ± 1.3	28.8 ± 1.6	<0.001 *	3.9 ± 0.6	5.7 ± 0.7	0.052
1 day	8.1 ± 1.0	7.0 ± 0.8	0.383	11.4 ± 1.1	12.5 ± 1.1	0.490	4.1 ± 0.6	3.0 ± 0.5	0.166

Timing	Painfulness during Procedure			Preference in a Future Endoscopy		
	CO_2	Air	*p* Value	CO_2	Air	*p* Value
2 h	33.5 ± 1.4	37.1 ± 1.3	0.059	-	-	-
1 day	-	-	-	19.1 ± 1.4	18.8 ± 1.3	0.844

Data was expressed as mean ± standard error. * shows significant difference between CO_2 and air insufflation at same timing.

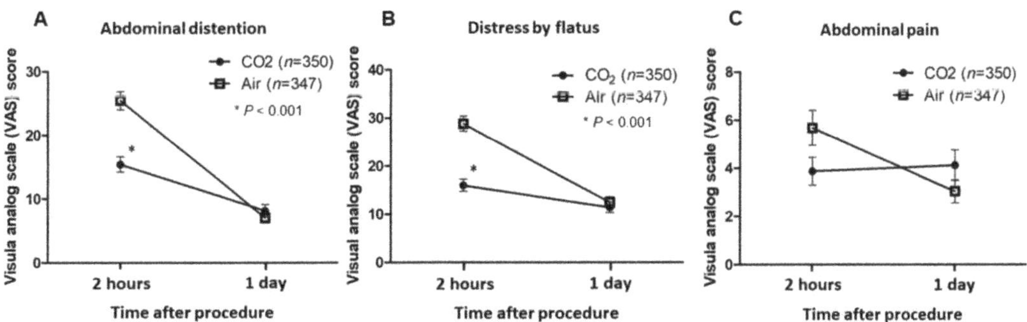

Figure 2. The change over time in the visual analog scale (VAS) score from 2 h to 1 day after the procedure. (**A**) VAS scores for abdominal distension. The VAS score for CO_2 insufflation was significantly lower than that for air insufflation (15.4 vs. 25.5; $p < 0.001$) at 2 h, but not at 1 day after the procedure. (**B**) VAS scores for distress due to flatus. The VAS score for CO_2 insufflation was significantly lower than that for air insufflation at 2 h after the procedure (16.0 vs. 28.8; $p < 0.001$). (**C**) VAS scores for abdominal pain. There was no significant difference in abdominal pain between the two groups.

Some examinees complained of nasal symptoms such as nasal pain and rhinorrhea in the free comments at both 2 h and 1-day post-procedure. The rate of nasal symptoms was compared between the groups (no data shown). However, there was no significant difference between CO_2 and air insufflation at both time points (9.4% vs. 9.8%; $p = 0.869$ at 2 h post-procedure and 4.9% vs. 3.5%; $p = 0.355$ at 1-day postprocedure, respectively).

3.4. Results of Endoscopist and Nurse Questionnaires

The results of the endoscopist and nurse questionnaires are summarized in Table 3. Ratings of overall scope handling by the endoscopist showed no significant difference between the CO_2 group and the air group (1.75 vs. 1.79; $p = 0.709$). The endoscopist and attending nurse evaluations of patient discomfort also showed no significant difference between the two groups (1.93 vs. 2.00; $p = 0.471$ by endoscopist, 1.29 vs. 1.32; $p = 0.794$ by nurse).

Table 3. Results of endoscopist and nurse questionnaires.

Evaluator	Parameter	CO_2 (*n* = 336)	Air (*n* = 338)	*p* Value
Endoscopist	Overall scope handling	1.75 ± 0.08	1.79 ± 0.08	0.709
	Examinee's discomfort	1.93 ± 0.08	2.00 ± 0.08	0.471
Nurse	Examinee's discomfort	1.29 ± 0.06	1.32 ± 0.06	0.794

Data was expressed as mean ± standard error. Each parameter was evaluated on a scale of 10.

3.5. Adverse Events

All procedures were safely completed according to the planned program, and there were no apparent adverse events requiring treatment or follow-up.

4. Discussion

4.1. Evaluation of the CO_2 Effect on Reducing Abdominal Discomfort

This prospective, double-blind, case-controlled study revealed that CO_2 insufflation during transnasal esophagogastroduodenoscopies reduced postprocedural abdominal discomfort, including abdominal distension and distress from flatus, compared to air insufflation. Initially, a randomized-control trial was planned, but the present study involved healthy people undergoing health checks, and a large number of examinees received endoscopies on the same day. Therefore, we were unable to take the time to randomize the subjects and double-blind them, and finally abandoned randomization. The VAS scores at 2 h post-procedure decreased by about 50 to 60% in the CO_2 insufflation group, although VAS scores at 1-day post-procedure were not significantly different. Many previous studies and meta-analyses have also reported that CO_2 insufflation reduces postprocedural abdominal pain compared to air insufflation. However, the targeted procedures were limited to colonoscopies and therapeutic endoscopies, such as double-balloon endoscopies, endoscopic retrograde cholangiopancreatoscopies, and ESDs. This is the first study to demonstrate the usefulness of CO_2 insufflation in a brief diagnostic endoscopy, the transnasal esophagogastroduodenoscopy. In the present study, pain during the procedure, abdominal distension, distress from flatus, and abdominal pain were used as indices to evaluate abdominal discomfort, almost the same as the parameters used in previous studies. Pain during the procedure tended to be lower with CO_2 insufflation, but the difference was not statistically significant. The difference between CO_2 and air seemed to be small because nasal pain and the vomiting reflex had greater effects than gas insufflation on patient discomfort from transnasal esophagogastroduodenoscopies. The examinees' discomfort was significantly different between the CO2 and air groups as assessed by the subjects themselves using the VAS scores but not by the nurses. These results indicate that the subjective evaluation of the examinees their selves is important for the discomfort from endoscopies because the objective evaluation by the surrounding medical personnel is not accurate.

4.2. Duration of the CO_2 Effect on Reducing Abdominal Discomfort

In the present study, CO_2 was observed to reduce abdominal discomfort at 2 h after the procedure but not on the next day. Rogers et al. analyzed the duration of the CO_2 effect on postprocedural pain in their meta-analysis [13]. This meta-analysis, which included 23 studies, revealed that patients receiving CO_2 insufflation consistently had less pain at 2 h postprocedure, and this effect persisted at 6 h postprocedure. However, there was no difference in abdominal pain between the CO_2 and air groups at 24 h postprocedure. Dollen et al. also reported that the CO_2 effect persisted to 6 h after the procedure in their meta-analysis [14]. The results of these meta-analyses match those of the present study. Therefore, the advantage of CO_2 insufflation in esophagogastroduodenoscopies can be expected to last for about 6 h after the procedure. The COVID-19 pandemic has become a worldwide concern in recent years, as has endoscopy-related transmission. CO_2 insufflation may reduce the length of the patient's hospital stay by reducing abdominal discomfort on the day of the test, and the reduced length of stay might help limit COVID-19 transmission.

4.3. CO_2 Effect on Procedure Time

Because the absorption of CO_2 from the gastrointestinal tract is much faster than that of air, there was concern that the amount and frequency of CO_2 insufflation required for the procedure would be greater, resulting in a longer procedure time. However, the procedure time did not differ between CO_2 insufflation and air insufflation (8.98 min. vs. 8.95 min, respectively; $p = 0.893$). Previous randomized controlled trials (RCTs) [15–17] and meta-analyses [13] showed similar results in colonoscopies. Therefore, CO_2 insufflation seems to have little effect on the procedure time of transnasal esophagogastroduodenoscopies.

4.4. Safety of CO_2 Insufflation during Transnasal Esophagogastroduodenoscopies

Carbon dioxide is easily eliminated by respiration after absorption from the gastrointestinal tract. Since the respiratory system is the main route of CO_2 excretion, most prospective studies, including the present study, excluded examinees with severe respiratory compromise or COPD with known CO_2 retention. Although severe respiratory compromise has been excluded, there have been no reports of adverse events with CO_2 insufflation in previous prospective studies. In the present study of 674 participants, no apparent adverse events were observed except for nasal hemorrhage that did not require treatment. Rogers et al. examined CO_2 concentration in the arterial blood before and after colonoscopic polypectomy with CO_2 insufflation and found that the increase in CO_2 partial pressure was limited (37.3–40.6 mmHg), and the pH value did not change (from 7.46 to 7.45) [18]. Bretthauer et al. evaluated end-tidal CO_2 under CO_2 insufflation in colonoscopies and revealed that end-tidal CO_2 decreased after the procedure with both CO_2 insufflation and air insufflation [19]. The results of these studies suggest that CO_2 insufflation during health check esophagogastroduodenoscopies is sufficiently safe.

4.5. Cost of CO_2 Insufflation for Esophagogastroduodenoscopies during Health Checks

Many RCTs and meta-analyses have examined the utility of CO_2 insufflation in diagnostic and therapeutic endoscopies, and its efficacy is now well established. However, in a 2009 survey of 580 European endoscopists, only 47% had heard of CO_2 insufflation. Moreover, among them, 87% were aware of the convincing evidence showing that CO_2 was superior to air, but only 4% were using CO_2 insufflation [20]. Cost is one of the reasons that CO_2 insufflation is not widely used [21]. Air insufflation does not cost money, but CO_2 insufflation does. No study addressed the additional cost of CO_2 use for endoscopic insufflation, and to date, no cost-effectiveness study has been performed. In practice, the cost of installing a CO_2 insufflator is about \$4000 to \$8000, but once it is installed, the running cost is negligible [22]. In this study, procedure time was about 9 min in the CO_2 group, and the amount of CO_2 used in one procedure was 16.2 L, even if CO_2 was delivered throughout the procedure. Given that liquid CO_2 can be purchased for about \$2 per kilogram, the cost of CO_2 per procedure can be calculated as about \$0.06. There was no significant difference in preference in a future endoscopy between CO_2 and air insufflation, so the likely impact of increasing the use of CO_2 seems to be minimal. In addition, in areas where medical resources are limited, the installation of CO_2 regulators and the stable supply of CO_2 could be difficult at present, and therefore, the use of CO_2 in routine clinical practice is limited in those areas. However, there is no reason to be reluctant to use CO_2, especially during health checks, because it can reduce abdominal discomfort on the day of the endoscopy at a low cost.

4.6. Limitations

First, it was conducted at a single center. Second, the subjects were not assigned randomly. The selection between CO_2 and air insufflation was changed weekly, and the schedule was already established before the study began. Although this technique is not randomization, bias is considered to be low. Third, the rate of obtaining consent was low, 38%, because the study was conducted with examinees having regular health checks.

While recognizing these limitations, we recommend CO_2 insufflation during transnasal esophagogastroduodenoscopies to reduce abdominal discomfort after the procedures.

5. Conclusions

CO_2 insufflation may reduce postprocedural abdominal discomfort in transnasal esophagogastroduodenoscopy.

Author Contributions: T.F. performed the study and drafted the article. S.I. and K.T. analyzed and interpreted the results. H.F., H.Y., M.S. and T.N. provided the health check clinic. N.S., M.H., A.N. and S.W. designed the study. H.I. modified and edited the manuscript. All authors have read and agreed to the published version of the manuscript.

Funding: This study was not funded by any organizations.

Institutional Review Board Statement: This study was carried out in accordance with relevant guidelines and regulations, and the study protocol was approved by the Hospital Ethics Committee of Juntendo University Hospital (No. 16-240).

Informed Consent Statement: We explained the study to all the participants, and written informed consent was obtained.

Data Availability Statement: The data sets used and/or analyzed during the current study are available from the corresponding authors on reasonable request. However, the data sets include personal information. Therefore, limited information without personal information is available.

Acknowledgments: We would like to express our appreciation to Fuzuki Iseki of the health check division, Kiyomi Nakamura, general manager and head nurse of the endoscopic division, and the staffs and nurses of the health check division and the endoscopic division, who kindly cooperated in this study. We also thank Tatsuo Ogiwara, Kyoko Fukuhara, Tomonori Aoyama, Kumiko Ueda, Shino Uchida, Hiroo Fukada, and Hirofumi Fukushima for performing the endoscopies.

Conflicts of Interest: The authors declare that they have no competing interests.

References

1. Saltzman, H.A.; Sieker, H.O. Intestinal response to changing gaseous environments: Normobaric and hyperbaric observations. *Ann. N. Y. Acad. Sci.* **1968**, *150*, 31–39. [CrossRef] [PubMed]
2. Stevenson, G.; Wilson, J.; Wilkinson, J.; Norman, G.; Goodacre, R. Pain following colonoscopy: Elimination with carbon dioxide. *Gastrointest. Endosc.* **1992**, *38*, 564–567. [CrossRef]
3. Sumanac, K.; Zealley, I.; Fox, B.M.; Rawlinson, J.; Salena, B.; Marshall, J.K.; Stevenson, G.W.; Hunt, R.H. Minimizing post-colonoscopy abdominal pain by using CO(2) insufflation: A prospective, randomized, double blind, controlled trial evaluating a new commercially available CO(2) delivery system. *Gastrointest. Endosc.* **2002**, *56*, 190–194. [CrossRef]
4. Bretthauer, M.; Lynge, A.B.; Thiis-Evensen, E.; Hoff, G.; Fausa, O.; Aabakken, L. Carbon Dioxide Insufflation in Colonoscopy: Safe and Effective in Sedated Patients. *Endoscopy* **2005**, *37*, 706–709. [CrossRef]
5. Domagk, D.; Bretthauer, M.; Lenz, P.; Aabakken, L.; Ullerich, H.; Maaser, C.; Domschke, W.; Kucharzik, T. Carbon dioxide insufflation improves intubation depth in double-balloon enteroscopy: A randomized, controlled, double-blind trial. *Endoscopy* **2007**, *39*, 1064–1067. [CrossRef]
6. Bretthauer, M.; Seip, B.; Aasen, S.; Kordal, M.; Hoff, G.; Aabakken, L. Carbon dioxide insufflation for more comfortable endoscopic retrograde cholangiopancreatography: A randomized, controlled, double-blind trial. *Endoscopy* **2007**, *39*, 58–64. [CrossRef]
7. Maple, J.T.; Keswani, R.N.; Hovis, R.M.; Saddedin, E.Z.; Jonnalagadda, S.; Azar, R.R.; Hagen, C.; Thompson, D.M.; Waldbaum, L.; Edmundowicz, S.A. Carbon dioxide insufflation during ERCP for reduction of postprocedure pain: A randomized, double-blind, controlled trial. *Gastrointest. Endosc.* **2009**, *70*, 278–283. [CrossRef]
8. Kuwatani, M.; Kawakami, H.; Hayashi, T.; Ishiwatari, H.; Kudo, T.; Yamato, H.; Ehira, N.; Haba, S.; Eto, K.; Kato, M.; et al. Carbon dioxide insufflation during endoscopic retrograde cholangiopancreatography reduces bowel gas volume but does not affect visual analogue scale scores of suffering: A prospective, double-blind, randomized, controlled trial. *Surg. Endosc.* **2011**, *25*, 3784–3790. [CrossRef]
9. Maeda, Y.; Hirasawa, D.; Fujita, N.; Obana, T.; Sugawara, T.; Ohira, T.; Harada, Y.; Yamagata, T.; Suzuki, K.; Koike, Y.; et al. A prospective, randomized, double-blind, controlled trial on the efficacy of carbon dioxide insufflation in gastric endoscopic submucosal dissection. *Endoscopy* **2013**, *45*, 335–341. [CrossRef]
10. Kim, S.Y.; Chung, J.-W.; Park, D.K.; Kwon, K.A.; Kim, K.O.; Kim, Y.J. Efficacy of carbon dioxide insufflation during gastric endoscopic submucosal dissection: A randomized, double-blind, controlled, prospective study. *Gastrointest. Endosc.* **2015**, *82*, 1018–1024. [CrossRef]
11. Alexandridis, E.; Inglis, S.; McAvoy, N.C.; Falconer, E.; Graham, C.; Hayes, P.C.; Plevris, J.N. Randomised clinical trial: Comparison of acceptability, patient tolerance, cardiac stress and endoscopic views in transnasal and transoral endoscopy under local anaesthetic. *Aliment. Pharmacol. Ther.* **2014**, *40*, 467–476. [CrossRef] [PubMed]
12. Moriarty, J.P.; Shah, N.D.; Rubenstein, J.H.; Blevins, C.H.; Johnson, M.; Katzka, D.A.; Wang, K.K.; Wongkeesong, L.M.; Ahlquist, D.A.; Iyer, P.G. Costs associated with Barrett's esophagus screening in the community: An economic analysis of a prospective randomized controlled trial of sedated versus hospital unsedated versus mobile community unsedated endoscopy. *Gastrointest. Endosc.* **2018**, *87*, 88–94.e2. [CrossRef] [PubMed]

13. Rogers, A.C.; Van De Hoef, D.; Sahebally, S.M.; Winter, D.C. A meta-analysis of carbon dioxide versus room air insufflation on patient comfort and key performance indicators at colonoscopy. *Int. J. Color. Dis.* **2020**, *35*, 455–464. [CrossRef] [PubMed]
14. Dellon, E.S.; Hawk, J.S.; Grimm, I.; Shaheen, N.J. The use of carbon dioxide for insufflation during GI endoscopy: A systematic review. *Gastrointest. Endosc.* **2009**, *69*, 843–849. [CrossRef]
15. Szura, M.; Pach, R.; Matyja, A.; Kulig, J. Carbon dioxide insufflation during screening unsedated colonoscopy: A randomised clinical trial. *Eur. J. Cancer Prev. Off. J. Eur. Cancer Prev. Organ. (ECP)* **2015**, *24*, 37–43. [CrossRef]
16. Falt, P.; Smajstrla, V.; Fojtik, P.; Hill, M.; Urban, O. Carbon dioxide insufflation during colonoscopy in inflammatory bowel disease patients: A double-blind, randomized, single-center trial. *Eur. J. Gastroenterol. Hepatol.* **2017**, *29*, 355–359. [CrossRef]
17. Chen, Y.-J.; Lee, J.; Puryear, M.; Wong, R.K.H.; Lake, J.M.; Maydonovitch, C.L.; Belle, L.; Moawad, F.J. A Randomized Controlled Study Comparing Room Air with Carbon Dioxide for Abdominal Pain, Distention, and Recovery Time in Patients Undergoing Colonoscopy. *Gastroenterol. Nurs.* **2014**, *37*, 273–278. [CrossRef]
18. Rogers, B.G. The safety of carbon dioxide insufflation during colonoscopic electrosurgical polypectomy. *Gastrointest. Endosc.* **1974**, *20*, 115–117. [CrossRef]
19. Bretthauer, M.; Thiis-Evensen, E.; Huppertz-Hauss, G.; Gisselsson, L.; Grotmol, T.; Skovlund, E.; Hoff, G. NORCCAP (Norwegian colorectal cancer prevention): A randomised trial to assess the safety and efficacy of carbon dioxide versus air insufflation in colonoscopy. *Gut* **2002**, *50*, 604–607. [CrossRef]
20. Janssens, F.; Deviere, J.; Eisendrath, P.; Dumonceau, J.-M. Carbon dioxide for gut distension during digestive endoscopy: Technique and practice survey. *World J. Gastroenterol.* **2009**, *15*, 1475–1479. [CrossRef]
21. Bretthauer, M.; Kalager, M.; Adami, H.-O.; Hoff, G. Who Is for CO2? Slow Adoption of Carbon Dioxide Insufflation in Colonoscopy. *Ann. Intern. Med.* **2016**, *165*, 145. [CrossRef] [PubMed]
22. Lo, S.K.; Fujii-Lau, L.L.; Enestvedt, B.K.; Hwang, J.H.; Konda, V.; Manfredi, M.A.; Maple, J.T.; Murad, F.M.; Pannala, R.; Woods, K.L.; et al. The use of carbon dioxide in gastrointestinal endoscopy. *Gastrointest. Endosc.* **2016**, *83*, 857–865. [CrossRef] [PubMed]

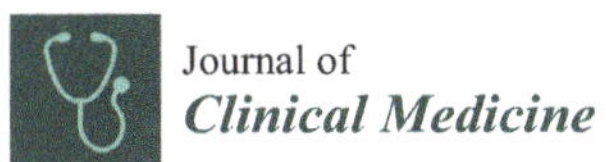

Journal of
Clinical Medicine

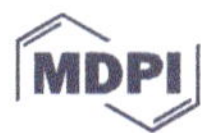

Article

Risk of Mortality among Patients with Gastrointestinal Bleeding with Early and Late Treatment with Tranexamic Acid: A Population-Based Cohort Study

Ke-Hsin Ting [1,2], Bei-Hao Shiu [2,3,4], Shun-Fa Yang [2,5], Pei-Lun Liao [2,5], Jing-Yang Huang [2,5], Yin-Yang Chen [2,3,*] and Chao-Bin Yeh [2,6,7,*]

[1] Division of Cardiology, Department of Internal Medicine, Changhua Christian Hospital, Yunlin Branch, Yunlin 648, Taiwan; patrickting3@kimo.com
[2] Institute of Medicine, Chung Shan Medical University, Taichung 402, Taiwan; shiubeihao@gmail.com (B.-H.S.); ysf@csmu.edu.tw (S.-F.Y.); liaopeilun0410@gmail.com (P.-L.L.); wchinyang@gmail.com (J.-Y.H.)
[3] Department of Surgery, Chung Shan Medical University Hospital, Taichung 402, Taiwan
[4] School of Medicine, Chung Shan Medical University, Taichung 402, Taiwan
[5] Department of Medical Research, Chung Shan Medical University Hospital, Taichung 402, Taiwan
[6] Department of Emergency Medicine, School of Medicine, Chung Shan Medical University, Taichung 402, Taiwan
[7] Department of Emergency Medicine, Chung Shan Medical University Hospital, Taichung 402, Taiwan
* Correspondence: jeff80329@hotmail.com (Y.-Y.C.); sky5ff@gmail.com (C.-B.Y.)

Citation: Ting, K.-H.; Shiu, B.-H.; Yang, S.-F.; Liao, P.-L.; Huang, J.-Y.; Chen, Y.-Y.; Yeh, C.-B. Risk of Mortality among Patients with Gastrointestinal Bleeding with Early and Late Treatment with Tranexamic Acid: A Population-Based Cohort Study. *J. Clin. Med.* 2022, 11, 1741. https://doi.org/10.3390/jcm11061741

Academic Editor: Hidekazu Suzuki

Received: 3 March 2022
Accepted: 18 March 2022
Published: 21 March 2022

Publisher's Note: MDPI stays neutral with regard to jurisdictional claims in published maps and institutional affiliations.

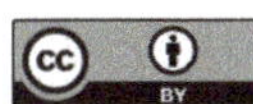

Abstract: Tranexamic acid (TXA) is an antifibrinolytic pharmacological agent, but its use in gastrointestinal bleeding remains contentious. Moreover, studies on the timing of TXA administration are limited. We examined whether early TXA administration reduced the risk of mortality in patients with gastrointestinal bleeding in a Taiwanese population. We used the National Health Insurance Research Database to identify patients diagnosed with gastrointestinal bleeding with early and late TXA treatment. We defined early treatment as initial TXA treatment in an emergency department and late treatment as initial TXA treatment after hospitalization. Mortality within 52 weeks was the primary outcome. A multivariable analysis using a multiple Cox regression model was applied for data analysis. Propensity score matching (PSM) was performed to reduce the potential for bias caused by measured confounding variables. Of the 52,949 selected patients with gastrointestinal bleeding, 5127 were assigned to either an early or late TXA treatment group after PSM. The incidence of mortality was significantly decreased during the first and fourth weeks (adjusted HR (aHR): 0.65, 95% CI: 0.56–0.75). A Kaplan–Meier curve revealed a significant decrease in cumulative incidence of mortality in the early TXA treatment group (log-rank test: $p < 0.0001$). Multiple Cox regression analysis revealed significantly lower mortality in the early TXA treatment group compared with the late treatment group (aHR: 0.64, 95% CI: 0.57–0.73). Thromboembolic events were not significantly associated with early or late TXA treatment (aHR: 1.03, 95% CI: 0.94–1.12). A Kaplan–Meier curve also revealed no significant difference in either venous or arterial events (log-rank test: $p = 0.3654$ and 0.0975, respectively). In conclusion, early TXA treatment was associated with a reduced risk of mortality in patients with gastrointestinal bleeding compared with late treatment, without an increase in thromboembolic events. The risk of rebleeding and need for urgent endoscopic intervention require further randomized clinical trials.

Keywords: tranexamic acid; gastrointestinal bleeding; mortality; thromboembolic events

1. Introduction

Acute gastrointestinal bleeding is a common cause of morbidity and mortality worldwide [1] with a reported mortality rate of 2–10% [2,3]. The bleeding can arise from both the upper and lower gastrointestinal tracts, including from peptic ulcers, esophageal or gastric varices, diverticulitis, colitis, or malignancy in the gastrointestinal tract. Clinical symptoms of acute gastrointestinal bleeding typically include hematemesis, melaena, or hematochezia. The initial management of gastrointestinal bleeding in emergency departments includes triage, supportive management, blood transfusion, fluid resuscitation, and endoscopic therapy, depending on the severity and hemodynamic status of patients.

Tranexamic acid (TXA) is an antifibrinolytic agent that reversibly inhibits the conversion of plasminogen to plasmin, resulting in a reduction in fibrinolysis. First introduced for menorrhagia in 1968 [4], TXA has the ability to reduce postoperative hemorrhage [5,6], postpartum hemorrhage [7], and mortality in patients with traumatic hemorrhage [8]. The role of TXA in acute gastrointestinal bleeding remains under debate, without clear recommendations for its clinical use.

However, studies have demonstrated its efficacy in reducing the mortality rate of patients with acute gastrointestinal bleeding [9,10]. A recent systemic review and meta-analysis including 13 randomized trials with a total of 2271 patients with acute gastrointestinal bleeding revealed that TXA significantly reduced the mortality rate (relative risk (RR) = 0.60; 95% CI, 0.45–0.80) and rates of continued bleeding (RR = 0.60; 95% CI, 0.43–0.84) [11]. In contrast, another randomized controlled trial (HALT-IT trial) revealed that TXA did not significantly reduce mortality in patients with gastrointestinal bleeding (RR = 0.99, 95% CI, 0.82–1.18) [12]. However, adverse venous thromboembolic events were higher in patients using TXA than in those not using it.

A possible confounding factor is the timing of TXA administration, which has rarely been considered in studies and could affect study outcomes. Hence, this nationwide cohort study aimed to identify whether early or late use of TXA reduced the mortality of patients with gastrointestinal bleeding in Taiwan. We hypothesized that patients with gastrointestinal bleeding receiving TXA early would have lower risk of mortality.

2. Materials and Methods

2.1. Study Design and Population

In this retrospective cohort study, we analyzed the administration of TXA for gastrointestinal bleeding and the risk of all-cause mortality. Taiwan adopted a National Health Insurance system in 1995, this system claims data as the National Health Insurance Research Database (NHIRD). The NHIRD provides real-world evidence for exploring the risk factors or effects of an intervention for specific diseases, and contains the insurance claims data of more than 99% of Taiwan's population. We used NHIRD data from between January 2000 and December 2017 to evaluate the risk of all-cause mortality among patients with gastrointestinal bleeding who received early or late TXA treatment. This study was approved by the Institutional Review Board of the Chung Shan Medical University Hospital (approval number CS2-20036).

2.2. Study Population

We initially included 52,949 hospitalized patients who went to an emergency department for gastrointestinal bleeding, as defined by the following International Classification of Diseases, Ninth Revision, Clinical Modification (ICD-9-CM) codes: 530.1, 530.2, 530.7, 531.0, 531.4, 531.9, 532.0, 532.4, 532.9, and 578. In addition, the following ICD-10-CM codes were applied: K20.0, K20.8, K20.9, K21.0, K22.10, K22.11, K22.6, K25.0, K25.4, K25.9, K26.0, K26.4, K26.9, K92.0, K92.1, and K92.2 (Supplementary Table S1). All the selected patients had a subsequent hospitalization record within 1 day of emergency care. The exclusion criteria were as follows: (1) an index date before 2000 or after 2016 (n = 6670); (2) lack of TXA treatment (ATC code: B02AA02) during emergency treatment or admission (n = 27,436); (3) cancer diagnosis before the index date (n = 4151); and (4) death before the index date (n = 6). This study included 14,686 patients with gastrointestinal bleeding who had received TXA treatment; among these patients, 9513 received early treatment, defined as initial TXA treatment in an emergency department, and 5173 received late treatment, defined as initial TXA treatment after hospitalization.

2.3. Characteristics, Comorbidities, and Study Outcomes

We identified the baseline (within 180 days of the index date) demographic characteristics, such as age and sex, and the comorbidities and medication of each participant to evaluate their health status. Comorbidities included hypertension, diabetes mellitus, hyperlipidemia, kidney disease, chronic pulmonary diseases, liver disease, ischemic heart diseases, ischemic stroke, hemorrhagic stroke, atrial fibrillation, congestive heart failure, dementia, and peripheral vascular disease. Medications included proton-pump inhibitors, hemostatic agents, drugs for constipation, furosemide, metoclopramide, silicon, magnesium oxide, aspirin, clopidogrel or ticagrelor, and nonsteroidal anti-inflammatory drugs.

The study's primary outcome was all-cause mortality within 52 weeks of the index date. The secondary outcomes were thromboembolic events (deep-vein thrombosis, pulmonary embolism, acute myocardial infarction, hemorrhagic stroke, and ischemic stroke). All the patients in the study were followed up from the index date until their withdrawal from the National Health Insurance program, the occurrence of a study event, or 52 weeks after the index date.

2.4. Statistical Analysis

Statistical analysis was performed using SAS software version 9.4 (SAS Institute, Cary, NC, USA), and a p value of < 0.05 was considered significant. The propensity score was the odds of gastrointestinal bleeding according to demographic data, including birth year, sex, age (± 1 year) on the index date, index year, comorbidities, and medication. To reduce potential confounding bias caused by measured factors, 1:1 propensity score matching (PSM) was performed using greedy nearest neighbor non-replacement matching with a caliper width of 0.1. The difference in covariates between the 2 study groups was evaluated using the absolute standardized difference (ASD), as an absolute ASD value of ASD < 0.1 indicated that the groups were balanced with their matched control.

Categorical data are presented as numbers and percentages, and the differences in categorical variables were compared using a chi-square test. The incidence rate with the corresponding CIs and crude hazard ratios (HRs) were calculated using Poisson regression. After the proportional hazards assumption was tested, a Cox proportional hazards model analysis was performed to estimate the HRs for mortality and 95% CIs. The cumulative probabilities of mortality were assessed using a Kaplan–Meier analysis, with statistical significance being determined using the results of a log-rank test.

3. Results

3.1. Characteristics of the Participants

The study flowchart is presented in Figure 1. Of the patients with gastrointestinal bleeding administered TXA, 9513 received early treatment and 5173 received late treatment. In total, 67% of the patients were male and 32% were female, and more than 40% were aged ≥ 71 years. Before PSM, the statistically significant differences between the two groups were index year and medication (including hemostatic agents, drugs for constipation, furosemide, metoclopramide, and silicon). After PSM, the two groups were balanced, as indicated by the ASD of the covariates (Table 1).

Table 1. Baseline characteristics among study groups.

	Before PSM			After PSM		
	Early Treatment	Late Treatment	ASD	Early Treatment	Late Treatment	ASD
N	9513	5173		5127	5127	
Index year			0.2488			0.0239
2000–2005	2064 (21.70%)	1596 (30.85%)		1516 (29.57%)	1551 (30.25%)	
2006–2010	2996 (31.49%)	1692 (32.71%)		1747 (34.07%)	1691 (32.98%)	
2011–2015	4453 (46.81%)	1885 (36.44%)		1864 (36.36%)	1885 (36.77%)	
Sex			0.0025			0.0042
Female	3060 (32.17%)	1658 (32.05%)		1633 (31.85%)	1643 (32.05%)	
Male	6453 (67.83%)	3515 (67.95%)		3494 (68.15%)	3484 (67.95%)	

Table 1. *Cont.*

	Before PSM			After PSM		
	Early Treatment	**Late Treatment**	**ASD**	**Early Treatment**	**Late Treatment**	**ASD**
Age			0.0405			0.0000
$\leq$50	2443 (25.68%)	1277 (24.69%)		1289 (25.14%)	1268 (24.73%)	
51–70	3060 (32.17%)	1591 (30.76%)		1570 (30.62%)	1583 (30.88%)	
$\geq$71	4010 (42.15%)	2305 (44.56%)		2268 (44.24%)	2276 (44.39%)	
CCI score			0.0885			0.0263
0	2225 (23.39%)	1009 (19.51%)		1043 (20.34%)	1006 (19.62%)	
1	2564 (26.95%)	1340 (25.90%)		1265 (24.67%)	1332 (25.98%)	
2	1848 (19.43%)	1101 (21.28%)		1056 (20.6%)	1088 (21.22%)	
$\geq$3	2876 (30.23%)	1723 (33.31%)		1763 (34.39%)	1701 (33.18%)	
Co-morbidity						
Hypertension	4608 (48.44%)	2518 (48.68%)	0.0047	2494 (48.64%)	2495 (48.66%)	0.0004
Diabetes mellitus	2862 (30.09%)	1577 (30.49%)	0.0087	1565 (30.52%)	1564 (30.51%)	0.0004
Hyperlipidemia	1373 (14.43%)	652 (12.60%)	0.0535	637 (12.42%)	650 (12.68%)	0.0077
Kidney disease	1441 (15.15%)	965 (18.65%)	0.0937	940 (18.33%)	946 (18.45%)	0.0030
Chronic pulmonary diseases	1715 (18.03%)	1086 (20.99%)	0.0749	1023 (19.95%)	1065 (20.77%)	0.0203
Liver disease	3233 (33.99%)	1858 (35.92%)	0.0405	1880 (36.67%)	1840 (35.89%)	0.0162
Ischemic heart diseases	1598 (16.80%)	839 (16.22%)	0.0156	810 (15.80%)	834 (16.27%)	0.0128
Ischemic stroke	1045 (10.98%)	615 (11.89%)	0.0284	634 (12.37%)	606 (11.82%)	0.0167
Hemorrhage stroke	239 (2.51%)	170 (3.29%)	0.0461	161 (3.14%)	166 (3.24%)	0.0055
Atrial fibrillation	487 (5.12%)	258 (4.99%)	0.0060	252 (4.92%)	257 (5.01%)	0.0045
Congestive heart failure	1103 (11.59%)	667 (12.89%)	0.0396	647 (12.62%)	656 (12.80%)	0.0053
Dementia	631 (6.63%)	384 (7.42%)	0.0309	386 (7.53%)	380 (7.41%)	0.0045
Peripheral vascular disease	434 (4.56%)	213 (4.12%)	0.0218	198 (3.86%)	212 (4.13%)	0.0139
Medication						
Proton-pump inhibitors	8140 (85.57%)	4430 (85.64%)	0.0020	4403 (85.88%)	4389 (85.61%)	0.0078
Hemostatic	3237 (34.03%)	2085 (40.31%)	0.1302	2069 (40.35%)	2049 (39.96%)	0.0080
Drugs for constipation	5973 (62.79%)	3554 (68.70%)	0.1249	3489 (68.05%)	3508 (68.42%)	0.0080
Furosemide	3329 (34.99%)	2326 (44.96%)	0.2046	2291 (44.69%)	2283 (44.53%)	0.0031
Metoclopramide	4008 (42.13%)	2598 (50.22%)	0.1628	2564 (50.01%)	2553 (49.80%)	0.0043
Silicon	4157 (43.70%)	2539 (49.08%)	0.1081	2502 (48.80%)	2500 (48.76%)	0.0008
Magnesium oxide	1512 (15.89%)	910 (17.59%)	0.0455	887 (17.30%)	890 (17.36%)	0.0016
Aspirin	2833 (29.78%)	1744 (33.71%)	0.0846	1679 (32.75%)	1708 (33.31%)	0.0120
Clopidogrel/Ticagrelor	772 (8.12%)	398 (7.69%)	0.0156	392 (7.65%)	397 (7.74%)	0.0037
NSAIDs	6403 (67.31%)	3638 (70.33%)	0.0652	3603 (70.28%)	3598 (70.18%)	0.0021

ASD: absolute standardized difference, PSM: propensity score matching, CCI score: Charlson Comorbidity Index score.

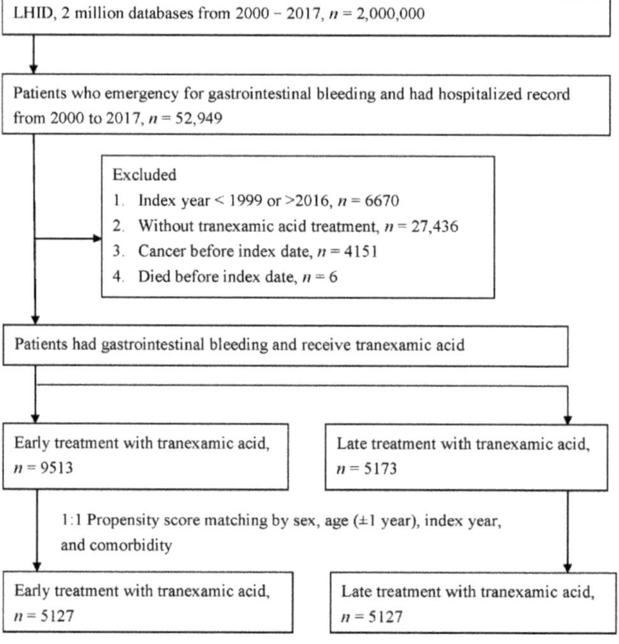

Figure 1. Study flowchart.

3.2. The Risk of Mortality in the TXA Treatment Group

Figure 2 presents the mortality incidence density (per 100 person month), which were 1.22 (95% CI: 1.09–1.37) and 1.86 (95% CI: 1.70–2.04) in the PSM early and late treatment groups, respectively; the adjusted HR for early treatment was 0.65 (95% CI: 0.56–0.75) during the first and fourth weeks. During the 13th and 52nd weeks, the mortality incidence density (per 100 person month) was 0.23 (95% CI: 0.21–0.25) and 0.25 (95% CI: 0.23–0.27) in the early and late treatment groups, respectively; the adjusted HR (aHR) for early treatment was 0.90 (95% CI: 0.80–1.00). A Kaplan–Meier survival analysis revealed significantly lower cumulative incidence of mortality in the early treatment group (log-rank test: $p < 0.0001$; Figure 3).

	Incidence density *(95% C.I.)			aHR *(95% C.I.)
	Early treatment	Late treatment		
Before PSM				
From index date to				
1-4weeks	1.01(0.92-1.11)	1.87(1.71-2.05)		0.65(0.57-0.74)
5-8weeks	0.22(0.19-0.26)	0.48(0.42-0.55)		0.57(0.46-0.69)
9-12weeks	0.15(0.13-0.17)	0.21(0.17-0.25)		0.88(0.70-1.11)
13-52 weeks	0.19(0.17-0.20)	0.25(0.23-0.27)		0.89(0.80-0.99)
After PSM				
From index date to				
1-4weeks	1.22(1.09-1.37)	1.86(1.70-2.04)		0.65(0.56-0.75)
5-8weeks	0.27(0.23-0.33)	0.47(0.41-0.55)		0.55(0.44-0.70)
9-12weeks	0.19(0.16-0.23)	0.20(0.17-0.24)		0.92(0.71-1.18)
13-52 weeks	0.23(0.21-0.25)	0.25(0.23-0.27)		0.90(0.80-1.00)

* Incidence rate, per 100 person months

* aHR, Adjusted Hazard Ratio, adjusted variable including age, sex, co-morbidities and medication

Figure 2. Incidence density of mortality.

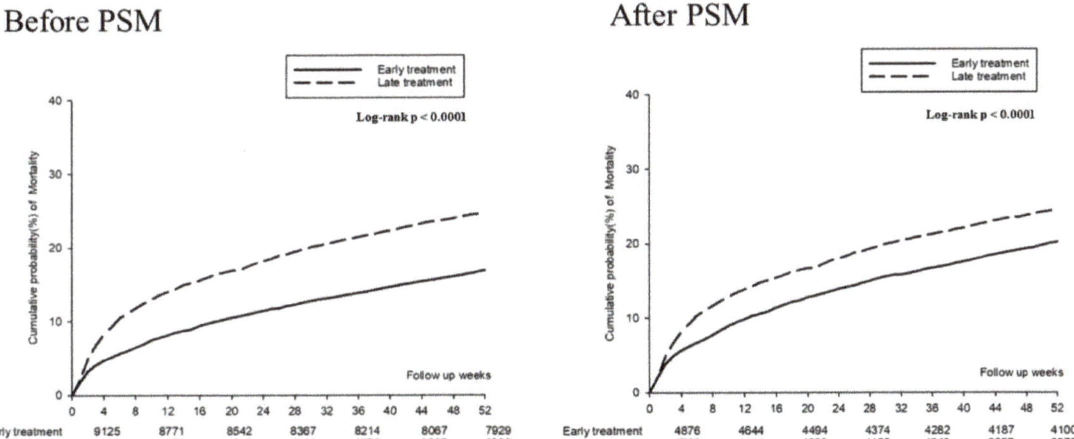

Figure 3. Kaplan–Meier curves for the 52 week mortality risk.

The patients who received early TXA treatment had a significantly lower risk of mortality during the first and eighth weeks compared with those who received late treatment (aHR: 0.64, 95% CI: 0.57–0.73). Other significant risk factors of mortality were age; comorbid kidney disease, liver disease, and hemorrhagic stroke; and prescription for hemostatic agents, drugs for constipation, furosemide, and metoclopramide (Table 2).

Table 2. Multiple Cox regression to estimate the hazard ratio for the 52 week mortality risk.

Variable	aHR (95% CI)	
	1–8 Weeks	**9–52 Weeks**
Study group		
Early treatment	0.64 (0.57–0.73)	0.90 (0.80–1.00)
Late treatment	Reference	Reference
Index year		
2000–2005	Reference	Reference
2006–2010	1.23 (1.05–1.45)	0.98 (0.85–1.14)
2011–2015	1.12 (0.95–1.32)	1.04 (0.90–1.20)
Sex		
Female	Reference	Reference
Male	1.09 (0.95–1.25)	1.24 (1.10–1.40)
Age		
≤ 50	Reference	Reference
51–70	1.18 (0.96–1.45)	0.98 (0.81–1.18)
≥ 71	2.09 (1.70–2.57)	1.81 (1.51–2.18)
Co-morbidity (ref: non)		
Hypertension	0.74 (0.64–0.85)	0.94 (0.83–1.07)
Diabetes mellitus	1.07 (0.93–1.23)	1.24 (1.10–1.39)
Hyperlipidemia	0.76 (0.61–0.94)	0.73 (0.61–0.88)
Kidney disease	1.41 (1.21–1.63)	1.52 (1.34–1.73)
Chronic pulmonary diseases	1.09 (0.94–1.26)	1.22 (1.08–1.39)
Liver disease	1.32 (1.14–1.52)	1.48 (1.31–1.68)
Ischemic heart diseases	0.95 (0.79–1.13)	0.86 (0.73–1.00)
Ischemic stroke	1.01 (0.84–1.21)	1.05 (0.90–1.23)
Hemorrhage stroke	1.88 (1.45–2.44)	1.64 (1.27–2.11)
Atrial fibrillation	0.88 (0.68–1.13)	1.08 (0.88–1.33)
Congestive heart failure	1.18 (0.99–1.40)	1.11 (0.95–1.29)
Dementia	1.17 (0.96–1.42)	1.43 (1.21–1.69)
Peripheral vascular disease	1.23 (0.94–1.61)	1.09 (0.85–1.40)
Medication (ref: non)		
Proton-pump inhibitors	0.93 (0.75–1.14)	1.00 (0.84–1.20)
Hemostatic	1.95 (1.71–2.22)	1.27 (1.13–1.42)
Drugs for constipation	1.22 (1.02–1.45)	2.32 (1.93–2.79)
Furosemide	2.71 (2.32–3.16)	2.41 (2.12–2.74)
Metoclopramide	1.43 (1.25–1.64)	1.50 (1.33–1.69)
Silicon	0.85 (0.75–0.97)	0.97 (0.87–1.09)
magnesium oxide	0.95 (0.81–1.12)	0.92 (0.80–1.05)
Aspirin	1.11 (0.97–1.28)	1.06 (0.94–1.20)
Clopidogrel/Ticagrelor	1.09 (0.87–1.36)	1.27 (1.06–1.53)
NSAIDs	0.93 (0.75–1.14)	1.00 (0.84–1.20)

We also classified the TXA treatment into three groups: (1) early TXA treatment in an emergency department; (2) late TXA treatment after hospitalization; and (3) both early and late TXA treatment. Figure 4 presents the risk of mortality in those who received early TXA treatment compared with those who only received late TXA treatment. Regarding risk during the first and fourth weeks, the aHR for early treatment was 0.55 (95% CI: 0.46–0.65), and the aHR for both early and late treatment was 0.74 (95% CI: 0.63–0.86). Regarding risk during the 13th and 52nd weeks, the aHR for early treatment was 0.89 (95% CI: 0.78–1.02), and the aHR for both early and late treatment was 0.89 (95% CI: 0.78–1.01).

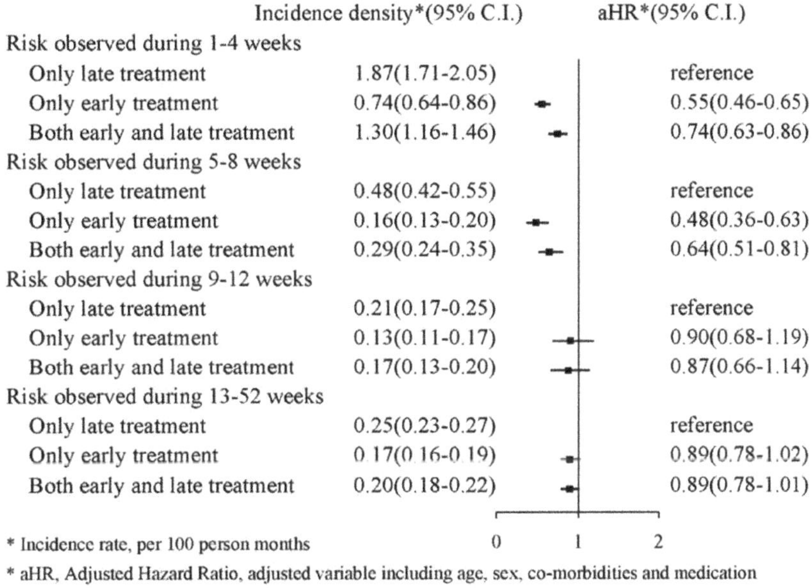

	Incidence density*(95% C.I.)	aHR*(95% C.I.)
Risk observed during 1-4 weeks		
Only late treatment	1.87(1.71-2.05)	reference
Only early treatment	0.74(0.64-0.86)	0.55(0.46-0.65)
Both early and late treatment	1.30(1.16-1.46)	0.74(0.63-0.86)
Risk observed during 5-8 weeks		
Only late treatment	0.48(0.42-0.55)	reference
Only early treatment	0.16(0.13-0.20)	0.48(0.36-0.63)
Both early and late treatment	0.29(0.24-0.35)	0.64(0.51-0.81)
Risk observed during 9-12 weeks		
Only late treatment	0.21(0.17-0.25)	reference
Only early treatment	0.13(0.11-0.17)	0.90(0.68-1.19)
Both early and late treatment	0.17(0.13-0.20)	0.87(0.66-1.14)
Risk observed during 13-52 weeks		
Only late treatment	0.25(0.23-0.27)	reference
Only early treatment	0.17(0.16-0.19)	0.89(0.78-1.02)
Both early and late treatment	0.20(0.18-0.22)	0.89(0.78-1.01)

* Incidence rate, per 100 person months

* aHR, Adjusted Hazard Ratio, adjusted variable including age, sex, co-morbidities and medication

Figure 4. Incidence density of mortality.

3.3. Thromboembolic Events in the TXA Treatment

The thromboembolic events (including deep-vein thrombosis, pulmonary embolism, acute myocardial infarction, hemorrhagic stroke, and ischemic stroke) are presented in Figure 5. The forest plot analysis indicated no significant association between thromboembolic events and early or late TXA treatment (aHR: 1.03, 95% CI: 0.94–1.12). The Kaplan–Meier survival analysis also identified no significant increased cumulative probability of either venous or arterial events (log-rank: *p* = 0.3654 and 0.0975, respectively, Figure 6).

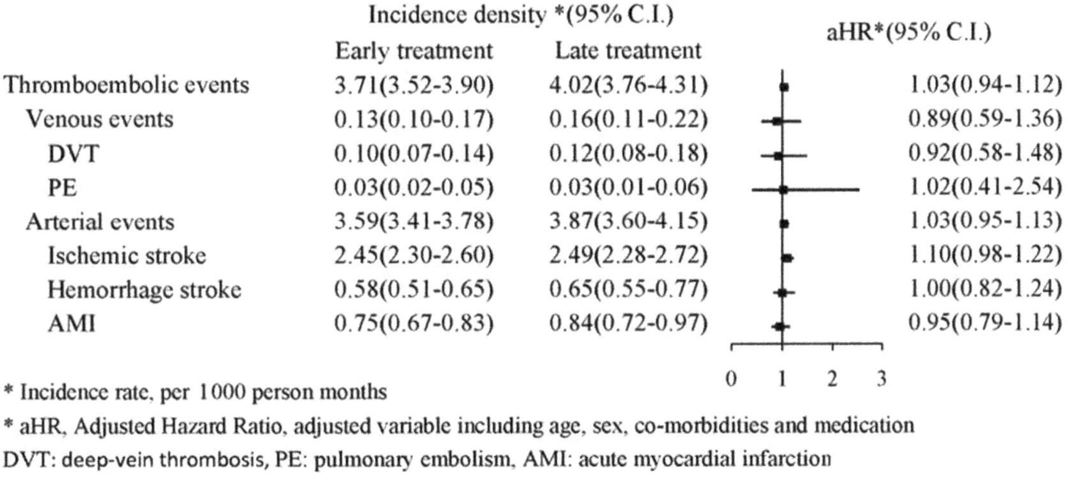

	Incidence density *(95% C.I.)		aHR*(95% C.I.)
	Early treatment	Late treatment	
Thromboembolic events	3.71(3.52-3.90)	4.02(3.76-4.31)	1.03(0.94-1.12)
Venous events	0.13(0.10-0.17)	0.16(0.11-0.22)	0.89(0.59-1.36)
DVT	0.10(0.07-0.14)	0.12(0.08-0.18)	0.92(0.58-1.48)
PE	0.03(0.02-0.05)	0.03(0.01-0.06)	1.02(0.41-2.54)
Arterial events	3.59(3.41-3.78)	3.87(3.60-4.15)	1.03(0.95-1.13)
Ischemic stroke	2.45(2.30-2.60)	2.49(2.28-2.72)	1.10(0.98-1.22)
Hemorrhage stroke	0.58(0.51-0.65)	0.65(0.55-0.77)	1.00(0.82-1.24)
AMI	0.75(0.67-0.83)	0.84(0.72-0.97)	0.95(0.79-1.14)

* Incidence rate, per 1000 person months

* aHR, Adjusted Hazard Ratio, adjusted variable including age, sex, co-morbidities and medication

DVT: deep-vein thrombosis, PE: pulmonary embolism, AMI: acute myocardial infarction

Figure 5. Flowchart of patient selection.

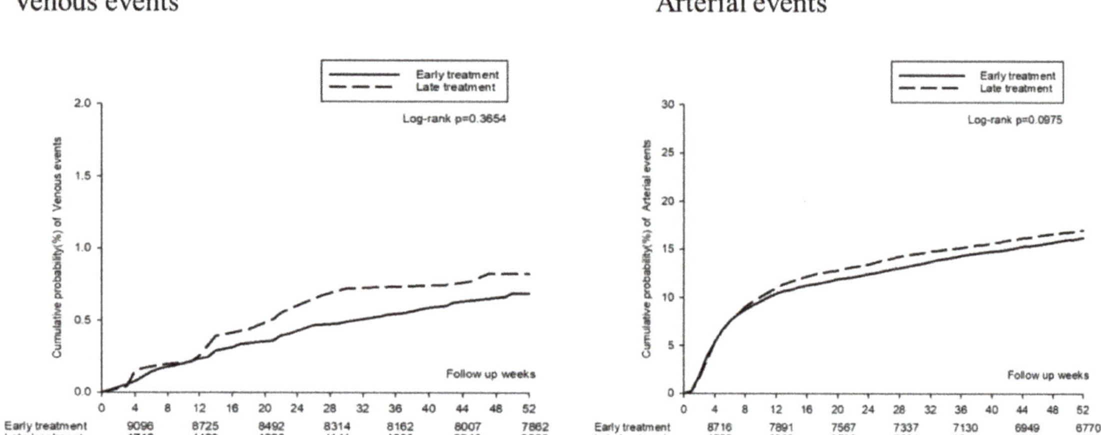

Figure 6. Kaplan–Meier curves for the 52 week thromboembolic events.

4. Discussion

In this population-based trial, which included 10,254 patients with gastrointestinal bleeding, early TXA treatment was associated with 36% and 12% lower mortality for a follow-up period of 1 to 8 and 9 to 52 weeks, respectively. Moreover, early TXA treatment did not increase the risk of either venous or arterial thromboembolic events compared with late treatment.

TXA use for gastrointestinal bleeding has been evaluated in randomized clinical trials. In the HALT-IT trial, compared with the equivalent infusion of saline, TXA administration resulted in a lower risk of death caused by bleeding and rebleeding within 24 h, 5 days, and 28 days. However, an increased risk of venous thromboembolic events was observed [12]. Another randomized clinical trial, focusing on lower gastrointestinal bleeding, revealed that TXA had no benefits in relation to blood loss and clinical outcomes [13]. However, the results for TXA and outcomes for gastrointestinal bleeding have been inconsistent in recent systematic reviews and meta-analyses. Burke et al. performed a systemic review of 8 studies that included 12,994 patients with upper gastrointestinal bleeding. Although no effect on mortality was noted, the beneficial effect of TXA on lower rebleeding risk and a decreased need for surgery was observed [14]. Another systematic review and meta-analysis, including 13 relevant randomized clinical trials and a total of 2271 patients, demonstrated lower mortality and continued bleeding and less need for urgent endoscopic intervention [11].

Most of the aforementioned studies failed to consider a potential confounding factor: the timing of TXA administration. TXA can be prescribed for patients with gastrointestinal bleeding in an emergency department along with other initial treatments, or during hospitalization. For traumatic or postpartum hemorrhage, immediate TXA administration is recommended for improved survival [15]. Similarly, the timing of TXA treatment might affect its benefits for gastrointestinal bleeding, and trial results may be influenced by this confounding factor. Furthermore, current TXA treatment guidelines for gastrointestinal bleeding include no clear timings [16,17].

Hence, in our study design, we defined early treatment as TXA administered in an emergency department and late treatment as TXA administered after hospitalization. The results demonstrated a significant decrease in mortality rates for early TXA treatment in patients with gastrointestinal bleeding compared with late treatment for both short-term and long-term follow-up, which is compatible with the results of a systematic review and meta-analysis [11]. In addition to reducing mortality, early TXA administration in an emergency department was associated with a significant decrease in the need for urgent endoscopy in a randomized clinical trial exploring the effect of TXA on the urgent endoscopy rate for gastrointestinal bleeding [18].

The length of hospital stay is also a key clinical outcome. Our study demonstrated that early TXA treatment and both early and late treatment resulted in a shorter length of hospital stay compared with late treatment alone. Similar to our results, Miyamoto et al., who conducted a nationwide observational study in Japan, reported that TXA reduced the length of stay for patients with colonic diverticular bleeding [19]. Other retrospective studies have also revealed a decreased hospital stay following TXA administration for patients with vascular trauma [20] or intraoperative administration [21].

In addition to the common adverse effects of nausea, diarrhea, and stomach pain, the risk of thromboembolic events is a major adverse effect of TXA use in clinical practice [22,23]. The HALT-IT trial revealed an increase in venous thromboembolic events with TXA use, but primarily in patients with underlying liver diseases [12]. In contrast, the CRASH-3 trial demonstrated that TXA reduced the risk of death, with a similar risk of thromboembolic events compared with placebo groups [8]. Regarding the timing of TXA treatment, our study revealed a similar risk of thromboembolic events in early and late TXA treatment.

Our study also demonstrated that patients older than 71 years and those with liver and kidney disease all had a significantly increased risk of mortality from gastrointestinal bleeding. These results are consistent with those of a UK population-based study, which reported that older age was the most crucial prognostic factor for gastrointestinal bleeding, with a mortality rate 53 times higher for patients aged over 85 years. Liver and renal comorbidities were also associated with a 7.9 and 3.9 times higher mortality rate [24]. Another meta-analysis evaluated the relationship between kidney disease and outcomes of gastrointestinal bleeding, revealing a higher mortality in the chronic kidney disease group (odds ratio (OR): 1.786, 95% CI: 1.689–1.888, $p < 0.001$) and the end-stage renal disease group (OR: 2.530, 95% CI: 1.386–4.616, $p = 0.002$) [25].

Studies have demonstrated that TXA use leads to improved clinical outcomes for other hemorrhagic conditions, such as traumatic [8,26], major obstetric [27], postpartum [7], and surgical hemorrhage [5,28–30]. Studies have also considered the effect of TXA use on cerebral hemorrhage. A systematic review and meta-analysis including 14 randomized controlled trials with 4703 patients with cerebral hemorrhage demonstrated no improvement in mortality by day 90 in patients receiving TXA (OR: 0.99, 95% CI: 0.84–1.18, $p = 0.95$) [31]. However, the risk of rebleeding and hematoma expansion was reduced and thromboembolic events were not increased. Furthermore, Rowell et al. performed a double-blinded, randomized clinical trial of out-of-hospital TXA use within 2 h for neurological outcomes in patients with severe traumatic brain injury [32]. No significant difference in neurologic function at 6 months or mortality and progression of intracranial hemorrhage was observed.

This study has some limitations. First, data on personal behaviors, such as smoking and alcohol consumption, are not available in the NHIRD; such personal behaviors are potential confounders. However, to address these factors, we included related comorbidities and performed PSM. Second, the cause and location of the gastrointestinal bleeding, disease severity, endoscopic intervention and TXA dosage are not included in the NHIRD. Different hemorrhage severity, endoscopic intervention and TXA dosages are potential confounders of our results. Third, no control group of patients with gastrointestinal bleeding but without TXA treatment was included because our study evaluated the timing of TXA treatment. Finally, further randomized clinical trials with a sufficient sample size, rigorous patient selection, and controlled intervention are required.

5. Conclusions

In this Taiwan population-based study, early TXA treatment was associated with lower mortality without increased thromboembolic events compared with late treatment in patients with gastrointestinal bleeding. Future research is required to clarify the outcomes in terms of continued bleeding, rebleeding, blood transfusion, and the need for urgent endoscopic intervention.

Supplementary Materials: The following supporting information can be downloaded at: https://www.mdpi.com/article/10.3390/10.3390/jcm11061741/s1, Table S1: Definition of study diseases related to ICD-9-CM and ICD-10-CM.

Author Contributions: Conceptualization, K.-H.T., Y.-Y.C. and C.-B.Y.; formal analysis, B.-H.S., S.-F.Y., P.-L.L. and J.-Y.H.; writing—original draft preparation, K.-H.T., Y.-Y.C. and C.-B.Y.; writing—review and editing, K.-H.T., Y.-Y.C. and C.-B.Y. All authors have read and agreed to the published version of the manuscript.

Funding: This research received no external funding.

Institutional Review Board Statement: The study was conducted according to the guidelines of the Declaration of Helsinki, and approved by the Ethical Review Board of the Chung Shan Medical University Hospital (CS2-20036) approved our study.

Informed Consent Statement: Patient consent was waived by both the National Health Insurance Administration and the Institutional Review Board of Chung Shan Medical University Hospital due to the database-processing nature of the current study.

Data Availability Statement: Restrictions apply to the availability of these data. Data was obtained from National Health Insurance database and are available from the authors with the permission of National Health Insurance Administration of Taiwan.

Acknowledgments: This study was supported by research grants from the Chung Shan Medical University Hospital, Taiwan (CSH-2022-C-010). This study was partly based on data from the NHIRD provided by the NHI Administration, Ministry of Health and Welfare, and managed by the Health and Welfare Data Science Center (HWDC) in Taiwan. The interpretation and conclusions contained herein do not represent those of the NHI Administration, Ministry of Health and Welfare, or National Health Research Institutes.

Conflicts of Interest: The authors declare no conflict of interest.

References

1. Van Leerdam, M.E. Epidemiology of acute upper gastrointestinal bleeding. *Best Pract. Res. Clin. Gastroenterol.* **2008**, *22*, 209–224. [CrossRef] [PubMed]
2. Rockall, T.A.; Logan, R.F.A.; Devlin, H.B.; Northfield, T.C. Incidence of and mortality from acute upper gastrointestinal haemorrhage in the United Kingdom. *BMJ* **1995**, *311*, 222–226. [CrossRef] [PubMed]
3. Sostres, C.; Lanas, A. Epidemiology and Demographics of Upper Gastrointestinal Bleeding: Prevalence, Incidence, and Mortality. *Gastrointest. Endosc. Clin. N. Am.* **2011**, *21*, 567–581. [CrossRef] [PubMed]
4. Vermylen, J.; Verhaegen-Declercq, M.L.; Fierens, F.; Verstraete, M. A double blind study of the effect of tranexamic acid in essential menorrhagia. *Bull. Soc. R. Belg. Gynecol. Obs.* **1968**, *38*, 385–390. [CrossRef]
5. Brown, J.R.; Birkmeyer, N.J.; O'Connor, G.T. Meta-analysis comparing the effectiveness and adverse outcomes of antifibrinolytic agents in cardiac surgery. *Circulation* **2007**, *115*, 2801–2813. [CrossRef] [PubMed]
6. Myles, P.S.; Smith, J.A.; Forbes, A.; Silbert, B.; Jayarajah, M.; Painter, T.; Cooper, D.J.; Marasco, S.; McNeil, J.; Bussières, J.S.; et al. Tranexamic Acid in Patients Undergoing Coronary-Artery Surgery. *N. Engl. J. Med.* **2016**, *376*, 136–148. [CrossRef]
7. Shakur, H.; Roberts, I.; Fawole, B.; Chaudhri, R.; El-Sheikh, M.; Akintan, A.; Qureshi, Z.; Kidanto, H.; Vwalika, B.; Abdulkadir, A.; et al. Effect of early tranexamic acid administration on mortality, hysterectomy, and other morbidities in women with post-partum haemorrhage (WOMAN): An international, randomised, double-blind, placebo-controlled trial. *Lancet* **2017**, *389*, 2105–2116. [CrossRef]
8. The CRASH-3 Trial Collaborators. Effects of tranexamic acid on death, disability, vascular occlusive events and other morbidities in patients with acute traumatic brain injury (CRASH-3): A randomised, placebo-controlled trial. *Lancet* **2019**, *394*, 1713–1723. [CrossRef]
9. Barer, D.; Ogilvie, A.; Henry, D.; Dronfield, M.; Coggon, D.; French, S.; Ellis, S.; Atkinson, M.; Langman, M. Cimetidine and tranexamic acid in the treatment of acute upper-gastrointestinal-tract bleeding. *N. Engl. J. Med.* **1983**, *308*, 1571–1575. [CrossRef]
10. Bennett, C.; Klingenberg, S.L.; Langholz, E.; Gluud, L.L. Tranexamic acid for upper gastrointestinal bleeding. *Cochrane Database Syst. Rev.* **2014**, *2014*, Cd006640. [CrossRef]
11. Lee, P.-L.; Yang, K.-S.; Tsai, H.-W.; Hou, S.-K.; Kang, Y.-N.; Chang, C.-C. Tranexamic acid for gastrointestinal bleeding: A systematic review with meta-analysis of randomized clinical trials. *Am. J. Emerg. Med.* **2021**, *45*, 269–279. [CrossRef] [PubMed]
12. Collaborators, H.-I.T. Effects of a high-dose 24-h infusion of tranexamic acid on death and thromboembolic events in patients with acute gastrointestinal bleeding (HALT-IT): An international randomised, double-blind, placebo-controlled trial. *Lancet* **2020**, *395*, 1927–1936. [CrossRef]

13. Smith, S.R.; Murray, D.; Pockney, P.G.; Bendinelli, C.; Draganic, B.D.; Carroll, R. Tranexamic Acid for Lower GI Hemorrhage: A Randomized Placebo-Controlled Clinical Trial. *Dis. Colon Rectum* **2018**, *61*, 99–106. [CrossRef]
14. Burke, E.; Harkins, P.; Ahmed, I. Is There a Role for Tranexamic Acid in Upper GI Bleeding? A Systematic Review and Meta-Analysis. *Surg. Res. Pract.* **2021**, *2021*, 8876991. [CrossRef]
15. Gayet-Ageron, A.; Prieto-Merino, D.; Ker, K.; Shakur, H.; Ageron, F.-X.; Roberts, I.; Kayani, A.; Geer, A.; Ndungu, B.; Fawole, B.; et al. Effect of treatment delay on the effectiveness and safety of antifibrinolytics in acute severe haemorrhage: A meta-analysis of individual patient-level data from 40 138 bleeding patients. *Lancet* **2018**, *391*, 125–132. [CrossRef]
16. Gralnek, I.M.; Dumonceau, J.-M.; Kuipers, E.J.; Lanas, A.; Sanders, D.S.; Kurien, M.; Rotondano, G.; Hucl, T.; Dinis-Ribeiro, M.; Marmo, R.; et al. Diagnosis and management of nonvariceal upper gastrointestinal hemorrhage: European Society of Gastrointestinal Endoscopy (ESGE) Guideline. *Endoscopy* **2015**, *47*, a1–a46. [CrossRef]
17. Stanley, A.J.; Laine, L. Management of acute upper gastrointestinal bleeding. *BMJ* **2019**, *364*, l536. [CrossRef] [PubMed]
18. Tavakoli, N.; Mokhtare, M.; Agah, S.; Azizi, A.; Masoodi, M.; Amiri, H.; Sheikhvatan, M.; Syedsalehi, B.; Behnam, B.; Arabahmadi, M.; et al. Comparison of the efficacy of intravenous tranexamic acid with and without topical administration versus placebo in urgent endoscopy rate for acute gastrointestinal bleeding: A double-blind randomized controlled trial. *United Eur. Gastroenterol. J.* **2017**, *6*, 46–54. [CrossRef]
19. Miyamoto, Y.; Ohbe, H.; Ishimaru, M.; Matsui, H.; Fushimi, K.; Yasunaga, H. Effect of tranexamic acid in patients with colonic diverticular bleeding: A nationwide inpatient database study. *J. Gastroenterol. Hepatol.* **2021**, *36*, 999–1005. [CrossRef]
20. GnanaDev, R.; Dong, F.; Ali, A.; Makkar, G.; Esiobu, P.; Vara, R.; Wong, D.; Neeki, M. RS12. Comparing Mortality and Hospital Length of Stay in the Setting of Truncal and Peripheral Vascular Trauma in Patients Treated with Tranexamic Acid on Initial Presentation. *J. Vasc. Surg.* **2019**, *69*, e188–e189. [CrossRef]
21. Saad, B.N.; Menken, L.G.; Elkattaway, S.; Liporace, F.A.; Yoon, R.S. Tranexamic acid lowers transfusion requirements and hospital length of stay following revision total hip or knee arthroplasty. *Patient Saf. Surg.* **2021**, *15*, 21. [CrossRef]
22. Calapai, G. Systematic Review of Tranexamic Acid Adverse Reactions. *J. Pharmacovigil.* **2015**, *3*, 171. [CrossRef]
23. Murdaca, G.; Greco, M.; Vassallo, C.; Gangemi, S. Tranexamic acid adverse reactions: A brief summary for internists and emergency doctors. *Clin. Mol. Allergy* **2020**, *18*, 16. [CrossRef] [PubMed]
24. Roberts, S.E.; Button, L.A.; Williams, J.G. Prognosis following Upper Gastrointestinal Bleeding. *PLoS ONE* **2012**, *7*, e49507. [CrossRef] [PubMed]
25. Hágendorn, R.; Farkas, N.; Vincze, Á.; Gyöngyi, Z.; Csupor, D.; Bajor, J.; Erőss, B.; Csécsei, P.; Vasas, A.; Szakács, Z.; et al. Chronic kidney disease severely deteriorates the outcome of gastrointestinal bleeding: A meta-analysis. *World J. Gastroenterol.* **2017**, *23*, 8415–8425. [CrossRef] [PubMed]
26. Roberts, I. Tranexamic acid in trauma: How should we use it? *J. Thromb. Haemost.* **2015**, *13*, S195–S199. [CrossRef] [PubMed]
27. Wellington, K.; Wagstaff, A.J. Tranexamic Acid. *Drugs* **2003**, *63*, 1417–1433. [CrossRef]
28. Cheriyan, T.; Maier, S.P., II; Bianco, K.; Slobodyanyuk, K.; Rattenni, R.N.; Lafage, V.; Schwab, F.J.; Lonner, B.S.; Errico, T.J. Efficacy of tranexamic acid on surgical bleeding in spine surgery: A meta-analysis. *Spine J.* **2015**, *15*, 752–761. [CrossRef]
29. Ker, K.; Edwards, P.; Perel, P.; Shakur, H.; Roberts, I. Effect of tranexamic acid on surgical bleeding: Systematic review and cumulative meta-analysis. *BMJ Br. Med. J.* **2012**, *344*, e3054. [CrossRef]
30. Sprigg, N.; Flaherty, K.; Appleton, J.P.; Salman, R.A.-S.; Bereczki, D.; Beridze, M.; Christensen, H.; Ciccone, A.; Collins, R.; Czlonkowska, A.; et al. Tranexamic acid for hyperacute primary IntraCerebral Haemorrhage (TICH-2): An international randomised, placebo-controlled, phase 3 superiority trial. *Lancet* **2018**, *391*, 2107–2115. [CrossRef]
31. Hu, W.; Xin, Y.; Chen, X.; Song, Z.; He, Z.; Zhao, Y. Tranexamic Acid in Cerebral Hemorrhage: A Meta-Analysis and Systematic Review. *CNS Drugs* **2019**, *33*, 327–336. [CrossRef] [PubMed]
32. Rowell, S.E.; Meier, E.N.; McKnight, B.; Kannas, D.; May, S.; Sheehan, K.; Bulger, E.M.; Idris, A.H.; Christenson, J.; Morrison, L.J.; et al. Effect of Out-of-Hospital Tranexamic Acid vs Placebo on 6-Month Functional Neurologic Outcomes in Patients with Moderate or Severe Traumatic Brain Injury. *JAMA* **2020**, *324*, 961–974. [CrossRef] [PubMed]

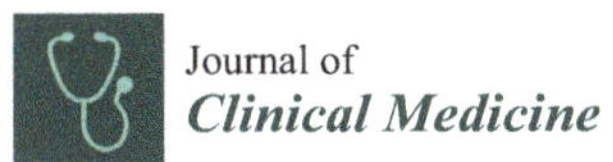

Journal of
Clinical Medicine

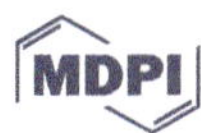

Article

Surgery for Liver Metastasis of Non-Colorectal and Non-Neuroendocrine Tumors

Shadi Katou [1], Franziska Schmid [1], Carolina Silveira [1], Lina Schäfer [1], Tizian Naim [1], Felix Becker [1],
Sonia Radunz [1], Mazen A. Juratli [1], Leon Louis Seifert [2], Hauke Heinzow [2,3], Benjamin Struecker [1],
Andreas Pascher [1] and M. Haluk Morgul [1,*]

[1] Department for General, Visceral and Transplant Surgery, University Hospital Muenster,
48149 Muenster, Germany; shadi.katou@ukmuenster.de (S.K.); franziska_schmid96@yahoo.de (F.S.);
c_silv01@uni-muenster.de (C.S.); linamariaschafer@gmail.com (L.S.); tizianamir.naim@ukmuenster.de (T.N.);
felix.becker@ukmuenster.de (F.B.); sonia.raduenz@ukmuenster.de (S.R.);
mazen.juratli@ukmuenster.de (M.A.J.); benjamin.struecker@ukmuenster.de (B.S.);
andreas.pascher@ukmuenster.de (A.P.)
[2] Department of Gastroenterology and Hepatology, University Hospital Muenster, 48149 Muenster, Germany;
leonlouis.seifert@ukmuenster.de (L.L.S.); h.heinzow@bk-trier.de (H.H.)
[3] Department of Internal Medicine I, Krankenhaus der Barmherzigen Brüder Trier, 54292 Trier, Germany
* Correspondence: haluk.morgul@gmail.com; Tel.: +49-251-83-56304

Abstract: Surgery has become well established for patients with colorectal and neuroendocrine liver metastases. However, the value of this procedure in non-colorectal and non-neuroendocrine metastases (NCRNNELMs) remains unclear. We analyzed the outcomes of patients that underwent liver surgery for NCRNNELMs and for colorectal liver metastases (CRLMs) between 2012 and 2017 at our institution. Prognostic factors of overall and recurrence-free survival were analyzed, and a comparison of survival between two groups was performed. Seventy-three patients (30 NCRNNELM and 43 CRLM) were included in this study. Although the mean age, extrahepatic metastases, and rate of reoperation were significantly different between the groups, recurrence-free survival was comparable. The 5-year overall survival rates were 38% for NCRNNELM and 55% for CRLM. In univariate analysis, a patient age of ≥60 years, endodermal origin of the primary tumor, and major complications were negative prognostic factors. Resection for NCRNNELM showed comparable results to resection for CRLM. Age, the embryological origin of the primary tumor, and the number of metastases might be the criteria for patient selection.

Keywords: liver metastases; colorectal liver metastases; non-colorectal and non-neuroendocrine liver metastases; liver resection

Citation: Katou, S.; Schmid, F.;
Silveira, C.; Schäfer, L.; Naim, T.;
Becker, F.; Radunz, S.; Juratli, M.A.;
Seifert, L.L.; Heinzow, H.; et al.
Surgery for Liver Metastasis of
Non-Colorectal and
Non-Neuroendocrine Tumors. *J. Clin.
Med.* **2022**, *11*, 1906. https://doi.org/
10.3390/jcm11071906

Academic Editor: Hidekazu Suzuki

Received: 10 February 2022
Accepted: 28 March 2022
Published: 29 March 2022

Publisher's Note: MDPI stays neutral
with regard to jurisdictional claims in
published maps and institutional affiliations.

1. Introduction

Surgical treatment of colorectal liver metastasis (CRLM) has been well established over the past few decades. Multimodal approaches, innovative surgical techniques, and inter-disciplinary therapy concepts have contributed to achieving better long-term survival rates in patients who were previously deemed palliative. In fact, recent analyses suggest 5- and 10-year survival rates of 40–58% and 12–36%, respectively, when radical resection (R0) was achieved [1–8]. In parallel to the implementation of surgical strategies for CRLM, hepatic neuroendocrine metastases have also become a field of interest. While hepatic metastases that originate from neuroendocrine tumors generally indicate a negative prognosis, resec-tion of the metastases has been shown to be beneficial for patients in both palliative and curative settings of the disease with a favorable influence on long-term outcomes [9–11].

Since colorectal cancers and neuroendocrine tumors mainly metastasize through the portal vein, the incidence of their metastasis in the liver is high. Nevertheless, the liver is a common metastatic site of various other primary tumors. The role of resection in such settings has been scarcely explored until recently, mainly due to the rarity of these diseases compared to CRLM [12–14]. An epidemiologic study from the Netherlands showed that 46% of adenocarcinoma liver metastases were colorectal in origin, whereas gastric, pancreatic, or esophageal metastases represented only 15%. Metastasis of breast cancer is the most common metastatic disease of a non-splanchnic organ, accounting for only 8.2% of all metastases [15].

Recent developments in surgical techniques, resulting in reduced postoperative morbidity following liver surgery, have increased the courage to offer hepatic resection to patients with non-colorectal non-endocrine liver metastases (NCRNNELMs). Thus, the indication for hepatic resection for NCRNNELM has to be redefined in-line with these developments. However, there is a current gap in knowledge regarding surgical outcomes, as most available data on this subject lack follow-up results of hepatic re-section and dismiss the comparison with CRLM.

The aim of this study was to analyze the outcomes of patients treated for liver metastasis of NCRNNE origin compared with patients suffering from CRLM and to identify prognostic factors of overall and recurrence-free survival in this cohort.

2. Materials and Methods

This study was carried out as an observational retrospective single-center trial, which analyzed all patients that underwent surgical resection for liver metastases between 2012 and 2017 at our tertiary center. The study was conducted in accordance with the Declaration of Helsinki and approved by our local ethics committee (ID: ID 2019-636-f-S). Due to the retrospective character of the analysis, patient consent was waived. Patient data were collected from hospital archives and electronic patient records.

The inclusion criteria were histologically proven liver metastases and surgical treatment of the metastases with curative intention. The exclusion criteria were age <18 years, palliative resections, and other tumor control therapies for liver metastasis, such as ablation, radiation, or embolization (Figure 1).

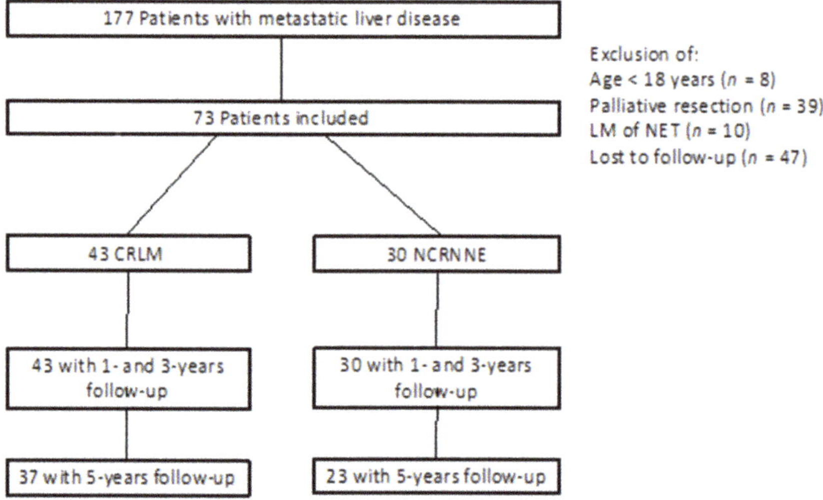

Figure 1. Flow chart of patient inclusion.

All patients were discussed at our local interdisciplinary tumor board prior to oncological procedures. Due to their unique biology, liver metastases of neuroendocrine tissues were excluded from our study. Patients with extrahepatic disease manifestations (beyond the primary lesion) were not excluded. Resection of four or more segments in one session was considered as major hepatectomy. Oligometastatic liver disease was defined as less than five metastases [16]. Synchronous metastases were those that were diagnosed within the first six months of primary diagnosis [17].

Two groups were defined based on the site of the primary tumor: the CRLM and NCRNNELM groups. In addition to the patients' demographic data, information regarding the primary disease, description of hepatic lesions, and surgical procedure was acquired. The patients' postoperative course was screened for complications and follow-up. The tumor burden score was calculated according to the formula A2 + B2 = C2 (A: maximum tumor diameter; B: number of tumors; C: Tumor Burden Score) [18]. To overcome the heterogeneity of primary cancers, tumors were categorized according to embryological origin: ectodermal, mesodermal, and endodermal.

Statistics

Statistical analysis was performed using SPSS (V. XX, IBM, Armonk, New York, NY, USA). Data were described as the mean and standard deviation or median and range. Paired and unpaired Student's t-tests were carried out for comparison of parameters, as appropriate. For multivariate analysis and group comparison, log-rank and Cox regression analyses were performed. Overall survival (OS) was calculated from the day of surgery to death or last follow-up. Recurrence-free survival (RFS) was calculated from the day of surgery to the first diagnosis of recurrence if radical resection of the liver and extrahepatic manifestations were initially achieved. Analyses of OS and RFS were obtained by using the Kaplan–Meier method. A p-value < 0.05 was considered statistically significant.

3. Results

3.1. Characteristic Data

A total of 73 patients were included in this study, of which 43 had CRLM and 30 had NCRNNELM (Figure 1). The median follow-up time of all patients after hepatic resection was 45 months.

Descriptive data of both groups are presented in Table 1. Female patients represented 60.5% and 50% of CRLM and NCRNNELM cases, respectively. The patients' mean age in the NCRNNELM group was 54.3 years, which was significantly younger than that in the CRLM group (64.6 years, p = 0.03). Extrahepatic manifestations and metastases were significantly more frequent in patients with NCRNNELMs than those with CRLM (5% vs. 30%, p = 0.003). There was no significant difference regarding sex, American Society of Anasthesiologists (ASA) state, pre-existing liver conditions, or synchronicity of metastases between the two groups. Solitary metastasis in the NCRNNELM group was more common (55% vs. 80%, whereas cases of oligo- and multiple metastases were more frequent in the CRLM group (30% vs. 16.7% and 15% vs. 3.3%, respectively, p = 0.02). However, the tumor burden score was similar in both groups (4.5 for CRLM; 3.9 NCRNNELM). The majority of lesions were smaller than 5 cm and located in the right lobe of the liver in both groups. However, bilobar lesions were more frequent in CRLM (25.6% vs. 6.7%, p = 0.03). Although a major hepatectomy was more commonly performed for CRLM, the operation time and extent of liver resection did not differ significantly between the groups. Margin-free resection (R0) was achieved in 93% and 90% of the CRLM and NCRNNELM groups, respectively (p = 0.67). None of the patients in the NCRNNELM group required reoperation or died in the first 30 days after surgery, whereas seven patients (16.3%) with CRLM underwent reoperation due to complications after liver re-section, of which one patient (2.3%) died on postoperative day 14 after extended right hepatectomy due to portal vein thrombosis and liver failure. Hence, the major complication rate in CRLM was higher than in the NCRNNELM group (Clavien–Dindo $\leq$ 3a were 37.2% and 46.7%, Clavien–Dindo > 3a were 18.6% and 6.7%, respectively).

Table 1. Patient characteristics.

Parameter	CRLM $n = 43$	NCRNNE $n = 30$	p (<0.05)
All patients	43 (100.0)	30 (100.0)	
Age (median and range)	64.5 (35–90)	54.3 (20–80)	0.03 [a]
Sex (n, %)			
Male	26 (60.5)	15 (50.0)	n.s.
Female	17 (39.5)	15 (50.0)	n.s.
BMI (kg/m^2, mean ± SD)	27.2	26.0	n.s.
ASA score (n, %)			
≤2	28 (65.1) *	22 (73.3)	n.s.
>2	12 (27.9)	8 (26.7)	
Synchronicity (n, %)			
synchronous	19 (44.2)	12 (40.0)	n.s.
metachronous	24 (55.8)	18 (60.0)	n.s.
Extrahepatic metastasis (n, %)			
Yes	2 (4.7)	9 (30.0)	0.003 [b]
No	41 (95.3)	21 (70.0)	
Number of metastases (n, %)			
Solitary	22 (51.1) *	24 (80.0)	
Oligo	12 (27.9)	5 (16.7)	0.02 [b]
Multiple	6 (13.9)	1 (3.3)	
Size of biggest lesion (n, %)			
≤5 cm	36 (83.7) *	25 (83.3)	n.s.
>5 cm	4 (9.3)	5 (16.7)	
TBS (mean ± SD)	4.5 ± 4.6	3.9 ± 3.4	n.s.
Location (n, %)			
Right lobe	25 (58.1)	17 (56.7)	
Left lobe	7 (16.3)	11 (36.7)	0.03
Bilobar	11 (25.6)	2 (6.7)	
Preoperative chemotherapy (n, %)			
Yes	28 (65.1)	17 (56.7)	n.s.
No	15 (34.9)	13 (43.3)	
Postoperative chemotherapy (n, %)			
Yes	21 (48.8) *	12 (40.0) *	n.s.
No	20 (46.5)	16 (53.3)	
Liver resection (n, %)			
minor	36 (83.7)	29 (96.7)	n.s.
major	7 (16.3)	1 (3.3)	
Surgery time (min, mean ± SD)	214	237.8	n.s.
ICU (day, mean ± SD)	5.6	4.1	n.s.
Blood Transfusion (n, %)			
Yes	7 (16.2) *	2 (6.66) *	n.s.
No	34 (79.0)	26 (86.6)	
R-status (n, %)			
R0	40 (93.0)	27 (90.0)	n.s.
R1	3 (7.0)	3 (10.0)	
Reoperation (n, %)			
Yes	7 (16.3)	0 (0)	0.02 [b]
No	36 (83.7)	30 (100.0)	

Table 1. *Cont.*

Parameter	CRLM $n = 43$	NCRNNE $n = 30$	p (<0.05)
Complications (*n*, %)			
none	18 (41.8) *	14 (46.7)	
CD ≤ 3a	16 (37.2)	14 (46.7)	n.s.
CD > 3a	8 (18.6)	2 (6.7)	
ICU readmission (*n*, %)			
yes	2 (5.0)	1 (3.3)	n.s.
no	41 (95.0)	29 (96.7)	

CRLMs: colorectal liver metastases, NCRNNE: non-colorectal non-neuroendocrine, ASA: American Society of Anesthesiologists, BMI: body mass index, TBS: tumor burden score, ICU: intensive care unit, CD: Clavien–Dindo score, n.s.: not signifcant, [a]: Student's *t*-test, [b]: Fischer's exact test, * missing patients' data.

Although the overall survival (OS) of patients after resection of CRLM was higher than that of the NCRNNELM group, this difference was not statistically significant (Figure 2). However, the 1- and 3-year survival rates were significantly higher in the CRLM group (93% vs. 60%, $p = 0.001$; 72% vs. 43%, $p = 0.01$). There was no significant difference in 5-year survival between the CRLM and NCRNNELM groups (55% vs. 38%, $p = 0.26$). In the CRLM group there were more patients having more than one liver lesion, but the tumor burden was similar in both groups. On the contrary, extrahapatic disease was more common in the NCRNNELM group. However, none of these parameters were significantly predictive of overall survival in NCRNNELM patients.

To estimate recurrence-free survival, we excluded patients with R1 resection and untreated extrahepatic disease. Of the remaining 22 patients in the NCRNNELM group, 12 patients (54.5%) developed disease recurrence during follow-up; in seven cases (25.9%), hepatic recurrence was reported, and in five cases (18.5%), extrahepatic disease recurrence was reported. The mean recurrence-free survival was 11.7 months. In the CRLM group, three patients were excluded due to R1 resection, and of the remaining 40, disease recurrence was reported in 29 cases (72.5%). There was no significant difference in recurrence-free survival between the two groups; however, after 1 year, patients with CRLM tended to develop recurrence more frequently than those with NCRNNELM (Table 2, Figure 2).

Table 2. Parameters on recurrence-free survival.

Variables	Recurrence-Free Survival					
	Univariate			Multivariante		
	HR	95% CI	p	HR	95% CI	p
ASA, ≤2 vs. >2	1.22	0.32–4.66	0.76			
Sex, male vs. female	0.56	0.16–1.89	0.35			
Age, ≤60 years vs. >60 years	1.36	0.41–4.45	0.60			
Primary embryology, mesoderm vs. ectoderm vs. endoderm	3.41	1.34–8.67	0.01	2.96	1.10–7.94	0.03
Extra-hepatic disease manifestation, yes vs. No	0.76	0.16–3.55	0.73			
Synchronicity, synchronous vs. metachronous	1.44	0.43–4.81	0.55			
Timing of metastases, ≤24 months vs. >24 months	0.99	0.29–3.35	0.99			
Number of metastases, solitary vs. Multiple	12.59	2.09–75.74	0.006	5.71	0.92–35.47	0.06
Location of metastases, right vs. Left vs. Bilobar	0.94	0.31–2.85	0.92			
Size of biggest lesion, ≤5 cm vs. >5 cm	0.26	0.31–2.21	0.21			
Neoadjuvant chemotherapy, yes vs. no	0.56	0.16–1.92	0.36			
Adjuvant chemotherapy, yes vs. no	0.75	0.19–2.83	0.67			
Clavien-Dindo, 0 vs. ≤3a vs. >3a	1.67	0.62–4.44	0.30			

ASA; American Society of Anesthesiologists, HR; hazard ratio, CI; confidence interval.

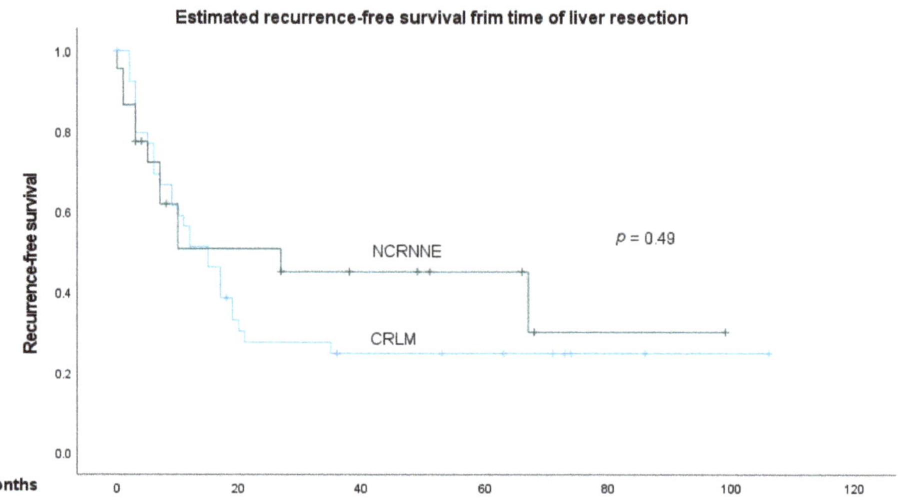

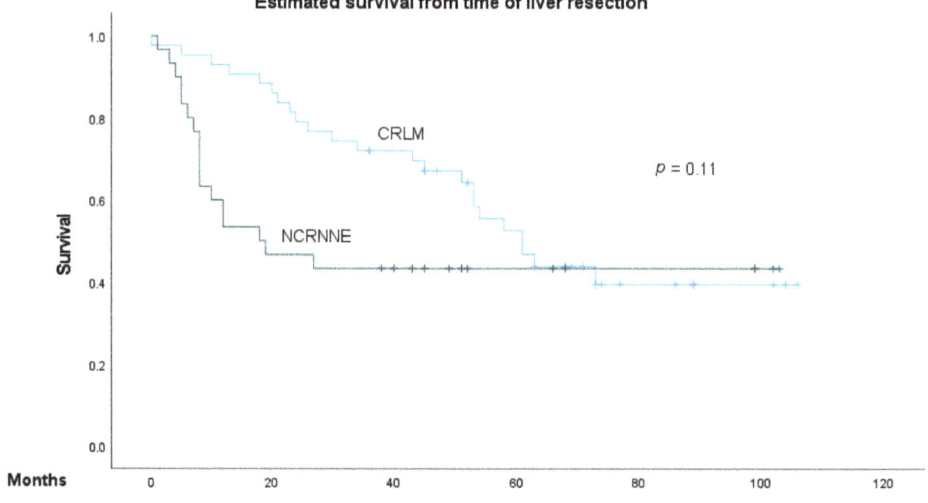

Figure 2. Kaplan–Meier analysis of the overall and recurrence-free survival of patients with NCRNNE and CRLM.

3.2. Predictive Factors of Overall Survival and Recurrence-Free Survival in NCRNNELM

Primary tumors for NCRNNCELM ($n = 30$) were pancreatic adenocarcinoma ($n = 4$), renal cell carcinoma ($n = 3$), esophageal cancer ($n = 3$), gastrointestinal stromal tumor ($n = 3$), melanoma ($n = 3$), sarcoma ($n = 3$), testicular cancer ($n = 3$), papillary adenocarcinoma ($n = 2$), ovarian cancer ($n = 2$), thyroid cancer ($n = 2$), breast cancer ($n = 1$), and gallbladder cancer ($n = 1$). Accordingly, metastases were of mesodermal, ectodermal, and endodermal origin in 46.7%, 13.3%, and 40% of cases, respectively. Overall survival (OS) in this group at 1, 3, and 5 years was 60%, 43.3%, and 38%, respectively, although it should be noted that 5-year survival was not applicable in patients treated after 2015. In univariate analysis, a patient age over 60 years of age and a primary tumor of endodermal origin were identified as negative prognostic factors for OS; however, none of these factors proved significant in multivariate analysis as independent factors (Table 3, Figure 3). Recurrence-free survival

(RFS) rates at 1, 3, and 5 years were 47.4%, 38.9%, and 23.5%, respectively, with a median RFS of 25.1 ± 28.9 (0–99) months. Embryology of the primary tumor stood out as a significant predictor for RFS in univariate and multivariate analyses, with endodermal origin demonstrating the poorest prognosis. Univariate analysis confirmed the number of liver lesions as a significant factor for RFS; however, the multivariate analyses on ASA, age, extrahepatic manifestation, synchronicity, location of metastases, size of the largest lesion, adjuvant or neoadjuvant chemotherapy, and postoperative complications did not show any significance.

Table 3. Parameters on overall survival.

Variables	Overall Survival					
	Univariate			Multivariate		
	HR	95% CI	p	HR	95% CI	p
ASA, <2 vs. >2	1.76	0.65–4.77	0.26			
Sex, male vs. female	0.74	0.28–1.92	0.53			
Age, ≤60 years vs. >60 years	4.03	1.48–10.99	0.006	1.90	0.51–7.01	0.33
Primary embryology, mesoderm vs. ectoderm vs. endoderm	2.46	1.37–4.41	0.003	1.93	0.91–4.08	0.08
Extra-hepatic disease manifestation, yes vs. no	0.88	0.30–2.50	0.81			
Synchronicity, synchronous vs. metachronous	0.80	0.30–2.12	0.66			
Timing of metastases, ≤24 months vs. >24 months	1.86	0.65–5.30	0.24			
Number of metastases, solitary vs. multiple	1.42	0.46–4.39	0.53			
Location of metastases, right vs. Left vs. bilobar	0.96	0.43–2.14	0.93			
Size of biggest lesion, <5 cm vs. >5 cm	1.02	0.29–3.56	0.97			
Neoadjuvant chemotherapy, yes vs. No	0.54	0.20–1.40	0.20			
Adjuvant chemotherapy, yes vs. No	0.65	0.23–1.79	0.40			
R status, R0 vs. R1	1.66	0.37–7.28	0.50			
Blood transfusion, yes vs. No	4.63	0.99–21.52	0.05			
Clavien-Dindo, 0 vs. ≤3a vs. >3a	1.83	0.89–3.78	0.09			

ASA: American Society of Anesthesiologists, HR: hazard ratio, CI: confidence interval.

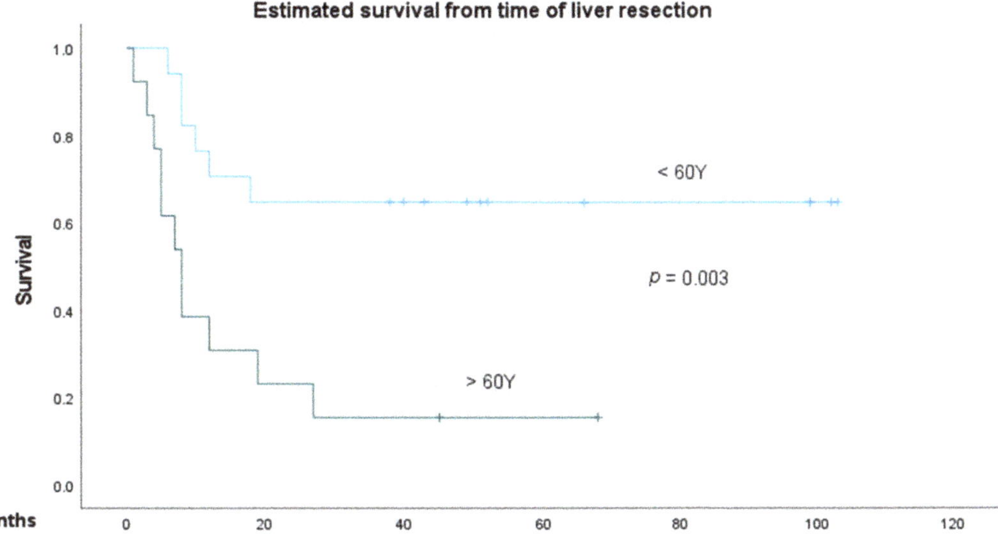

Figure 3. *Cont.*

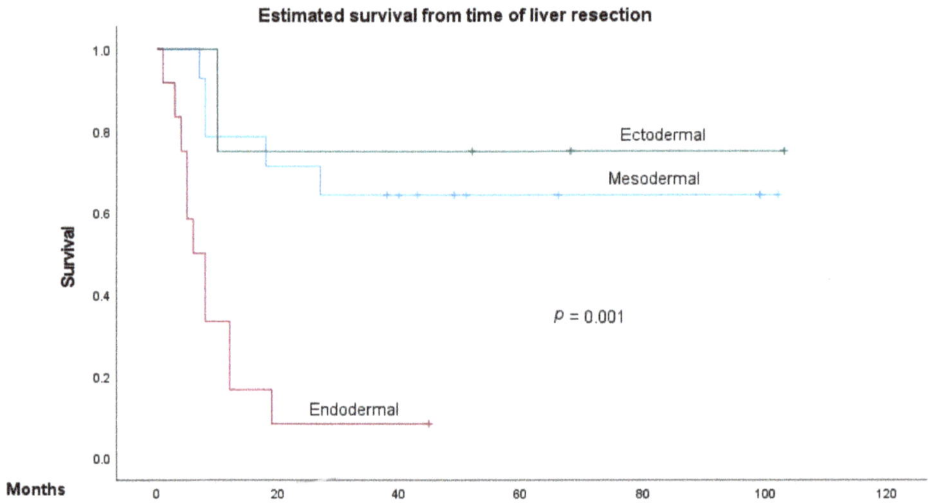

Figure 3. Kaplan–Meier analysis of the age (above and below 60 years) and embryological origin of the primary tumor on overall survival of the patient with NCRNNE.

4. Discussion

To date, the role of radical surgical treatment of NCRNNELM is a topic of ongoing debate. Currently, many patients with NCRNNELM are treated as palliative despite modern advances in liver surgery and improvement of multimodal therapy concepts. Our study analyzed the 5-year survival of patients after liver resection for NCRNNELM and compared them to a cohort of surgically treated patients with CRLM. In addition, we focused on prognostic predictors in NCRNNE liver metastasis patients.

Adam et al. shed light in 2006 on resection of NCRNNELM in a multicenter study including 1452 patients and developed an algorithm to assist selecting patients and predicting their outcomes [19]. This was a milestone in this field, yet a decade later, some of those factors might be outdated [20]. In their population, they identified an age of over 60 years, extrahepatic metastases, and major hepatectomy as negative prognostic factors. In a more recent study with 100 patients, Holzner et al. found residual disease, female sex, endodermal origin, and onset of metastatic disease within 24 months of primary diagnosis to have a negative prognostic effect on outcome [21]. However, in their data, they excluded patients with extrahepatic or extra-abdominal disease and selected only patients with "curative" intent surgery. We explicitly did not exclude patients with extrahepatic disease in our cohort and found no negative correlation with either OS or RFS. We were only able to reproduce two of the previously suggested negative prognostic factors on OS in our results: patient age over 60 years and endodermal origin of the primary tumor. On the other hand, the number of metastases in addition to the origin of the primary tumor was found to be a further prognostic factor of recurrence-free survival.

There have been several previous publications on the surgical treatment of various metastatic liver diseases, many of which reported breast or genitourinary cancer as the most common primary [22–24]. In particular, metastases of genitourinary primaries have shown a more favorable outcome in comparison to those of the gastrointestinal tract, and a median survival time as much as three times longer has been described [25,26]. In our cohort, the most common primary site was the gastrointestinal tract (33.3%). Fewer metastases of genitourinary primaries were observed, and only one case of breast cancer was included. The contrast with some other studies was due to different geography and distribution of primary disease, which might have had an effect on different outcomes. Wakabayashi et al. showed in a recent multicentric analysis a 5-year survival rate of 41% in 205 patients after curative resection of non-colorectal liver metastases of the stomach and pancreas as the most common primary sites, which was similar to our results [27].

The establishment of liver resection in CRLM has come a long way, and the initial results 20 years ago on surgical treatment of CRLM showed comparable results to the most recent data on surgical resection of NCRNNELM cases [28]. Therefore, one must assume that there is room for improvement in this field. In particular, the implementation and improvement of minimally invasive liver resection for NCRNNELM might lead to further improvement in this area as it did in surgical treatment of CRLM [29,30]. Furthermore, minimally invasive treatment of the primary tumor would lead to a better postoperative performance score of patients. Thus, several patients would be suitable for additive surgery in terms of liver metastasis [31]. On the other hand, in the last decade, significant progress in the multidisciplinary treatment of oncological diseases was seen. Thus, neoadjuvant concepts have been widely investigated in gastrointestinal malignancies, showing encouraging results for tumor shrinkage and improved survival [32,33].

In our cohort, the liver resection of the metastasis of tumors with endodermal origin showed a significantly worse prognosis. The sample size would not allow the comparison of all the entities. However, i.e., the liver metastases of pancreatic adenocarcinoma were only solitary tumors. In one patient, the resection of the metastasis was conducted simultaneously during the primary operation for pancreatic cancer. Three patients underwent hepatic surgery following primary pancreas surgery and additive chemotherapy. Recently, Shao et al. showed the feasibility of simultaneous pancreas and liver resection in the oligometastatic concept due to pancreatic cancer, and it showed a significant benefit for the patients following resection and (neo)adjuvant chemotherapy and surgery in comparison to patients that underwent palliative regimens only [34]. Although they included nine patients without neoadjuvant chemotherapy due to the intraoperative diagnosis of liver lesions, they favored chemotherapy for oligometastatic diseases. We also propose that the NCRNELM should be rapidly evaluated for aggressive systemic therapy, since there are encouraging steps in the oncological treatment of, especially, pancreatic [33], esophageal, gastric [35], and renal cell cancer [36]. Taking all these developments into consideration, it is more likely that more patients with liver metastasis of NCRNNE could be candidates for hepatic resection.

Although our data were not able to detect independent prognostic factors for outcomes after liver resection of NCRNNELM, as demonstrated in previous studies, we found that age and embryological origin of primary tumors had an effect in univariate analysis. This was probably due to the relatively small sample of patients in our study. Moreover, although the short-term survival of patients after liver resection for CRLM was better, the overall and 5-year survival results showed no significant difference between the CRLM and NCRNNELM groups. Thus, we were not able to identify any factors that significantly impaired overall survival following surgery on NCRNNELM. This finding was in line with the recent publications of Patkar et al. and Lok et al. with similar sample sizes [37,38]. This suggested that patients with NCRNNELM could benefit from radical treatment in the long run. Therefore, patients with NCRNNELM should be evaluated for surgical treatment in terms of the concept of oligometastases, before palliative regimens are introduced.

As a retrospective study with a small number of patients, due to the rarity of such surgically treated cases, even in a high-volume single center, our data had certain limitations. Primary diseases were heterogeneous in our cohort, and comparisons of those diseases were mostly carried out in other studies according to histology. We deliberately did not categorize subgroups depending on histology or site of primary tumor because the number of patients in each subgroup would have been too small for statistical comparison. Instead, the embryonic origin of the primary tumor was considered. Furthermore, outcome data beyond 5 years were missing in this study, since we only analyzed patients treated between 2012 and 2017.

Since the occurrence of liver surgery for NCRNNELM is rare, attempts have to be made to build collaborations to achieve bigger cohorts. However, the indication, surgical strategy, and the treatments in terms of adjuvant and neoadjuvant chemotherapy for NCRNNELM may differ between centers, thus it still would be challenging to define the objective criteria for NCRNNELM. On the other hand, as stated by a Dutch group recently, even in a nationwide data analysis, variation on outcomes following liver surgery can occur [39].

5. Conclusions

Despite the heterogeneous distribution of the primary disease, our results concluded that hepatic resection of NCRNNELM might be feasible for patients under 60 years of age and with metastasis of non-endodermal primaries, and showing satisfying 5-year survival results. For recurrence-free survival, multiple metastases and endodermal origin of the primary tumor appeared to have an unfavorable influence. However, in multivariate analyses, our data did not identify any significant factor that affected overall survival. Hence, cases of NCRNNELM should be individually discussed by multidisciplinary boards with an experienced liver surgeon, and surgical treatment should be considered. To establish a treatment algorithm for these patients, further prospective and multicentric studies are needed.

Author Contributions: Conceptualization, S.K., B.S. and M.H.M.; data curation, S.K., F.B., S.R., M.A.J., L.L.S., B.S. and M.H.M.; formal analysis, S.K., L.L.S. and M.H.M.; funding acquisition, A.P. and M.H.M.; investigation, S.K., F.S., C.S., L.S. and T.N.; methodology, S.K., H.H., B.S. and M.H.M.; project administration, B.S., A.P. and M.H.M.; resources, H.H. and A.P.; software, S.K., F.S., C.S., L.S. and T.N.; supervision, A.P.; validation, S.K., F.S., C.S. and F.B.; visualization, S.K. and M.H.M.; writing—original draft, S.K. and M.H.M.; writing—review and editing, S.K., F.S., C.S., L.S., T.N., F.B., S.R., M.A.J., L.L.S., H.H., B.S., A.P. and M.H.M. All authors were informed about each step of manuscript processing including submission, revision, revision reminder, etc. via emails from our system or assigned Assistant Editor. All authors have read and agreed to the published version of the manuscript.

Funding: This research received no external funding.

Institutional Review Board Statement: The trial was conducted in accordance with the Declaration of Helsinki. The study was approved by the local ethics committee of the Westfälische Wilhelms-University of Muenster, Germany (NO.: 2019-636-f-S).

Informed Consent Statement: Due to the retrospective character of this trial informed consent of patients was not obtained.

Data Availability Statement: The data presented in this study are available on request from the corresponding author. The data are not publicly available due to the approval of the ethic committee.

Acknowledgments: We acknowledge support by Open Access Publication Fund of University Münster.

Conflicts of Interest: The authors declare no conflict of interest.

References

1. Abbas, S.; Lam, V.; Hollands, M. Ten-year survival after liver resection for colorectal metastases: Systematic review and meta-analysis. *ISRN Oncol.* **2011**, *2011*, 763245. [CrossRef]
2. Creasy, J.M.; Sadot, E.; Koerkamp, B.G.; Chou, J.F.; Gonen, M.; Kemeny, N.E.; Balachandran, V.P.; Kingham, T.P.; DeMatteo, R.P.; Allen, P.J.; et al. Actual 10-year survival after hepatic resection of colorectal liver metastases: What factors preclude cure? *Surgery* **2018**, *163*, 1238–1244. [CrossRef]
3. Engstrand, J.; Nilsson, H.; Stromberg, C.; Jonas, E.; Freedman, J. Colorectal cancer liver metastases—A population-based study on incidence, management and survival. *BMC Cancer* **2018**, *18*, 78. [CrossRef]
4. Hackl, C.; Neumann, P.; Gerken, M.; Loss, M.; Klinkhammer-Schalke, M.; Schlitt, H.J. Treatment of colorectal liver metastases in Germany: A ten-year population-based analysis of 5772 cases of primary colorectal adenocarcinoma. *BMC Cancer* **2014**, *14*, 810. [CrossRef]
5. Kanas, G.P.; Taylor, A.; Primrose, J.N.; Langeberg, W.J.; Kelsh, M.A.; Mowat, F.S.; Alexander, D.D.; Choti, M.A.; Poston, G. Survival after liver resection in metastatic colorectal cancer: Review and meta-analysis of prognostic factors. *Clin Epidemiol.* **2012**, *4*, 283–301.

6. Rees, M.; Tekkis, P.P.; Welsh, F.K.; O'Rourke, T.; John, T.G. Evaluation of long-term survival after hepatic resection for metastatic colorectal cancer: A multifactorial model of 929 patients. *Ann. Surg.* **2008**, *247*, 125–135. [CrossRef]
7. Dorr, N.M.; Bartels, M.; Morgul, M.H. Current treatment of colorectal liver metastasis as a chronic disease. *Anticancer Res.* **2020**, *40*, 1–7. [CrossRef]
8. Petrowsky, H.; Fritsch, R.; Guckenberger, M.; De Oliveira, M.L.; Dutkowski, P.; Clavien, P.A. Modern therapeutic approaches for the treatment of malignant liver tumours. *Nat. Rev. Gastroenterol. Hepatol.* **2020**, *17*, 755–772. [CrossRef]
9. Frilling, A.; Clift, A.K. Therapeutic strategies for neuroendocrine liver metastases. *Cancer* **2015**, *121*, 1172–1186. [CrossRef]
10. Mayo, S.C.; de Jong, M.C.; Pulitano, C.; Clary, B.M.; Reddy, S.K.; Gamblin, T.C.; Celinksi, S.A.; Kooby, D.A.; Staley, C.A.; Stokes, J.B.; et al. Surgical management of hepatic neuroendocrine tumor metastasis: Results from an international multi-institutional analysis. *Ann. Surg. Oncol.* **2010**, *17*, 3129–3136. [CrossRef]
11. Fairweather, M.; Swanson, R.; Wang, J.; Brais, L.K.; Dutton, T.; Kulke, M.H.; Clancy, T.E. Management of neuroendocrine tumor liver metastases: Long-term outcomes and prognostic factors from a large prospective database. *Ann. Surg Oncol.* **2017**, *24*, 2319–2325. [CrossRef]
12. Yedibela, S.; Gohl, J.; Graz, V.; Pfaffenberger, M.K.; Merkel, S.; Hohenberger, W.; Meyer, T. Changes in indication and results after resection of hepatic metastases from noncolorectal primary tumors: A single-institutional review. *Ann. Surg Oncol.* **2005**, *12*, 778–785. [CrossRef]
13. Kassahun, W.T. Controversies in defining prognostic relevant selection criteria that determine long-term effectiveness of liver resection for noncolorectal nonneuroendocrine liver metastasis. *Int. J. Surg.* **2015**, *24 Pt A*, 85–90. [CrossRef]
14. Takemura, N.; Saiura, A. Role of surgical resection for non-colorectal non-neuroendocrine liver metastases. *World J. Hepatol.* **2017**, *9*, 242–251. [CrossRef]
15. De Ridder, J.; De Wilt, J.H.; Simmer, F.; Overbeek, L.; Lemmens, V.; Nagtegaal, I. Incidence and origin of histologically confirmed liver metastases: An explorative case-study of 23,154 patients. *Oncotarget* **2016**, *7*, 55368–55376. [CrossRef]
16. Chiapponi, C.; Berlth, F.; Plum, P.S.; Betzler, C.; Stippel, D.L.; Popp, F.; Bruns, C.J. Oligometastatic Disease in Upper Gastrointestinal Cancer—How to Proceed? *Visc. Med.* **2017**, *33*, 31–34. [CrossRef]
17. Leporrier, J.; Maurel, J.; Chiche, L.; Bara, S.; Segol, P.; Launoy, G. A population-based study of the incidence, management and prognosis of hepatic metastases from colorectal cancer. *Br. J. Surg.* **2006**, *93*, 465–474. [CrossRef]
18. Sasaki, K.; Margonis, G.A.; Andreatos, N.; Zhang, X.F.; Buettner, S.; Wang, J.; Deshwar, A.; He, J.; Wolfgang, C.L.; Weiss, M.; et al. The prognostic utility of the "Tumor Burden Score" based on preoperative radiographic features of colorectal liver metastases. *J. Surg. Oncol.* **2017**, *116*, 515–523. [CrossRef]
19. Adam, R.; Chiche, L.; Aloia, T.; Elias, D.; Salmon, R.; Rivoire, M.; Jaeck, D.; Saric, J.; Le Treut, Y.P.; Belghiti, J.; et al. Hepatic resection for noncolorectal nonendocrine liver metastases: Analysis of 1452 patients and development of a prognostic model. *Ann. Surg.* **2006**, *244*, 524–535.
20. Bohlok, A.; Lucidi, V.; Bouazza, F.; Daher, A.; Germanova, D.; Van Laethem, J.L.; Hendlisz, A.; Donckier, V. The lack of selection criteria for surgery in patients with non-colorectal non-neuroendocrine liver metastases. *World J. Surg Oncol.* **2020**, *18*, 106. [CrossRef]
21. Holzner, P.A.; Makowiec, F.; Klock, A.; Glatz, T.; Fichtner-Feigl, S.; Lang, S.A.; Neeff, H.P. Outcome after hepatic resection for isolated non-colorectal, non-neuroendocrine liver metastases in 100 patients—The role of the embryologic origin of the primary tumor. *BMC Surg.* **2018**, *18*, 89. [CrossRef]
22. Parisi, A.; Trastulli, S.; Ricci, F.; Regina, R.; Cirocchi, R.; Grassi, V.; Gemini, A.; Pironi, D.; D'Andrea, V.; Santoro, A.; et al. Analysis of long-term results after liver surgery for metastases from colorectal and non-colorectal tumors: A retrospective cohort study. *Int. J. Surg.* **2016**, *30*, 25–30. [CrossRef] [PubMed]
23. O'Rourke, T.R.; Tekkis, P.; Yeung, S.; Fawcett, J.; Lynch, S.; Strong, R.; Wall, D.; John, T.G.; Welsh, F.; Rees, M. Long-term results of liver resection for non-colorectal, non-neuroendocrine metastases. *Ann. Surg Oncol.* **2008**, *15*, 207–218. [CrossRef] [PubMed]
24. Groeschl, R.T.; Nachmany, I.; Steel, J.L.; Reddy, S.K.; Glazer, E.S.; de Jong, M.C.; Pawlik, T.M.; Geller, D.A.; Tsung, A.; Marsh, J.W.; et al. Hepatectomy for noncolorectal non-neuroendocrine metastatic cancer: A multi-institutional analysis. *J. Am. Coll. Surg.* **2012**, *214*, 769–777. [CrossRef] [PubMed]
25. Uggeri, F.; Ronchi, P.A.; Goffredo, P.; Garancini, M.; Degrate, L.; Nespoli, L.; Gianotti, L.; Romano, F. Metastatic liver disease from non-colorectal, non-neuroendocrine, non-sarcoma cancers: A systematic review. *World J. Surg. Oncol.* **2015**, *13*, 191. [CrossRef] [PubMed]
26. Sano, K.; Yamamoto, M.; Mimura, T.; Endo, I.; Nakamori, S.; Konishi, M.; Miyazaki, M.; Wakai, T.; Nagino, M.; Kubota, K.; et al. Outcomes of 1639 hepatectomies for non-colorectal non-neuroendocrine liver metastases: A multicenter analysis. *J. Hepatobiliary Pancreat Sci.* **2018**, *25*, 465–475. [CrossRef]
27. Wakabayashi, T.; Hibi, T.; Yoneda, G.; Iwao, Y.; Sawada, Y.; Hoshino, H.; Uemura, S.; Ban, D.; Kudo, A.; Takemura, T.; et al. Predictive model for survival after liver resection for noncolorectal liver metastases in the modern era: A Japanese multicenter analysis. *J. Hepatobiliary Pancreat Sci.* **2019**, *26*, 441–448. [CrossRef] [PubMed]
28. Schiergens, T.S.; Luning, J.; Renz, B.W.; Thomas, M.; Pratschke, S.; Feng, H.; Lee, S.M.L.; Engel, J.; Rentsch, M.; Guba, M.; et al. Liver resection for non-colorectal non-neuroendocrine metastases: Where do we stand today compared to colorectal cancer? *J. Gastrointest. Surg.* **2016**, *20*, 1163–1172. [CrossRef]

29. Aghayan, D.L.; Kalinowski, P.; Kazaryan, A.M.; Fretland, A.A.; Sahakyan, M.A.; Rosok, B.I.; Pelanis, E.; Bjørnbeth, B.A.; Edwin, B. Laparoscopic liver resection for non-colorectal non-neuroendocrine metastases: Perioperative and oncologic outcomes. *World J. Surg. Oncol.* **2019**, *17*, 156. [CrossRef]
30. Knitter, S.; Andreou, A.; Kradolfer, D.; Beierle, A.S.; Pesthy, S.; Eichelberg, A.-C.; Kästner, A.; Feldbrügge, L.; Krenzien, F.; Schulz, M.; et al. Minimal-invasive versus open hepatectomy for colorectal liver metastases: Bicentric analysis of postoperative outcomes and long-term survival using propensity score matching analysis. *J. Clin. Med.* **2020**, *9*, 4027. [CrossRef]
31. Feldbrügge, L.; Ortiz Galindo, S.A.; Frisch, O.; Benzing, C.; Krenzien, F.; Riddermann, A.; Kästner, A.; Nevermann, N.F.; Malinka, T.; Schöning, W.; et al. Safety and feasibility of robotic liver resection after previous abdominal surgeries. *Surg. Endosc.* **2021**. [CrossRef] [PubMed]
32. Zhao, X.; Ren, Y.; Hu, Y.; Cui, N.; Wang, X.; Cui, Y. Neoadjuvant chemotherapy versus neoadjuvant chemoradiotherapy for cancer of the esophagus or the gastroesophageal junction: A meta-analysis based on clinical trials. *PLoS ONE* **2018**, *13*, e0202185. [CrossRef] [PubMed]
33. Rangarajan, K.; Pucher, P.H.; Armstrong, T.; Bateman, A.; Hamady, Z. Systemic neoadjuvant chemotherapy in modern pancreatic cancer treatment: A systematic review and meta-analysis. *Ann. R. Coll. Surg. Engl.* **2019**, *101*, 453–462. [CrossRef] [PubMed]
34. Shao, Y.; Feng, J.; Hu, Z.; Wu, J.; Zhang, M.; Shen, Y.; Zheng, S. Feasibility of pancreaticoduodenectomy with synchronous liver metastasectomy for oligometastatic pancreatic ductal adenocarcinoma—A case-control study. *Ann. Med. Surg.* **2020**, *62*, 490–494. [CrossRef] [PubMed]
35. Turgeman, I.; Ben-Aharon, I. Evolving treatment paradigms in esophageal cancer. *Ann. Transl. Med.* **2021**, *9*, 903. [CrossRef] [PubMed]
36. Hau, H.M.; Thalmann, F.; Lübbert, C.; Morgul, M.H.; Schmelzle, M.; Atanasov, G.; Benzing, C.; Lange, U.; Ascherl, R.; Ganzer, R.; et al. The value of hepatic resection in metastasic renal cancer in the Era of Tyrosinkinase Inhibitor Therapy. *BMC Surg.* **2016**, *16*, 49. [CrossRef]
37. Lok, H.; Fung, A.; Chong, C.; Lee, K.; Wong, J.; Cheung, S.; Lai, P.; Ng, K. Comparison of long-term survival outcome after curative hepatectomy between selected patients with non-colorectal and colorectal liver metastasis: A propensity score matching analysis. *Asian J. Surg.* **2021**, *44*, 459–464. [CrossRef]
38. Patkar, S.; Niyogi, D.; Parray, A.; Goel, M. Is resection for noncolorectal, nonneuroendocrine liver metastases justified? *J. Surg. Oncol.* **2021**, *123*, 957–962. [CrossRef]
39. Elfrink, A.; Kok, N.; Swijnenburg, R.; den Dulk, M.; van den Boezem, P.; Hartgrink, H.; te Riele, W.W.; Patijn, G.; Leclercq, W.; Lips, D.; et al. Nationwide oncological networks for resection of colorectal liver metastases in the Netherlands: Differences and postoperative outcomes. *Eur. J. Surg. Oncol.* **2021**, *48*, 435–448. [CrossRef]

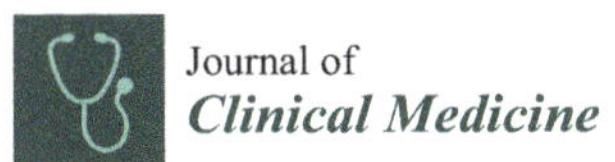

Journal of
Clinical Medicine

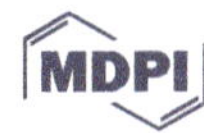

Systematic Review

Health-Related Quality of Life of Patients Treated with Biological Agents and New Small-Molecule Drugs for Moderate to Severe Crohn's Disease: A Systematic Review

Hasan Aladraj [1,*], Mohamed Abdulla [1], Salman Yousuf Guraya [2] and Shaista Salman Guraya [2]

[1]   School of Medicine, Royal College of Surgeons Ireland-Bahrain, RCSI-Medical University of Bahrain (MUB), Adliya P.O. Box 15503, Bahrain; 19201165@rcsi.com
[2]   Clinical Sciences Department, College of Medicine, University of Sharjah, Sharjah 27272, United Arab Emirates; salmanguraya@gmail.com (S.Y.G.); ssalman@rcsi.com (S.S.G.)
*   Correspondence: 19200005@rcsi.com; Tel.: +973-33377350

Abstract: Crohn's disease (CD) leads to a poor health-related quality of life (HRQoL). This review aimed to investigate the effect of biological agents and small-molecule drugs in improving the HRQoL of patients with moderate to severe CD. We adopted a systematic protocol to search PubMed and Cochrane Central Register of Controlled Trials (CENTRAL), which was supplemented with manual searches. Eligible studies were RCTs that matched the research objective based on population, intervention, comparison and outcomes. Studies in paediatric populations, reviews and conference abstracts were excluded. Covidence was used for screening and data extraction. We assessed all research findings using RoB2 and reported them narratively. We included 16 multicentre, multinational RCTs in this review. Of the 15 studies that compared the effect of an intervention to a placebo, 9 were induction studies and 6 investigated maintenance therapy. Of these, 13 studies showed a significant ($p < 0.05$) improvement in the HRQoL of patients with CD. One non-inferiority study compared the intervention with another active drug and favoured the intervention. This systematic review reported a substantial improvement in the HRQoL of patients with CD using biological agents and small-molecule drugs. These pharmaceutical substances have the potential to improve the HRQoL of patients with CD. However, further large clinical trials with long-term follow-up are essential to validate these findings.

Keywords: Crohn's disease; biologics; small-molecule drugs; health-related quality of life (HRQoL)

Citation: Aladraj, H.; Abdulla, M.; Guraya, S.Y.; Guraya, S.S. Health-Related Quality of Life of Patients Treated with Biological Agents and New Small-Molecule Drugs for Moderate to Severe Crohn's Disease: A Systematic Review. *J. Clin. Med.* **2022**, *11*, 3743. https://doi.org/10.3390/jcm11133743

Academic Editors: Hidekazu Suzuki and Christian Selinger

Received: 14 May 2022
Accepted: 14 June 2022
Published: 28 June 2022

Publisher's Note: MDPI stays neutral with regard to jurisdictional claims in published maps and institutional affiliations.

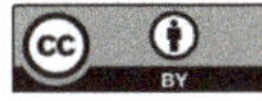

1. Introduction

Crohn's disease (CD) is a debilitating inflammatory disease that affects any part of the gastrointestinal tract, resulting in intestinal and systemic manifestations. It is a chronic disease characterised by alternating periods of disease relapse and remission. The chronic nature, early age of onset and incapacitating intestinal and systemic manifestations account for major social and financial stressors. Some distressing factors in patients with CD include frequent hospital visits, long-term medications with their side effects, bowel stenosis, possible surgical interventions and the fear of developing cancer [1,2]. A major burden on healthcare systems is related to the management of the CD-specific chronic internal and perianal fistulas, which need special attention in highly specialised colorectal surgery centres. The most dreadful complication of CD remains colorectal cancer, with a reported incidence of 746,000 cases (10.0% of the total cancer burden in men) and 614,000 cases (9.2% of the cancer incidence in women) [3,4].

HRQoL is a multidimensional concept which pertains to vitality, social energy and physical wellbeing [5–8]. To determine the effect of disease activity on HRQoL, several disease-specific HRQoL questionnaires have been used, such as the McMaster inflammatory bowel disease questionnaire (IBDQ) [9], the short IBDQ [10], the rating form of inflammatory bowel disease patient concerns (RFIPC) [11] and the sickness impact profile (SIP) [12]. All such tools measure specific elements of the HRQoL of patients with a focus on the certain characteristics of vitality and mental and social wellbeing.

To improve HRQoL, traditionally, the contemporary management of CD was driven by a progressive, stepwise therapeutic intensification with a re-review of the clinical response according to symptoms. This approach did not improve the long-term clinical outcomes in patients with CD [13], leading to the introduction of a "treat to target" CD management strategy, which guides physicians in the regular assessment of disease activity using objective clinical and biological outcome measures and subsequent treatment modifications [14]. The STRIDE-II initiative, an Update on the Selecting Therapeutic Targets in Inflammatory Bowel Disease (STRIDE) Initiative, confirmed that the restoration of QoL is the most important long-term treatment target in CD, irrespective of other objective markers of inflammation [15].

In the last two decades, biological agents (generally large, complex molecules manufactured by biotechnology[16]) have emerged as novel therapeutic agents for CD. Since the approval of infliximab in 1999, five other agents have been approved. These drugs work by inhibiting TNF-alpha, integrin-alpha4 or IL23/12p40 [17,18]. Due to a rising number of non-responders to treatment and a deeper understanding of the pathophysiological mechanisms of CD, new drugs are being developed to target IL23p19 and the JAK/STAT mechanisms or to regulate gut leukocyte trafficking [18]. As a primary outcome measure of therapy and a key factor of consideration for decision-makers, HRQoL has become a frequently measured outcome in clinical trials.

In 2009, a systematic review reported that the then-approved biologics (infliximab, adalimumab, certolizumab and natalizumab) demonstrated clinical improvement in the HRQoL of patients with inflammatory bowel disease (IBD) [19]. Since then, despite a staggering upsurge in CD management strategies and the availability of novel biological agents, there has been a scarcity of literature that could validate their efficacy using the best clinical evidence. Therefore, this systematic review aimed to evaluate the outcomes of the currently approved and promising in-development biological agents and small-molecule agents in improving the HRQoL of patients with moderate to severe CD.

2. Methods

2.1. Objective

Our review targeted studies of patients with moderate to severe CD, measured using a Crohn's Disease Activity Index (CDAI) score of 221 to 450 points or equivalent, being treated with biological agents and small-molecule agents such as TNF-alpha, integrin-alpha4 or IL23/12p40 inhibitors or those regulating the JAK/STAT mechanism or gut leukocyte trafficking. We included studies that compared interventions with placebos or any other drug. The co-primary outcomes of this review were the number of patients achieving clinically meaningful improvements in HRQoL using the inflammatory bowel disease questionnaire (IBDQ) or the SF-36 questionnaires and the mean change in IBDQ total score or the physical component summary (PCS) and mental component summary (MCS) of the SF-36. Only studies that reported the targeted outcomes were included.

2.2. The HRQoL Scales

The IBDQ is the most frequently used disease-specific HRQoL tool [20]. The IBDQ is a 32-item questionnaire with 4 domains: bowel symptoms, systemic symptoms, emotional functioning and social functioning. The IBDQ total score is the sum of responses to all the items, which use a 7-point Likert scale grading system with 1 reflecting a severe problem and 7, no problem at all. The total score ranges between 32 (very poor HRQoL) and 224 (perfect HRQoL) [19,21].

The SF-36 is a generic HRQOL tool mainly used in IBD clinical trials [20]. The SF-36 has two summary components, the PCS and the MCS, derived from scores in eight individual scales (physical functioning, role—physical, bodily pain, general health, vitality, social functioning, role—emotional and mental health). A scale of 0 to 100 is used to score eight scales, with better HRQoL indicated by a higher score [19].

2.3. Inclusion and Exclusion Criteria

All double- or triple-blinded randomised controlled trials (RCTs) published in English that met the objective of our review were included. We excluded studies regarding adolescents and children (under 18 years of age). Conference proceedings, systematic reviews and non-English studies were also excluded.

2.4. Search Strategy

On 25 January 2022, a literature search, designed in conjunction with a senior librarian, was carried out on the databases of PubMed and Cochrane Central Register of Controlled Trials (CENTRAL). No limits were placed on the time span. Our search did not include grey literature. The capture–recapture method was used to verify the completeness of the search strategy results [22]. Keywords of Crohn's disease, HRQoL, IBDQ, SF-36, anti-TNF and infliximab were used. To narrow our results towards RCTs, we used a search strategy suggested by the Cochrane handbook that is highly sensitive for identifying results of RCTs [23]. A manual search of the reference lists and www.clinicaltrials.gov (29 January 2022) was also conducted independently. Details of the search strategy are shown in Appendix A.

2.5. Data Extraction

The screening of titles, abstracts and full-text articles was conducted by two independent reviewers (H.A. and M.A.) using the Covidence software, using the defined inclusion and exclusion criteria as benchmarks. Any discrepancies were discussed and resolved by the two reviewers. The same software was used for the extraction of data. A customised template containing fields such as general information (title, study ID and registration number), the characteristics of the included studies (aim, date conducted and funding) and the results was used.

2.6. Risk of Bias Assessment

To ascertain the risk of bias, Cochrane collaboration's risk of bias tool 2 (RoB2, 22 August 2019 version) was used independently by two reviewers (H.A. and M.A.) [24]. Any discrepancies were discussed, and then, a third researcher was consulted to secure a consensus. RoB2 is an outcome-based tool examining five domains which may lead to bias (bias arising from the randomisation process, deviations from intended interventions, missing outcome data, measurement of the outcome and the selection of the reported result). Studies that were rated high in one domain or raised some concerns in multiple domains that substantially lowered the confidence in the results were rated high overall. The risk of bias in relevant outcomes was reported, and those studies with a high risk of bias were not excluded based on those results.

2.7. Strategy for Data Synthesis

The extracted data were categorised according to the interventions used. The results were reported narratively using descriptive statistics, with the addition of tables and graphs where appropriate. If a study showed a statistically significant improvement ($p < 0.05$) in at least one dose group at the end of the study period, the intervention was considered to be effective in improving HRQoL.

This review was reported according to The Preferred Reporting Items for Systematic reviews and Meta-Analyses (PRISMA) guidelines [25]. This review is registered with The International Prospective Register of Systematic Reviews (PROSPERO), an open-access online database of systematic review protocols, with the registration number CRD42022306394 [26].

3. Results

Our first search retrieved 306 and 303 records from PubMed and CENTRAL, respectively. A further 38 records were retrieved by hand searching www.clinicaltrails.gov and reference lists. After the removal of 95 duplicates, 552 title/abstracts were screened, which showed 433 irrelevant reports. Furthermore, 44 reports did not have retrievable full-text articles, 9 were ongoing studies and 44 were excluded for other reasons, as depicted in the flowchart. Finally, 22 reports of 16 studies were included (Figure 1). Four studies met the inclusion criteria. However, we excluded those studies as there was no data about HRQoL outcomes [27–30].

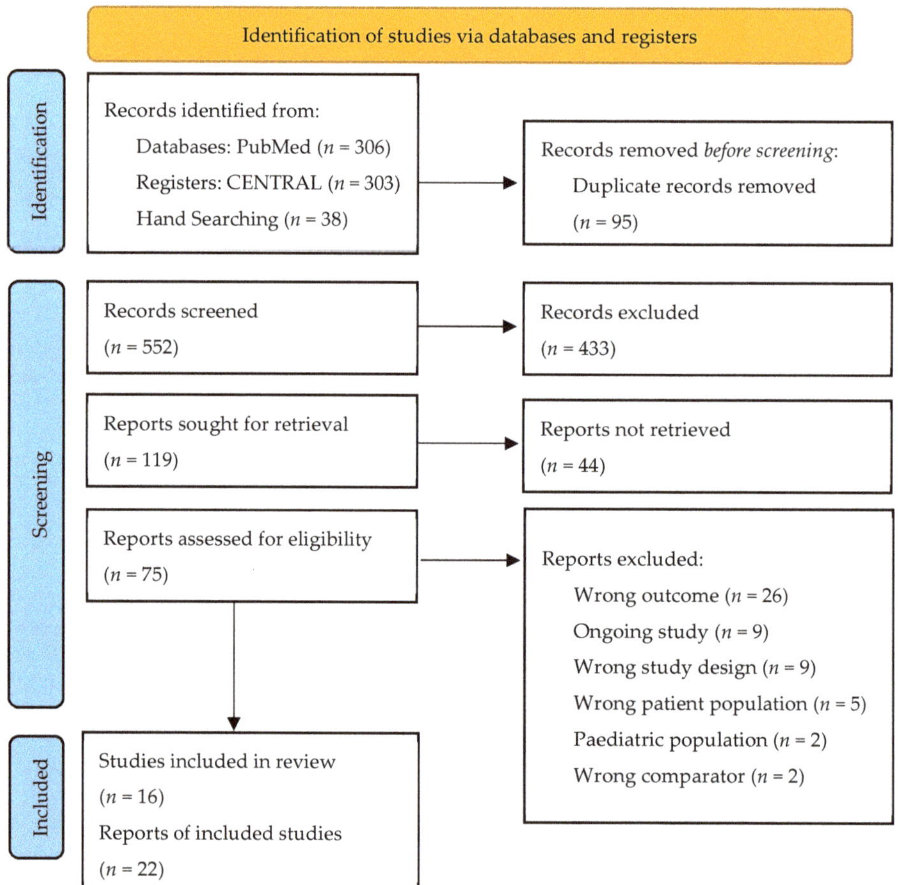

Figure 1. PRISMA flowchart for the stepwise screening and final selection of studies.

3.1. Characteristics of the Included Studies

Our systematic review identified 16 studies. Fifteen compared their investigated interventions to a placebo. Only SONIC compared its intervention (infliximab) to another active drug (azathioprine) [31]. All included studies were multinational, multicentre RCTs. The total number of participants in this review was 7463 and ranged between 108 and 1281. Three studies investigated infliximab [31–33], three studies investigated certolizumab pegol [34–36], three studies investigated ustekinumab [37], two studies investigated natalizumab [38,39] and one study each investigated adalimumab [40], filgotinib [41], upadacitinib [42], tofacitinib [43] and apilimod mesylate [44]. Nine were induction studies, and six were maintenance studies. SONIC was an induction study with a maintenance extension [31].

A clinically meaningful improvement (MCID) in HRQoL is defined as an increase of ≥16 points in the IBDQ total score and an increase of 3 to 5 points in the SF-36 PCS and MCS scores. [45] Based on these values, nine studies defined MCID in the IBDQ as ≥16 points. Three studies defined MCID in the SF-36 PCS and MCS as ≥5 points. Only the PRECiSE 2 trial defined MCID in the PCS and MCS as 4.1 and 3.9 points, respectively [35].

3.2. Risk of Bias

A total of 157 outcomes were assessed. Of these, 104 (66%), 1 (0.6%) and 52 (33%) were rated as having high risks, some concerns or low risks of bias overall, respectively. As many as 9.5% of outcomes [33,44] were rated has having some concerns in domain 1: randomisation process. Meanwhile, 22.3% of outcomes [38,39,43] were rated as having a high risk in domain 2: deviations from intended interventions. A total of 88 (56%) [32–35,37,39,40,44] outcomes were rated as having a high risk in missing outcome data (domain 3), while 14% [36,37] of outcomes were rated as having some concerns. In domain 5: selection of the reported results, 38 (24.2%) [32–34,40] and 41 outcomes (26.1%) [33,35,39] were rated as having a high risk and some concerns, respectively. All outcomes were rated as having low risks in domain 4 (Table 1 and Figure 2).

Table 1. The estimated risk of bias in the studies recruited for this systematic review (*n* = 16).

Study ID	Experimental	No. of Participants	Group Favoured	Outcome	Weight	Risk of Bias					
						D1	D2	D3	D4	D5	O
SONIC [31]	Infliximab	508	Intervention	All HRQoL outcomes	8	+	+	+	+	+	+
Targan et al. [32]	CA2	108	Intervention	All HRQoL outcomes	3	+	+	−	+	−	−
ACCENT I [33]	Infliximab	573	Intervention	All IBDQ outcomes	5	!	+	−	+	−	−
				All PCS and MCS outcomes	10	!	+	−	+	!	−
CHARM [40]	Adalimumab	499	Intervention	All HRQoL outcomes	15	+	+	−	+	−	−
PRECiSE 1 [34]	Certolizumab pegol	662	Intervention	All HRQoL outcomes	2	+	+	−	+	−	−
PRECiSE 2 [35]	Certolizumab pegol	428	Intervention	All HRQoL outcomes	7	+	+	−	+	!	−
Rutgeerts et al. [36]	Certolizumab pegol	292	Intervention	All HRQoL outcomes	5	+	+	!	+	−	−
UNITI I and II [37]	Ustekinumab	742 and 628	Intervention	All IBDQ outcomes	8	+	+	+	+	+	+
				All PCS and MCS outcomes	16	+	+	!	+	+	+
IM UNITI [37]	Ustekinumab	1281	Intervention	All HRQoL outcomes	18	+	+	−	+	+	−
ENCORE [38]	Natalizumab	509	Intervention	All HRQoL outcomes	3	+	−	+	+	+	−
ENACT 2 [39]	Natalizumab	339	Intervention	All HRQoL outcomes	24	+	−	−	+	!	−
FITZROY [41]	Filgotinib	174	Intervention	All HRQoL outcomes	1	+	+	!	+	+	!
CELEST [42]	Upadacitinib	220	Intervention	All HRQoL outcomes	20	+	+	+	+	+	+
Tofacitinib [43]	Tofacitinib	280	Not reported	All HRQoL outcomes	8	+	−	+	+	−	−
Sands et al. [44]	Apilimod mesylate	220	Not significant	All HRQoL outcomes	4	!	+	−	+	+	−

D1: randomisation process, D2: deviations from the intended interventions, D3: missing outcome data, D4: measurement of the outcome, D5: selection of the reported result. + low risk, ! some concerns, − high risk.

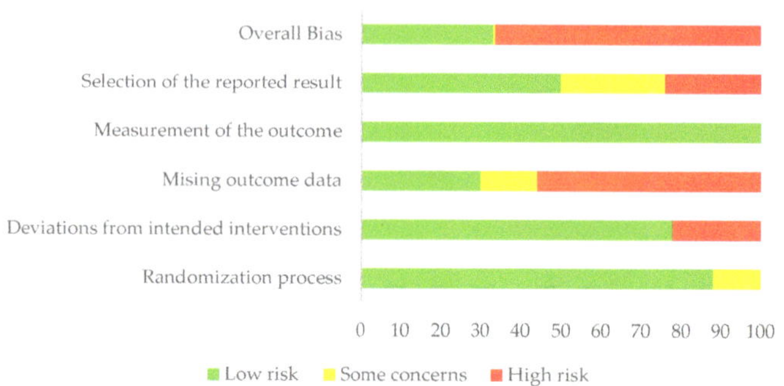

Figure 2. Risk of bias in the included study outcomes.

All studies used random allocation sequences except ACCENT I [33] and Sands et al. [44]. Their outcomes raised some concerns in domain 1, as the allocation sequence was concealed, and the baseline characteristics were consistent with randomisation. All studies used the intention to treat (ITT) or modified intention to treat (mITT) populations for analysis, except ENCORE [38], ENACT-2 [39] and Tofacitinib [43], in which there was no information available about the analysed population. Hence, their outcomes were rated as high risk in domain 2. The outcomes of PRECiSE 1 [34] and PRECiSE 2 [35] (more withdrawals in the placebo groups) and Targan et al. [32], ACCENT I [33], CHARM [40], IM UNITI [37], ENACT-2 [39] and Sands et al. [44] (lack of information about the number of or reason for withdrawals) were rated as high risk in domain 3. The major reason for withdrawal in Rutgeerts et al. [36], UNITI I and II [37] and Filgotinib [41] was a lack of efficacy. However, their outcomes showed some concerns, as the number of withdrawn participants was balanced between the study groups. In UNITI I and II, [37] unlike the IBDQ outcomes (which had low risk), PCS and MCS outcomes were rated as having some concerns due to missing outcome data. The protocols of PRECiSE- 2 [35] and ENACT-2 [39] (in which there were some concerns that results were selected), Targan et al. [32], CHARM [40], PRECISE 1 [34], Rutgeerts et al. [36] and Tofacitinib [43] (in which it was likely that results were selected; high risk of bias) were not found. The IBDQ results were likely selected (high risk) in ACCENT I [33], but selection was not suspected in PCS and MCS results (some concerns). The full details of the RoB2 assessment can be found in Appendix B.

3.3. Effect of Interventions on HRQoL

The effect of interventions on HRQoL is summarised in Table 2 for the SONIC [31] study and Table 3 for the placebo-controlled trials. The tables include the study ID/registration number, intervention, dosage, results and conclusion.

Table 2. The summary of findings for the SONIC [31] study. Results of the SONIC trials. All values are in means (SD).

Study Id and Registration Number	Intervention and Comparator	Dosage and Frequency	Results for	Intervention	Azathioprine	*p* Value	Conclusion
SONIC [31] NCT00094458	Infliximab (IV) and azathioprine (oral)	Infliximab 5mg/kg given at week 2,4,6 and then every 8 weeks OR azathioprine 2.5 mg/kg	Mean IBDQ at baseline	126.7 (30.3)	128 (29)	-	Non-inferiority trial favoured infliximab over azathioprine in improving HRQoL.
			Change at week 2	27.2 (26.1)	20.1 (24.3)	0.007	
			Change at week 6	34.8 (31.8)	28.3 (31.3)	0.10	
			Change at week 10	37.8 (35.6)	31.0 (31.7)	0.10	
			Change at week 18	39.9 (34.2)	30.3 (33.9)	0.01	
			Change at week 26	39.9 (36.6)	31.4 (35.4)	0.05	
			Change at week 32 *	55.8 (33.6)	39.1 (32.9)	0.001	
			Change at week 42 *	51.4 (32.8)	40.3 (32.1)	0.04	
			Change at week 50 *	51.6 (32.9)	43.0 (33.4)	0.09	

* SONIC extension for maintenance therapy.

Table 3. Summary of findings of the placebo-controlled studies ($n = 15$).

Study Id and Registration Number	Intervention	Dosage and Frequency	Results for	Intervention	Placebo	p Value	Conclusion
Targan et al. [32] NCT00269854	Infliximab (IV)	5 mg/kg single dose	**Mean IBDQ at baseline**	122 (29)	128 (29)	-	Infliximab significantly improved IBDQ in the short term.
			Mean at week 4	168 (36)	133 (28)	<0.001	
		10 mg/kg single dose	**Mean IBDQ at baseline**	116 (23)	128 (29)	-	
			Mean at week 4	146 (41)	133 (28)	0.02	
		15 mg/kg single dose	**Mean IBDQ at baseline**	118 (28)	128 (29)	-	
			Mean at week 4	149 (35)	133 (28)	0.03	
ACCENT I [33] NCT00207662	Infliximab (IV)	5 mg/kg every 8 weeks	**Mean IBDQ at baseline**	170 (26)	170 (29)	-	Both doses of infliximab maintenance maintained a significant increase in mean IBDQ and PCS at all time points. Mean MCS difference was not significant except at week 50 in the 10 mg/kg dose.
			Change at week 10	37.8	28.9	<0.05	
			Change at week 30	27.1	14.0	<0.05	
			Change at week 50	22.1	8.9	<0.05	
			Mean PCS at baseline	NR	NR	-	
			Change at week 10	8.6	4.9	<0.001	
			Change at week 30	7.3	3.1	<0.01	
			Change at week 50	6.1	2.5	<0.05	
			Mean MCS at baseline	NR	NR	-	
			Change at week 10	6.5	3.8	≥0.05	
			Change at week 30	4.6	2.9	≥0.05	
			Change at week 50	5.1	2.0	≥0.05	
		10 mg/kg every 8 weeks	**Mean IBDQ at baseline**	168 (31)	170 (29)	-	
			Change at week 30	31.7	14	<0.01	
			Change at week 50	30.2	8.9	<0.001	
			Mean PCS at baseline	NR	NR	-	
			Change at week 30	7.3	3.1	<0.01	
			Change at week 50	7.2	2.5	<0.01	
			Mean MCS at baseline	NR	NR	-	
			Change at week 30	4.9	2.9	≥0.05	
			Change at week 50	5.8	2.0	<0.05	

Table 3. *Cont.*

Study Id and Registration Number	Intervention	Dosage and Frequency	Results for	Intervention	Placebo	*p* Value	Conclusion
CHARM [40] NCT00077779	Adalimumab (SC)	40 mg every other week	**Mean IBDQ at baseline**	NR	NR	-	Both doses of adalimumab maintained a significant increase in mean IBDQ at week 56. Adalimumab every other week maintained a significant increase in mean PCS. Increase in mean MCS reached significance at week 56 in the every other week group. Adalimumab weekly showed no significance in SF-36 outcomes compared to placebo.
			Mean at week 56	176	NR	<0.001	
			Mean PCS at baseline	37.1 (7.9)	36.8 (8.0)	-	
			Mean at week 4 (OL)	44.5 (7.8)	44.3 (8.9)	-	
			Mean at week 12	46.9 (8.6)	44.5 (9.0)	<0.01	
			Mean at week 26	47.4 (9.2)	44.7 (8.6)	<0.01	
			Mean at week 56	47.5 (8.5)	45.3 (8.6)	<0.01	
			Mean MCS at baseline	38.2 (11.0)	38.6 (10.9)	-	
			Mean at week 4 (OL)	46.2 (10.4)	47.4 (10.4)	-	
			Mean at week 12	48.4 (10.7)	46.2 (11.0)	NS	
			Mean at week 26	48.2(10.6)	45.8 (11.4)	NS	
			Mean at week 56	48.7 (10.5)	45.9 (11.2)	<0.05	
			PCS MCID ** at week 56	77	61	<0.01	
			MSC MCID ** at week 56	67	54	<0.05	
		40 mg weekly	**Mean IBDQ at baseline**	NR	NR	-	
			Mean at week 56	171	NR	<0.05	
			Mean PCS at baseline	36.9 (9.6)	36.8 (8.0)	-	
			Mean at week 4 (OL)	43.7 (8.4)	44.3 (8.9)	-	
			Mean at week 12	46.0 (8.6)	44.5 (9.0)	NS	
			Mean at week 26	46.1 (8.7)	44.7 (8.6)	NS	
			Mean at week 56	47.1 (9.4)	45.3 (8.6)	NS	
			Mean MCS at baseline	36.3 (10.5)	38.6 (10.9)	-	
			Mean at week 4 (OL)	45.7 (9.3)	47.4 (10.4)	-	
			Mean at week 12	46.1 (11.9)	46.2 (11.0)	NS	
			Mean at week 26	46.1 (11.3)	45.8 (11.4)	NS	
			Mean at week 56	46.5 (12.4)	45.9 (11.2)	NS	
PRECiSE 1 [34] NCT00152490	Certolizumab pegol (SC)	400 mg every 4 weeks	**Mean IBDQ at baseline**	NR	NR	-	
			Change at week 26	26.4 (35.1)	20.5 (33.1)	0.03	
			IBDQ MCID * at week 26	42.0	33.0	0.01	
PRECiSE 2 [35] NCT00152425	Certolizumab pegol (SC)	400 mg every 4 weeks	**Mean IBDQ at baseline**	NR	NR	-	Certolizumab maintained significant increases in mean IBDQ, PCS and MCS after 26 weeks.
			Mean at week 16	170.0	162	0.008	
			Mean at week 26	175.7 (29.94)	167.9 (23.19)	<0.001	
			Mean PCS at baseline	NR	NR	-	
			Mean at week 26	48.1 (8.17)	46.4 (7.69)	0.014	
			Mean MCS at baseline	NR	NR	-	
			Mean at week 26	46.9 (11.53)	45.2 (11.83)	0.001	
			IBDQ MCID * at week 26	60.6	42.9	<0.001	
			PCS MCID $_a$ at week 26	51.2	33.8	<0.001	
			MCS MCID $_b$ at week 26	44.2	32.4	0.016	

Table 3. *Cont.*

Study Id and Registration Number	Intervention	Dosage and Frequency	Results for	Intervention	Placebo	p Value	Conclusion
Rutgeerts et al. [36]	Certolizumab pegol (SC)	100 mg every 4 weeks	**Mean IBDQ at baseline**	132.2 (30.60)	122.9 (26.60)	-	Induction with certolizumab (400 mg) significantly improved IBDQ.
			Change at week 2	16.6	10.6	NS	
		200 mg every 4 weeks	**Mean IBDQ at baseline**	122.9 (27.07)	122.9(26.60)	-	
			Change at week 2	21.8	10.6	<0.05	
		400 mg every 4 weeks	**Mean IBDQ at baseline**	126.5(25.20)	122.9(26.60)	-	
			Change at week 2	22.8	10.6	<0.05	
			Change at week 10	32.2	18.6	<0.05	
			Mean at week 12	156.4 (37.36)	140.5 (35.88)	<0.05	
			IBDQ MCID * at week 2	52.8	NR	NR	
			IBDQ MCID * at week 12	66.7	NR	NR	
UNITI I [37] NCT01369329	Ustekinumab (IV)	130 mg single infusion	**Mean IBDQ at baseline**	119.5 (29.47)	120.0 (29.27)	-	Both doses of induction ustekinumab significantly increased mean IBDQ in patients who previously failed treatment with TNF-alpha inhibitors. In this population, ustekinumab showed no significance in improving PCS. Only 6 mg/kg ustekinumab significantly improved MCS.
			Change at week 8	18.1 (28.02)	11.9 (26.51)	<0.05	
			Mean PCS at baseline	37.8 (7.12)	37.8 (7.12)	-	
			Change at week 8	3.2 (6.43)	2.6 (6.50)	NS	
			Mean MCS at baseline	37.3 (9.98)	37.8 (10.64)	-	
			Change at week 8	3.3 (9.41)	2.2 (8.47)	NS	
			IBDQ MCID * at week 8	46.9	36.5	0.019	
			PCS MCID ** at week 8	33.3	30	NS	
			MCS MCID ** at week 8	36.4	30	NS	
		6 mg/kg single infusion	**Mean IBDQ at baseline**	118.2 (26.64)	120.0 (29.27)	-	
			Change at week 8	22.1(28.59)	11.9 (26.51)	<0.001	
			Mean PCS at baseline	37.2 (7.09)	37.8 (7.12)	-	
			Change at week 8	3.6 (6.75)	2.6 (6.50)	NS	
			Mean MCS at baseline	36.4 (9.89)	37.8 (10.64)	-	
			Change at week 8	4.9(9.28)	2.2 (8.47)	0.006	
			IBDQ MCID * at week 8	54.8	36.5	<0.001	
			PCS MCID ** at week 8	34.9	30	NS	
			MCS MCID ** at week 8	42.4	30	0.007	

Table 3. *Cont.*

Study Id and Registration Number	Intervention	Dosage and Frequency	Results for	Intervention	Placebo	p Value	Conclusion
UNITI II [37] NCT01369342	Ustekinumab (IV)	130 mg single infusion	Mean IBDQ at baseline	118.2 (30.99)	122.7 (31.32)	-	Both doses of induction ustekinumab significantly increased mean IBDQ, PCS and MCS in patients who previously failed conventional treatment. Ustekinumab groups had a significantly higher proportion of patients achieving MCID.
			Change at week 8	29.1 (33.82)	29.1 (33.82)	<0.001	
			Mean PCS at baseline	38.9 (7.52)	39.7 (7.19)	-	
			Change at week 8	5.1 (7.24)	2.6 (5.88)	<0.010	
			Mean MCS at baseline	37.2 (10.81)	37.1 (10.75)	-	
			Change at week 8	5.9 (10.55)	3.3 (9.47)	<0.010	
			IBDQ MCID * at week 8	58.7	41.1	<0.001	
			PCS MCID ** at week 8	44	31.2	0.009	
			MCS MCID ** at week 8	49.2	38.6	0.036	
		6 mg/kg single infusion	Mean IBDQ at baseline	122.8 (31.62)	122.7 (31.32)	-	
			Change at week 8	35.3 (36.05)	14.7 (26.96)	<0.001	
			Mean PCS at baseline	38.9 (7.05)	39.7 (7.19)	-	
			Change at week 8	6.0 (7.70)	2.6 (5.88)	<0.001	
			Mean MCS at baseline	37.9 (11.15)	37.1 (10.75)	-	
			Change at week 8	6.8 (11.34)	3.3 (9.47)	<0.001	
			IBDQ MCID * at week 8	68.1	41.1	<0.001	
			PCS MCID ** at week 8	49.2	31.2	<0.001	
			MCS MCID ** at week 8	51.3	38.6	0.014	
IM UNITI [37] NCT01369355	Ustekinumab (SC)	90 mg every 12 weeks (q12w)	Mean IBDQ at baseline	165.8 (32.82)	163.6 (31.76)	-	By the end of the study, ustekinumab (q8w) maintained significant improvement across all outcomes. The q12w group maintained improvement in mean IBDQ and MCS.
			Change at week 20	−6.3 (37.04)	−12.8 (34.05)	0.035	
			Change at week 44	−8.9 (43.08)	−21.5 (39.26)	<0.001	
			Mean PCS at baseline	47.1 (8.10)	46.3 (8.21)	-	
			Change at week 20	−1.7 (7.18)	−1.7 (7.67)	NS	
			Change at week 44	−2.3 (9.31)	−3.6 (9.33)	NS	
			Mean MCS at baseline	46.4 (10.66)	45.7 (10.89)	-	
			Change at week 20	−1.3 (11.53)	−2.7 (10.78)	NS	
			Change at week 44	−1.9 (12.68)	−4.4 (11.06)	<0.050	
			IBDQ MCID * at week 44	61.3	50.4	NS	
			PCS MCID ** at week 44	41.7	34.7	NS	
			MCS MCID ** at week 44	46.7	28.9	0.005	
		90 mg every 8 weeks (q8w)	Mean IBDQ at baseline	170.5 (29.33)	163.6 (31.76)	-	
			Change at week 20	−8.9 (31.46)	−12.8 (34.05)	NS	
			Change at week 44	−9.9 (34.83)	−21.5 (39.26)	<0.010	
			Mean PCS at baseline	47.4 (7.52)	46.3 (8.21)	-	
			Change at week 20	−0.6 (6.37)	−1.7 (7.67)	NS	
			Change at week 44	−0.9 (7.14)	−3.6 (9.33)	<0.010	
			Mean MCS at baseline	47.3 (9.91)	45.7 (10.89)	-	
			Change at week 20	−1.7 (9.01)	−2.7 (10.78)	NS	
			Change at week 44	−1.7 (9.76)	−4.4 (11.06)	<0.010	
			IBDQ MCID * at week 44	67.9	50.4	0.014	

Table 3. *Cont.*

Study Id and Registration Number	Intervention	Dosage and Frequency	Results for	Intervention	Placebo	p Value	Conclusion
			PCS MCID ** at week 44	52.1	34.7	0.008	
			MCS MCID ** at week 44	47.9	28.9	0.003	
ENCORE [38] NCT00078611	Natalizumab (IV)	300 mg every 4 weeks	Mean IBDQ at baseline	123.6 (31.06)	122.5 (28.44)	-	Natalizumab induction significantly increased mean IBDQ and PCS but not MCS.
			Change at week 12	26.7 (32.34)	15.2 (28.92)	<0.001	
			Mean PCS at baseline	34.7 (8.7)	34.6 (8.4)	-	
			Change at week 12	5.8 (8.2)	2.7 (6.7)	<0.001	
			Mean MCS at baseline	37.9 (10.8)	4.9 (10.5)	-	
			Change at week 12	4.9 (10.5)	2.6 (9.6)	0.052	
ENACT-2 [39] NCT00032786	Natalizumab (IV)	300 mg every 4 weeks	Mean IBDQ at ENACT 1 baseline	125 (30)	121 (30)	-	By week 60, the natalizumab group had a higher mean and proportion of patients achieving MCID in all three outcomes. Increase in mean IBDQ and PCS was significant at all timepoints, while mean MCS reached significance at week 48.
			Change at the end of ENACT-1	58.6 (30.0)	NG	-	
			Change at week 24	51.6 (31.4)	43.8 (35.0)	<0.01	
			Change at week 36	53.4 (32.9)	39.4 (38.9)	<0.001	
			Change at week 48	52.3 (32.9)	36.5 (39.6)	<0.001	
			Change at week 60	53.9 (33.6)	35.5 (40.3)	<0.001	
			MCID * at the end of ENACT-1	93.2	NG	-	
			IBDQ MCID * at week 24	85.8	77.9	NS	
			IBDQ MCID * at week 36	87.5	70.5	<0.01	
			IBDQ MCID * at week 48	86.7	65.1	<0.001	
			IBDQ MCID * at week 60	86.7	65.1	<0.001	
			Mean PCS at ENACT 1 baseline	33 (8)	34 (3)	-	
			Change at the end of ENACT-1	12.5(8.5)	NG	-	
			Change at week 24	12.5 (8.5)	8.8 (8.9)	<0.01	
			Change at week 36	13.4 (9.4)	7.6 (9.6)	<0.001	
			Change at week 48	12.9 (9.4)	6.9 (9.2)	<0.001	
			Change at week 60	12.6 (9.4)	6.8 (9.5)	<0.001	
			PCS MCID ** at the end of ENACT-1	78.5	NG	-	
			PCS MCID ** at week 24	79.1	63.0	<0.05	
			PCS MCID ** at week 36	82.4	54.8	<0.001	
			PCS MCID ** at week 48	77.9	53.4	<0.001	
			PCS MCID ** at week 60	75.7	53.4	<0.001	
			Mean MCS at ENACT 1 baseline	39 (11)	37 (11)	-	
			Change at the end of ENACT-1	10.5 (10.5)	NG	-	
			Change at week 24	8.6 (10.5)	8.0 (11.0)	NS	
			Change at week 36	8.3 (11.4)	7.2 (11.0)	NS	
			Change at week 48	8.9 (10.2)	6.3 (12.1)	<0.01	
			Change at week 60	9.7 (10.5)	6.8 (12.4)	<0.001	
			MCS MCID ** at the end of ENACT-1	68.7	NG	-	
			MCS MCID ** at week 24	59.7	62.6	NS	
			MCS MCID ** at week 36	61.0	53.0	<0.05	
			MCS MCID ** at week 48	61.8	53.4	<0.001	
			MCS MCID ** at week 60	64.7	52.6	<0.001	

Table 3. *Cont.*

Study Id and Registration Number	Intervention	Dosage and Frequency	Results for	Intervention	Placebo	p Value	Conclusion
FITZROY [41] NCT02048618	Filgotinib (oral)	200 mg once daily	**Mean IBDQ at baseline**	123.0 (2.8)	120.8 (3.6)	-	Filgotinib significantly improved mean IBDQ.
			Change at week 10	33.8 (3.0)	17.6 (5.1)	0.0046	
CELEST [42] NCT02365649	Upadacitinib (oral)	3 mg twice daily (BID)	**IBDQ mean at baseline**	115.2 (27.5)	118.0 (28.5)	-	Upadacitinib (6 mg and 24 mg BID) significantly increased mean IBDQ. By the end of the study, all doses had a higher proportion of patients achieving MCID in IBDQ compared to placebo.
			Change at week 8	19	17	NS	
			Change at week 16	21	13	NS	
			IBDQ MCID * at week 8	41	38	NS	
			IBDQ MCID * at week 16	46	24	≤0.05	
		6 mg twice daily (BID)	**IBDQ mean at baseline**	113.7 (25.9)	118.0 (28.5)	-	
			Change at week 8	35	17	≤0.05	
			Change at week 16	39	13	≤0.01	
			IBDQ MCID * at week 8	62	38	≤0.05	
			IBDQ MCID * at week 16	57	24	≤0.01	
		12 mg twice daily (BID)	**IBDQ mean at baseline**	115.2 (36.1)	118.0 (28.5)	-	
			Change at week 8	25	17	NS	
			Change at week 16	27	13	≤0.1	
			IBDQ MCID * at week 8	58	38	≤0.1	
			IBDQ MCID * at week 16	50	24	≤0.05	
		24 mg twice daily (BID)	**IBDQ mean at baseline**	113.8 (36.0)	118.0 (28.5)	-	
			Change at week 8	40	17	≤0.01	
			Change at week 16	41	13	≤0.01	
			IBDQ MCID * at week 8	53	38	NS	
			IBDQ MCID * at week 16	56	24	≤0.01	
		24 mg once daily (QID)	**IBDQ mean at baseline**	120.7 (36.3)	118.0 (28.5)	-	
			Change at week 8	23	17	NS	
			Change at week 16	22	13	NS	
			IBDQ MCID * at week 8	57	38	≤0.1	
			IBDQ MCID * at week 16	49	24	≤0.05	
Tofacitinib [43] NCT01393626	Tofacitinib (oral)	5 mg twice daily	**Mean IBDQ at baseline**	117.89 (27.98)	118.50 (28.48)	-	P-values were not reported; we cannot determine the significance of the results.
			Change at week 8	41.20 (3.90)	26.58 (3.76)	NR	
			Mean PCS at baseline	38.49 (6.78)	37.12 (7.66)	-	
			Change at week 8	8.07 (0.956)	3.72 (0.927)	NR	
			Mean MCS at baseline	34.85 (11.68)	36.50 (12.26)	-	
			Change at week 8	7.88 (1.178)	6.47 (1.143)	NR	
			IBDQ MCID * at week 8	75	61.4	NR	
		10 mg twice daily	**Mean IBDQ at baseline**	113.67 (28.45)	118.50(28.48)	-	
			Change at week 8	40.05 (3.90)	26.58 (3.76)	NR	
			Mean PCS at baseline	35.28 (8.49)	37.12 (7.66)	-	
			Change at week 8	7.28 (0.967)	3.72 (0.927)	NR	

Table 3. *Cont.*

Study Id and Registration Number	Intervention	Dosage and Frequency	Results for	Intervention	Placebo	*p* Value	Conclusion
			Mean MCS at baseline	35.84 (10.68)	36.50 (12.26)	-	
			Change at week 8	7.13 (1.180)	6.47 (1.143)	NR	
			IBDQ MCID * at week 8	76.5	61.4	NR	
Sands et al. [44] NCT00138840	Apilimod mesylate (oral)	50 mg daily	**Mean IBDQ at baseline**	NR	NR	-	There were no significant differences between the intervention and placebo groups.
			Change at day 29	17.0	18.7	0.76	
			Change at day 43	17.7	23.2	0.33	
		100 mg daily	**Mean IBDQ at baseline**	NR	NR	-	
			Change at day 29	17.0	18.7	0.73	
			Change at day 43	19.5	23.2	0.48	

NR: not reported, NG: the drug was not administered, IV: intravenous, SC: subcutaneous, IBDQ: inflammatory bowel disease questionnaire, PCS: physical component summary, MCS: mental component summary. A clinically meaning full improvement (MCID) was defined as an increase of $\geq$ 16 points in the IBDQ score and an increase of 3–5 points in SF-36 PCS and MCS. All mean change values are in mean (SD). All MCID values are percentages (%). MCID *: proportion of patients achieving an improvement of $\geq$ 16 in the IBDQ score. MCID **: proportion of patients achieving an improvement of [3]5 points in the SF-36 PCS or MCS score. MCID [a]: proportion of patients achieving an improvement of $\geq$ 4.1 points in the SF-36 PCS score. MCID [b]: proportion of patients achieving an improvement of $\geq$3.9 points in the SF-36 MCS score.

3.3.1. Infliximab vs. Azathioprine

SONIC [31] compared infliximab with azathioprine. In the induction period, the difference in the mean change in the IBDQ total score in the infliximab group was significantly higher than the azathioprine group at weeks 2, 18 and 26 ($p < 0.05$), but not at weeks 6 and 10 ($p = 0.10$). In the maintenance phase, the difference was statistically significant at weeks 34 and 42 but not at week 50 ($p = 0.001$, $p = 0.04$ and $p = 0.09$, respectively).

3.3.2. Infliximab vs. Placebo

Two studies, Targan et al. [32] and ACCENT I [33], compared infliximab with placebo.

Targan et al. [32] compared three groups using 5, 10 or 15 mg/kg infliximab induction with a placebo. Patients had a statistically higher mean IBDQ score in all infliximab groups at week 4 ($p < 0.05$, compared to placebo).

ACCENT 1 [33] examined the effect of two infliximab maintenance regimens, 5 mg/kg or 10 mg/kg infliximab, following a 5 mg/kg three-dose induction and compared them with a single dose of 5 mg/kg induction followed by a placebo. At week 10, the three-dose group had a higher mean IBDQ score compared to the single-dose induction group ($p < 0.05$). Higher IBDQ scores were maintained for both maintenance groups (5 mg/kg and 10 mg/kg infliximab) at week 30 ($p < 0.05$ and $p < 0.01$) and week 50 ($p < 0.05$ and $p < 0.001$), respectively, compared to the single-dose induction group. Up to week 14, all treatment groups had an increase exceeding the MCID. Following week 14, the infliximab maintenance groups maintained this increase, while it decreased to below 16 points in the induction-only group. The PCS scores were significantly greater ($p < 0.05$) for both maintenance groups at weeks 10, 30 and 52 compared to the single-dose induction group. The difference in MCS scores was only significant at week 54, comparing the 10mg/kg maintenance group with the single-dose group ($p < 0.05$).

3.3.3. Adalimumab vs. Placebo

The CHARM trial compared adalimumab maintenance, 40 mg every other week or weekly, with adalimumab induction only (placebo maintenance) [40].

Following a significant increase of 44.3 points ($p < 0.0001$, week 4 vs. baseline) in the mean IBDQ in the open-label induction phase, IBDQ scores continued to increase in the adalimumab maintenance groups (approximately 5 points), while IBDQ scores deteriorated in the induction-only group. There were statistically significant differences in the mean IBDQ total scores at all visits after week 4 between adalimumab maintenance groups and the induction-only group ($p < 0.001$ for adalimumab every other week and $p < 0.05$ for adalimumab weekly). After a year of maintenance (at week 56), patients in the adalimumab group had an IBDQ score of 18 points higher than those in the placebo group, a difference that exceeded the MCID of 16 points.

The differences in PCS scores were statistically significant at all visits following week 4 in the adalimumab-every-other-week maintenance group compared to the induction-only group ($p < 0.05$), while differences in the MCS were only significant at week 56 ($p < 0.05$). In total, 77% of adalimumab-every-other-week patients achieved an MCID of ≥ 5 points in the PCS compared to 61% in the induction-only group ($p < 0.01$). In the MCS, improvement was achieved by 67% and 54% of adalimumab-every-other-week and placebo patients, respectively ($p < 0.05$). Differences in the mean PCS and MCS between the adalimumab-weekly group and the placebo group were not statistically significant.

3.3.4. Certolizumab Pegol vs. Placebo

Three studies compared certolizumab pegol and a placebo. One study [36,46] had four arms comparing certolizumab (100 mg), certolizumab (200 mg) or certolizumab (400 mg) with a placebo. The PRECiSE 1 study had two groups comparing 400 mg of certolizumab with a placebo (administered at weeks 0, 2 and 4 and then every 4 weeks) [34]. In PRECiSE 2 [35,47], following an open-label induction of 400 mg of certolizumab at weeks 0, 2 and 4, patients received either maintenance certolizumab (400 mg) or a placebo.

Rutgeerts et al. and Schreiber et al. [36,46] reported statistically significant changes in the mean IBDQ at all reported timepoints for the 400 mg group compared to the placebo group, with the greatest change at week 10 (certolizumab pegol (400 mg): 32.2 points vs. 18.6 points for placebo; $p \leq 0.05$). The 200 mg group had significant changes at weeks 2 and 4 compared to the placebo group ($p \leq 0.05$), while changes in the 100 mg group were not statistically significant. Differences in the mean IBDQ between the certolizumab pegol and placebo arms were statistically significant at week 26 in both PRECiSE 1 and PRECiSE 2 ($p = 0.03$ and $p < 0.001$, respectively). PRECiSE 2 also reported significant differences in the IBDQ means at week 16 ($p = 0.008$). The percentages of patients achieving an MCID in the IBDQ at week 26 were significantly greater in the certolizumab groups in both PRECiSE 1 and 2 ($p = 0.01$ and $p < 0.001$, respectively) compared to the placebo groups.

Only PRECiSE 2 used the SF-36 tool for the estimation of HRQoL. Patients in the certolizumab group showed statistically significant ($p < 0.05$) differences at week 26 in the mean change and proportion achieving an MCID compared to the placebo group.

3.3.5. Ustekinumab vs. Placebo

The UNITI trials compared ustekinumab and a placebo [37,48]. UNITI I and UNITI II induction studies compared a single intravenous infusion of 130 mg of ustekinumab or 6 mg/kg ustekinumab to a placebo. Patients had an inadequate response or intolerance to tumour necrosis factor (TNF) antagonists (UNITI I) or conventional therapy (UNITI II). Patients with a clinical response were re-randomised to maintenance therapy with subcutaneous ustekinumab (90 mg) every 12 weeks (q12w) or every 8 weeks (q8w) for 44 weeks and compared to the placebo in IM UNITI.

In both induction studies, the mean change and proportion of patients achieving an MCID in the IBDQ total score in both ustekinumab groups were statistically significant at week 8 compared to the placebo groups ($p < 0.05$). In the maintenance study at week 20, the mean decrease from the maintenance baseline was significantly less in the q12w group but not in the q8w group compared to the placebo group ($p = 0.035$ and $p = 0.183$, respectively). The mean decrease at week 44 was significantly less in both ustekinumab maintenance groups ($p < 0.001$ and $p = 0.003$, q12w and q8w compared to the placebo group, respectively). A significantly greater proportion of patients achieved MCIDs in the IBDQ in the ustekinumab (q8w) but not the ustekinumab (q12w) group ($p = 0.014$ and $p = 0.140$, respectively, compared to the placebo group).

In UNITI II, the mean change from baseline in the PCS and MCS scores was significant for both ustekinumab doses at week 8 compared to the placebo dose ($p < 0.05$). In UNITI I, the only significant change at week 8 in the mean score was in the MCS of the ustekinumab 6 mg/kg group compared to the placebo group ($p = 0.006$). The same pattern was seen in MCID proportions, significant ($p < 0.05$) in UNITI II for the MCS and PCS in both doses but only significant in the MCS for the 6 mg/kg group in UNITI I.

In the maintenance study at week 44, the mean decrease in the PCS and MCS from the maintenance baseline was significantly less in the ustekinumab (q8w) group compared to the placebo group ($p < 0.01$), while it was only significantly less in the MCS in the ustekinumab (q12w) group compared to the placebo group ($p < 0.05$). Changes in the means of MCS and PCS were not significant at week 20 for both groups. Both groups had significantly ($p < 0.05$) higher proportions of patients with MCID improvements at week 44 in the PCS and MCS, except for the PCS in the q12w group.

3.3.6. Natalizumab vs. Placebo

Two studies compared natalizumab and a placebo. The ENCORE trial compared natalizumab as induction therapy to a placebo [38,49]. The ENACT-2 trial compared maintenance natalizumab with a placebo in patients who responded to natalizumab induction in ENACT-1 [39].

Induction treatment with natalizumab in the ENCORE trial showed a statistically significant ($p < 0.001$) increase in the mean IBDQ total score and the mean PCS score (compared to the placebo) but not in the MCS ($p = 0.052$).

Maintenance natalizumab in ENACT-2 maintained increases in the mean IBDQ total score, PCS and MCS scores achieved from the induction therapy in ENACT-1. The decrease from the change achieved in week 12 (randomisation of ENACT-2) was significantly less in the natalizumab group compared to the placebo group ($p < 0.01$) for all subsequent weeks in the IBDQ total score and PCS. MCS scores were not significant at weeks 24 and 36 but reached significance at weeks 48 and 60 ($p < 0.01$ and $p < 0.001$, respectively, compared to the placebo). The proportion of patients with MCIDs was significantly greater at weeks 36, 48 and 60 in the IBDQ and MCS and at all weeks in the PCS in the natalizumab group ($p < 0.05$, compared to the placebo).

3.3.7. Filgotinib vs. Placebo

The FITZROY study compared oral filgotinib to a placebo [41]. There was a 16-point difference favouring the filgotinib group compared to the placebo in the mean change from baseline of the IBDQ total score. This difference was statistically significant ($p = 0.0046$) and clinically meaningful.

3.3.8. Upadacitinib vs. Placebo

The CELEST study compared five doses of oral upadacitinib (3 mg, 6 mg, 12 mg or 24 mg twice daily or 24 mg once daily) with a placebo as induction therapy [42,50]. Changes in the mean IBDQ total score at weeks 8 and 16 were only statistically significant in the 6 mg and 24 mg twice-daily groups ($p \leq 0.05$, compared to the placebo). A significantly greater proportion of patients achieved clinically meaningful improvement in the IBDQ in all upadacitinib groups at week 16 and only the 6 mg twice-daily group at week 8 ($p \leq 0.05$, compared to placebo).

3.3.9. Tofacitinib vs. Placebo

One study compared three doses of tofacitinib (5 mg, 10 mg or 15 mg twice daily) with a placebo [43]. The 15 mg arm was closed early after the enrolment of only 16 participants. Therefore, this arm was not included in the efficacy analysis. Statistical significance was not calculated for HRQoL outcomes, and thus we could not determine the implications of the clinical evidence.

3.3.10. Apilimod Mesylate vs. Placebo

Sands et al. compared two doses of apilimod mesylate (50 mg and 100 mg daily) as induction therapy with a placebo [44]. No statistically significant differences were found between either of the apilimod groups and the placebo at both time points ($p > 0.3$).

4. Discussion

The overarching goal of treatment for moderate to severe CD using biological agents and small-molecule drugs is the achievement of clinical remission and the arrestment or stabilisation of chronic intestinal inflammation. Our systematic review reported evidence-based clinical data from 16 RCTs and endorsed a superior role of biological agents and small-molecule drugs in improving the HRQoL outcomes in patients with CD. Out of the 16 studies identified in this systematic review, 15 studies compared their investigated interventions to a placebo. Only SONIC compared its intervention (infliximab) to another active drug (azathioprine) and favoured the intervention in the induction phase [31]. Excluding the SONIC study (as it had a different comparator) and one study [43], which did not report the statistical significance. A total of 8/14 studies used the intervention as induction therapy. In contrast, the remaining six RCTs studied maintenance therapy. All studies reported a significant difference in the mean change in the total IBDQ score, favouring the intervention group by the end of the study in at least one dose group, except for Sands et al. [44], who did not report a statistically significant difference. Essentially, three out of eight induction studies and five out of six maintenance studies reported mean changes in the PCS and MCS. Of the induction studies, two out of three studies showed a significant difference in the mean change in the PCS and MCS favouring the intervention group, while all maintenance studies had a significantly greater change in the mean PCS and MCS in their intervention groups.

In our systematic review, two induction and four maintenance studies reported the proportion of patients achieving MCIDs in the IBDQ, and all reported significantly higher proportions in the intervention groups. The only induction studies that reported MCIDs in the PCS and MCS were UNITI I and UNITI II. UNITI I had a significantly higher proportion of patients with MCIDs in the MCS, while UNITI II had a higher proportion in both the MCS and PCS [37]. Furthermore, two out of six maintenance studies reported MCIDs in the PCS and MCS. Both studies had significant findings in favour of the intervention group.

In the systematic review conducted by Vogelaar et al., the researchers found that biologics (infliximab, adalimumab, certolizumab and natalizumab) improved HRQoL [19]. Comparably, the findings of our systematic review are in corroboration with Vogelaar et al. and showed significant improvements in HRQoL using other biologics (ustekinumab) and small-molecule drugs (upadacitinib and filgotinib). A Cochrane review of biologics in ulcerative colitis (another form of inflammatory bowel disease) found that infliximab and adalimumab significantly improved HRQoL [45]. This review argued that the studies on CD have also shown significant improvement in HRQoL. Another systematic review has reported that adalimumab improved fatigue, an aspect of HRQoL [51].

Our systematic review could not measure all of the relevant HRQoL outcomes, including the proportion of patients achieving MCIDs. Due to the missing data and inconsistency in the results from the analysed studies, appropriate statistical analyses could not be used. Some interventions showed inconsistencies in the improvement between physical and mental aspects of HRQoL. Lastly, most studies did not report both co-primary outcomes in both the IBDQ and SF-36 PCS and MCS summary scales. Despite these shortcomings, this systematic review diligently provided valuable data from RCTs which scientifically proves the efficacy of biological agents and small-molecule drugs in improving the HRQoL outcomes in patients with moderate to severe CD.

5. Limitations

There are some limitations to this review. The search strategy was conducted on two databases and only on English-language articles. Several studies that may have affected the results of this review were excluded because they did not report the targeted outcomes, or they were ongoing studies, including a trial for vedolizumab (a common biologic in current use). Effect measures were not calculated, nor were statistical analyses, including a meta-analysis conducted. Thus, the overall effect was not calculated. Owing to inconsistent clinical data from some of the selected studies, the possibility of unintentional research bias cannot be excluded. Nevertheless, during the systematic review process, for the accuracy and verification of results, the researchers arranged periodic meetings for mutual discussions, data cross-verifications and consensuses.

6. Conclusions

The cutting-edge advancements in drug research and biotechnology have introduced novel biologics and small-molecule drugs for the treatment of CD. Our systematic review demonstrated clear evidence of the efficacy of biological agents and small-molecule drugs in improving HRQoL outcomes in patients with moderate to severe CD. Due to the paucity of the comparative analysis of biologics and small-molecule drugs with other agents in the published literature, this study may potentially guide physicians in positioning and relocating drugs in management algorithms for patients with CD.

Supplementary Materials: The following supporting information can be downloaded at: https://drive.google.com/drive/folders/1IIraGwQGod8JjCyno07Rz-SdqUTthrtP?usp=sharing, Appendix B: Quality assessment instrument, Appendix C: Data extraction file, Appendix D: PRISMA checklist.

Author Contributions: H.A. and M.A. jointly developed the protocol and the search strategy of this review. The same authors independently screened the references and extracted the data. Both authors synthesised the data and wrote the report collaboratively. S.S.G. supervised the review from start to finish and supported H.A. and M.A. through training, advice and encouragement. S.Y.G. reviewed the raw and final data, edited the final draft of the article and cross-verified all files to ensure consistency and scientific rigor. All authors have read and agreed to the published version of the manuscript.

Funding: The APC was funded by the Royal College of Surgeons in Ireland—Bahrain.

Institutional Review Board Statement: Not applicable.

Informed Consent Statement: Not applicable.

Data Availability Statement: The data presented in this study are available in this article.

Acknowledgments: We would like to thank Bindhu Nair for her support in developing the search strategy.

Conflicts of Interest: The authors declare no conflict of interest.

Appendix A

A literature search, designed in conjunction with a senior librarian, was used on the following databases: PubMed and Cochrane Central Register of Controlled Trials (CENTRAL). A manual search of reference lists of relevant studies was also conducted for papers that met the inclusion criteria. No limits were set regarding language or date restrictions. We did not to search grey literature, and we did not contact study investigators. The aim of this systematic review was to evaluate the effect of currently approved and promising in-development biological agents and small-molecule agents in improving HRQOL in individuals with moderate to severe Crohn's disease. To answer this question, our search strategy was developed to find publications that are randomised controlled trials reporting on elements of our PICO. We used Boolean operators to combine the terms in Table A1 (both in the title/abstract field and using MeSH terms where applicable). In terms of narrowing our search to randomised control trails, no addition to the CENTRAL search strategy was needed, as it has a separate section for trails. For our PubMed search, with the AND operator, we added a search strategy suggested by the Cochrane handbook that is highly sensitive for identifying randomised controlled trials [23]. Our search was limited to only two databases, in reference to Cochrane guidance [52].

Table A1. Table of keywords used.

Population	Crohn Disease Crohn *
Intervention/Control	• Infliximab • Adalimumab • Certolizumab pegol • Ustekinumab • Vedolizumab • Natalizumab • Etrolizumab • Abrilumab • Risankizumab • Mirikizumab • Brazikumab • Guselkumab • Spesolimab • Filgotinib • Upadacitinib

Table A1. *Cont.*

Population	Crohn Disease Crohn *
	• TD-1473 • Deucravacitinib • Ontamalimab • Ozanimod • Etrasimod • Anti-tnf • Il-23 • Il-12 • Anti α4-integrin • JAK • Sphingosine 1-phosphate
Outcome	Quality of life "Health related quality of life" HRQOLQoLIBDQ "Inflammatory bowel disease questionnaire" SF-36 "36-item Short-Form Health Survey"

Appendix A.1. PubMed (n = 306) 25 January 2022

("crohn*"[Title/Abstract] OR "Crohn Disease"[MeSH Terms]) AND ("GLPG0634"[Supplementary Concept] OR "upadacitinib"[Supplementary Concept] OR "Janus Kinase Inhibitors"[Pharmacological Action] OR "td 1473"[Supplementary Concept] OR "deucravacitinib"[Supplementary Concept] OR "ontamalimab"[Supplementary Concept] OR "ozanimod"[Supplementary Concept] OR "etrasimod"[Supplementary Concept] OR "spesolimab"[Supplementary Concept] OR ("Infliximab"[MeSH Terms] OR "Tumor Necrosis Factor-alpha"[MeSH Terms] OR ("Adalimumab"[MeSH Terms] OR "adalimumab biosimilar HS016"[Supplementary Concept]) OR "Certolizumab Pegol"[MeSH Terms] OR "antibodies, monoclonal"[MeSH Terms] OR "Ustekinumab"[MeSH Terms] OR "vedolizumab"[Supplementary Concept] OR "Natalizumab"[MeSH Terms] OR "Integrin alpha4"[MeSH Terms] OR "etrolizumab"[Supplementary Concept] OR "abrilumab"[Supplementary Concept] OR "risankizumab"[Supplementary Concept] OR "mirikizumab"[Supplementary Concept] OR "guselkumab"[Supplementary Concept]) OR ("jak inhibitor"[Title/Abstract] OR "anti alpha4"[Title/Abstract] OR "sphingosine 1 phosphate"[Title/Abstract] OR "etrasimod"[Title/Abstract] OR "ozanimod"[Title/Abstract] OR "ontamalimab"[Title/Abstract] OR "deucravacitinib"[Title/Abstract] OR "td 1473"[Title/Abstract] OR "upadacitinib"[Title/Abstract] OR "Filgotinib"[Title/Abstract] OR "spesolimab"[Title/Abstract] OR "guselkumab"[Title/Abstract] OR "brazikumab"[Title/Abstract] OR "mirikizumab"[Title/Abstract] OR "risankizumab"[Title/Abstract] OR "abrilumab"[Title/Abstract] OR "etrolizumab"[Title/Abstract] OR "Natalizumab"[Title/Abstract] OR "vedolizumab"[Title/Abstract] OR "Ustekinumab"[Title/Abstract] OR "Certolizumab Pegol"[Title/Abstract] OR "Adalimumab"[Title/Abstract] OR "Infliximab"[Title/Abstract]) OR "tnf-alpha inhibitor"[Title/Abstract] OR ("interleukin 23"[MeSH Terms] OR "interleukin 23 subunit p19"[MeSH Terms] OR "Interleukin-12 Subunit p40"[MeSH Terms]) OR "Infliximab-qbtx"[Title/Abstract]) AND ("36-item Short-Form Health Survey"[Title/Abstract] OR "SF-36"[Title/Abstract] OR "Inflammatory bowel disease questionnaire"[Title/Abstract] OR "IBDQ"[Title/Abstract] OR "Health related quality of life"[Title/Abstract] OR "HRQoL"[Title/Abstract] OR "QoL"[Title/Abstract] OR "Quality of Life"[MeSH Terms] OR "Quality of Life"[Title/Abstract] OR "SF-36V2"[Title/Abstract]) AND (("trial"[Title/Abstract] OR "randomized controlled trial"[Publication Type] OR "controlled clinical trial"[Publication Type] OR "randomized"[Title/Abstract] OR "placebo"[Title/Abstract] OR "drug therapy"[MeSH Subheading] OR "randomly"[Title/Abstract] OR "groups"[Title/Abstract]) NOT ("animals"[MeSH Terms] NOT "humans"[MeSH Terms]))

Appendix A.2. CENTRAL

Date Run:	25 January 2022 04:24:08	
Comment:		
ID	Search	Hits
#1	MeSH descriptor: [Crohn Disease] explode all trees	1700
#2	(crohn*):ti,ab,kw	5202
#3	("36-item Short-Form Health Survey"):ti,ab,kw	1418
#4	("SF-36"):ti,ab,kw	11,356
#5	("SF-36v2"):ti,ab,kw	447
#6	("SF-36 v2"):ti,ab,kw	93
#7	("Inflammatory bowel disease questionnaire"):ti,ab,kw	424
#8	("IBDQ"):ti,ab,kw	550
#9	("Health related quality of life"):ti,ab,kw	18,967
#10	("HRQoL"):ti,ab,kw	6295
#11	("QoL"):ti,ab,kw	22,738
#12	("Quality of Life"):ti,ab,kw	124,127
#13	MeSH descriptor: [Quality of Life] explode all trees	27,298
#14	#1 OR #2	5202
#15	#3 OR #4 OR #5 OR #6 OR #7 OR #8 OR #9 OR #10 OR #11 OR #12 OR #13	131,938
#16	MeSH descriptor: [Janus Kinase Inhibitors] explode all trees	76
#17	MeSH descriptor: [Infliximab] explode all trees	776
#18	MeSH descriptor: [Tumor Necrosis Factor-alpha] explode all trees	3196
#19	MeSH descriptor: [Adalimumab] explode all trees	820
#20	MeSH descriptor: [Certolizumab Pegol] explode all trees	184
#21	MeSH descriptor: [Antibodies, Monoclonal] explode all trees	14,870
#22	MeSH descriptor: [Ustekinumab] explode all trees	227
#23	MeSH descriptor: [Natalizumab] explode all trees	90
#24	MeSH descriptor: [Integrin alpha4] explode all trees	25
#25	("jak inhibitor"):ti,ab,kw	437
#26	("anti alpha4"):ti,ab,kw	4
#27	("sphingosine 1 phosphate"):ti,ab,kw	307
#28	("etrasimod"):ti,ab,kw	53
#29	("ozanimod"):ti,ab,kw	125
#30	("ontamalimab"):ti,ab,kw	5
#31	("deucravacitinib"):ti,ab,kw	11
#32	("td 1473"):ti,ab,kw	14
#33	("upadacitinib"):ti,ab,kw	423
#34	("Filgotinib"):ti,ab,kw	242
#35	("spesolimab"):ti,ab,kw	10
#36	("guselkumab"):ti,ab,kw	369
#37	("brazikumab"):ti,ab,kw	10
#38	("mirikizumab"):ti,ab,kw	100
#39	("risankizumab"):ti,ab,kw	159
#40	("abrilumab"):ti,ab,kw	7
#41	("etrolizumab"):ti,ab,kw	61
#42	("Natalizumab"):ti,ab,kw	433
#43	("vedolizumab"):ti,ab,kw	460
#44	("Ustekinumab"):ti,ab,kw	981
#45	("Certolizumab Pegol"):ti,ab,kw	667
#46	("Adalimumab"):ti,ab,kw	3532
#47	("Infliximab"):ti,ab,kw	2501
#48	("tnf-alpha inhibitor"):ti,ab,kw	55
#49	MeSH descriptor: [Interleukin-23] explode all trees	100
#50	MeSH descriptor: [Interleukin-23 Subunit p19] explode all trees	21
#51	MeSH descriptor: [Interleukin-12 Subunit p40] explode all trees	19
#52	("Infliximab-qbtx"):ti,ab,kw	0
#53	#16 OR #17 OR #18 OR #19 OR #20 OR #21 OR #22 OR #23 OR #24 OR #25 OR #26 OR #27 OR #28 OR #29 OR #30 OR #31 OR #32 OR #33 OR #34 OR #35 OR #36 OR #37 OR #38 OR #39 OR #40 OR #41 OR #42 OR #43 OR #44 OR #45 OR #46 OR #47 OR #48 OR #49 OR #50 OR #51 OR #52	24,764
#54	#14 AND #15 AND #53	312 (303 trials)

References

1. Jawad, N.; Direkze, N.; Leedham, S.J. Inflammatory bowel disease and colon cancer. In *Inflammation and Gastrointestinal Cancers*; Springer: Berlin/Heidelberg, Germany, 2011; pp. 99–115.
2. Keller, D.; Windsor, A.; Cohen, R.; Chand, M. Colorectal cancer in inflammatory bowel disease: Review of the evidence. *Tech. Coloproctol.* **2019**, *23*, 3–13. [CrossRef] [PubMed]
3. Guraya, S.Y. Pattern, stage, and time of recurrent colorectal cancer after curative surgery. *Clin. Colorectal Cancer* **2019**, *18*, e223–e228. [CrossRef] [PubMed]
4. Guraya, S.Y.; Murshid, K.R. Malignant duodenocolic fistula. Various therapeutic surgical modalities. *Saudi Med. J.* **2004**, *25*, 1111–1114. [PubMed]
5. Casellas, F.; López-Vivancos, J.; Casado, A.; Malagelada, J.R. Factors affecting health related quality of life of patients with inflammatory bowel disease. *Qual. Life Res.* **2002**, *11*, 775–781. [CrossRef] [PubMed]
6. Min Ho, P.Y.; Hu, W.; Lee, Y.Y.; Gao, C.; Tan, Y.Z.; Cheen, H.H.; Wee, H.L.; Lim, T.G.; Ong, W.C. Health-related quality of life of patients with inflammatory bowel disease in Singapore. *Intest. Res.* **2019**, *17*, 107–118. [CrossRef]
7. Moradkhani, A.; Beckman, L.J.; Tabibian, J.H. Health-related quality of life in inflammatory bowel disease: Psychosocial, clinical, socioeconomic, and demographic predictors. *J. Crohns. Colitis* **2013**, *7*, 467–473. [CrossRef]
8. Umanskiy, K.; Fichera, A. Health related quality of life in inflammatory bowel disease: The impact of surgical therapy. *World J. Gastroenterol.* **2010**, *16*, 5024–5034. [CrossRef]
9. Guyatt, G.; Mitchell, A.; Irvine, E.J.; Singer, J.; Williams, N.; Goodacre, R.; Tompkins, C. A new measure of health status for clinical trials in inflammatory bowel disease. *Gastroenterology* **1989**, *96*, 804–810. [CrossRef]
10. Irvine, E.; Zhou, Q.; Thompson, A. The Short Inflammatory Bowel Disease Questionnaire: A Quality of Life Instrument for Community Physicians Managing Inflammatory Bowel Disease. *Am. J. Gastroenterol.* **1996**, *91*, 1571–1578.
11. Drossman, D.A.; Leserman, J.; Li, Z.; Mitchell, C.M.; Zagami, E.A.; Patrick, D.L. The rating form of IBD patient concerns: A new measure of health status. *Psychosom. Med.* **1991**, *53*, 701–712. [CrossRef]
12. Bergner, M.; Bobbitt, R.A.; Carter, W.B.; Gilson, B.S. The Sickness Impact Profile: Development and final revision of a health status measure. *Med. Care* **1981**, *19*, 787–805. [CrossRef]
13. Rutgeerts, P.; Feagan, B.G.; Lichtenstein, G.R.; Mayer, L.F.; Schreiber, S.; Colombel, J.F.; Rachmilewitz, D.; Wolf, D.C.; Olson, A.; Bao, W. Comparison of scheduled and episodic treatment strategies of infliximab in Crohn's disease. *Gastroenterology* **2004**, *126*, 402–413. [CrossRef]
14. Bouguen, G.; Levesque, B.G.; Feagan, B.G.; Kavanaugh, A.; Peyrin–Biroulet, L.; Colombel, J.F.; Hanauer, S.B.; Sandborn, W.J. Treat to target: A proposed new paradigm for the management of Crohn's disease. *Clin. Gastroenterol. Hepatol.* **2015**, *13*, 1042–1050. [CrossRef] [PubMed]
15. Turner, D.; Ricciuto, A.; Lewis, A.; D'Amico, F.; Dhaliwal, J.; Griffiths, A.M.; Bettenworth, D.; Sandborn, W.J.; Sands, B.E.; Reinisch, W.; et al. STRIDE-II: An Update on the Selecting Therapeutic Targets in Inflammatory Bowel Disease (STRIDE) Initiative of the International Organization for the Study of IBD (IOIBD): Determining Therapeutic Goals for Treat-to-Target strategies in IBD. *Gastroenterology* **2021**, *160*, 1570–1583. [CrossRef] [PubMed]
16. Food and Drug Administration. Definition of Biological Products. Silver Spring: Food and Drug Administration. 2022. Available online: https://www.fda.gov/files/drugs/published/Biological-Product-Definitions.pdf (accessed on 25 January 2022).
17. Gade, A.K.; Douthit, N.T.; Townsley, E. Medical Management of Crohn's Disease. *Cureus* **2020**, *12*, e8351. [CrossRef] [PubMed]
18. D'Amico, F.; Peyrin-Biroulet, L.; Danese, S.; Fiorino, G. New drugs in the pipeline for the treatment of inflammatory bowel diseases: What is coming? *Curr. Opin. Pharm.* **2020**, *55*, 141–150. [CrossRef]
19. Vogelaar, L.; Spijker, A.V.; van der Woude, C.J. The impact of biologics on health-related quality of life in patients with inflammatory bowel disease. *Clin. Exp. Gastroenterol.* **2009**, *2*, 101–109. [CrossRef]
20. Williet, N.; Sandborn, W.J.; Peyrin-Biroulet, L. Patient-reported outcomes as primary end points in clinical trials of inflammatory bowel disease. *Clin. Gastroenterol. Hepatol.* **2014**, *12*, 1246–1256.e1246. [CrossRef]
21. Irvine, E.J.; Feagan, B.; Rochon, J.; Archambault, A.; Fedorak, R.N.; Groll, A.; Kinnear, D.; Saibil, F.; McDonald, J.W. Quality of life: A valid and reliable measure of therapeutic efficacy in the treatment of inflammatory bowel disease. Canadian Crohn's Relapse Prevention Trial Study Group. *Gastroenterology* **1994**, *106*, 287–296. [CrossRef]
22. Lefebvre, C.; Glanville, J.; Briscoe, S.; Featherstone, R.; Littlewood, A.; Marshall, C.; Metzendorf, M.-I.; Noel-Storr, A.; Paynter, R.; Rader, T.; et al. Chapter 4: Searching for and selecting studies. In *Cochrane Handbook for Systematic Reviews of Interventions Version 6.3*; Higgins, J.P.T., Thomas, J., Chandler, J., Cumpston, M., Li, T., Page, M.J., Welch, V.A., Eds.; Cochrane: Hoboken, NJ, USA, 2022; (updated February 2022); Available online: www.training.cochrane.org/handbook (accessed on 20 January 2022).
23. Lefebvre, C.; Glanville, J.; Manheimer, E. Chapter 6: Searching for studies. In *Cochrane Handbook for Systematic Reviews of Interventions Version 5.1*; Higgins, J.P.T., Green, S., Eds.; Cochrane: Hoboken, NJ, USA, 2022; (updated March 2011); Available online: https://handbook-5-1.cochrane.org/chapter_6/6_4_11_1_the_cochrane_highly_sensitive_search_strategies_for.htm (accessed on 20 January 2022).
24. Sterne, J.A.C.; Page, M.J.; Elbers, R.G.; Blencowe, N.S.; Boutron, I.; Cates, C.J.; Cheng, H.-Y.; Corbett, M.S.; Eldridge, S.M.; Hernán, M.A.; et al. RoB 2: A revised tool for assessing risk of bias in randomised trials. *BMJ* **2019**, *366*, l4898. [CrossRef]

25. Page, M.J.; McKenzie, J.E.; Bossuyt, P.M.; Boutron, I.; Hoffmann, T.C.; Mulrow, C.D.; Shamseer, L.; Tetzlaff, J.M.; Akl, E.A.; Brennan, S.E.; et al. The PRISMA 2020 statement: An updated guideline for reporting systematic reviews. *BMJ* **2021**, *372*, n71. [CrossRef] [PubMed]

26. Guraya, S.S.; AlAdraj, H.R.M.H.A.; Abdulla, M.J.A.E. Health Related Quality of Life of Patients Treated with Biological Agents and New Small-Molecule Drugs for Moderate to Severe Crohn's Disease, a Systematic Review. PROSPERO 2022 CRD42022306394. Available online: https://www.crd.york.ac.uk/prospero/display_record.php?ID=CRD42022306394 (accessed on 25 February 2022).

27. Hanauer, S.B.; Sandborn, W.J.; Rutgeerts, P.; Fedorak, R.N.; Lukas, M.; MacIntosh, D.; Panaccione, R.; Wolf, D.; Pollack, P. Human anti-tumor necrosis factor monoclonal antibody (adalimumab) in Crohn's disease: The CLASSIC-I trial. *Gastroenterology* **2006**, *130*, 323–333. [CrossRef] [PubMed]

28. Sandborn, W.J.; Hanauer, S.B.; Rutgeerts, P.; Fedorak, R.N.; Lukas, M.; MacIntosh, D.G.; Panaccione, R.; Wolf, D.; Kent, J.D.; Bittle, B.; et al. Adalimumab for maintenance treatment of Crohn's disease: Results of the CLASSIC II trial. *Gut* **2007**, *56*, 1232–1239. [CrossRef] [PubMed]

29. Sandborn, W.J.; Feagan, B.G.; Rutgeerts, P.; Hanauer, S.; Colombel, J.F.; Sands, B.E.; Lukas, M.; Fedorak, R.N.; Lee, S.; Bressler, B.; et al. Vedolizumab as induction and maintenance therapy for Crohn's disease. *N. Engl. J. Med.* **2013**, *369*, 711–721. [CrossRef] [PubMed]

30. Sands, B.E.; Peyrin-Biroulet, L.; Kierkus, J.; Higgins, P.D.R.; Fischer, M.; Jairath, V.; Hirai, F.; D'Haens, G.; Belin, R.M.; Miller, D.; et al. Efficacy and Safety of Mirikizumab in a Randomized Phase 2 Study of Patients with Crohn's Disease. *Gastroenterology* **2022**, *162*, 495–508. [CrossRef]

31. Colombel, J.F.; Sandborn, W.J.; Reinisch, W.; Mantzaris, G.J.; Kornbluth, A.; Rachmilewitz, D.; Lichtiger, S.; D'Haens, G.; Diamond, R.H.; Broussard, D.L.; et al. Infliximab, azathioprine, or combination therapy for Crohn's disease. *N. Engl. J. Med.* **2010**, *362*, 1383–1395. [CrossRef]

32. Targan, S.R.; Hanauer, S.B.; van Deventer, S.J.; Mayer, L.; Present, D.H.; Braakman, T.; DeWoody, K.L.; Schaible, T.F.; Rutgeerts, P.J. A short-term study of chimeric monoclonal antibody cA2 to tumor necrosis factor alpha for Crohn's disease. Crohn's Disease cA2 Study Group. *N. Engl. J. Med.* **1997**, *337*, 1029–1035. [CrossRef]

33. Feagan, B.G.; Yan, S.; Bala, M.; Bao, W.; Lichtenstein, G.R. The effects of infliximab maintenance therapy on health-related quality of life. *Am. J. Gastroenterol* **2003**, *98*, 2232–2238. [CrossRef]

34. Sandborn, W.J.; Feagan, B.G.; Stoinov, S.; Honiball, P.J.; Rutgeerts, P.; Mason, D.; Bloomfield, R.; Schreiber, S. Certolizumab pegol for the treatment of Crohn's disease. *N Engl. J. Med.* **2007**, *357*, 228–238. [CrossRef]

35. Feagan, B.G.; Coteur, G.; Tan, S.; Keininger, D.L.; Schreiber, S. Clinically meaningful improvement in health-related quality of life in a randomized controlled trial of certolizumab pegol maintenance therapy for Crohn's disease. *Am. J. Gastroenterol* **2009**, *104*, 1976–1983. [CrossRef]

36. Rutgeerts, P.; Schreiber, S.; Feagan, B.; Keininger, D.L.; O'Neil, L.; Fedorak, R.N. Certolizumab pegol, a monthly subcutaneously administered Fc-free anti-TNFalpha, improves health-related quality of life in patients with moderate to severe Crohn's disease. *Int. J. Colorectal. Dis.* **2008**, *23*, 289–296. [CrossRef] [PubMed]

37. Sands, B.E.; Han, C.; Gasink, C.; Jacobstein, D.; Szapary, P.; Gao, L.L.; Lang, Y.; Targan, S.; Sandborn, W.J.; Feagan, B.G. The Effects of Ustekinumab on Health-related Quality of Life in Patients with Moderate to Severe Crohn's Disease. *J. Crohns. Colitis* **2018**, *12*, 883–895. [CrossRef] [PubMed]

38. Dudley-Brown, S.; Nag, A.; Cullinan, C.; Ayers, M.; Hass, S.; Panjabi, S. Health-related quality-of-life evaluation of crohn disease patients after receiving natalizumab therapy. *Gastroenterol. Nurs.* **2009**, *32*, 327–339. [CrossRef] [PubMed]

39. Feagan, B.G.; Sandborn, W.J.; Hass, S.; Niecko, T.; White, J. Health-related quality of life during natalizumab maintenance therapy for Crohn's disease. *Am. J. Gastroenterol.* **2007**, *102*, 2737–2746. [CrossRef]

40. Loftus, E.V.; Feagan, B.G.; Colombel, J.F.; Rubin, D.T.; Wu, E.Q.; Yu, A.P.; Pollack, P.F.; Chao, J.; Mulani, P. Effects of adalimumab maintenance therapy on health-related quality of life of patients with Crohn's disease: Patient-reported outcomes of the CHARM trial. *Am. J. Gastroenterol.* **2008**, *103*, 3132–3141. [CrossRef]

41. Vermeire, S.; Schreiber, S.; Petryka, R.; Kuehbacher, T.; Hebuterne, X.; Roblin, X.; Klopocka, M.; Goldis, A.; Wisniewska-Jarosinska, M.; Baranovsky, A.; et al. Clinical remission in patients with moderate-to-severe Crohn's disease treated with filgotinib (the FITZROY study): Results from a phase 2, double-blind, randomised, placebo-controlled trial. *Lancet* **2017**, *389*, 266–275. [CrossRef]

42. Peyrin-Biroulet, L.; Louis, E.; Loftus, E.V.; Lacerda, A.; Zhou, Q.; Sanchez Gonzalez, Y.; Ghosh, S. Quality of Life and Work Productivity Improvements with Upadacitinib: Phase 2b Evidence from Patients with Moderate to Severe Crohn's Disease. *Adv. Ther.* **2021**, *38*, 2339–2352. [CrossRef]

43. Euctr, H.R. A Randomized, Double-Blind, Placebo-Controlled, Parallel Group, Multi-Centre Study to Investigate the Safety and Efficacy of CP-690,550 for Induction Therapy in Subjects with Moderate to Severe Crohn's Disease. 2014. Available online: https://trialsearch.who.int/Trial2.aspx?TrialID=EUCTR2011-001733-16-HR (accessed on 1 February 2022).

44. Sands, B.E.; Jacobson, E.W.; Sylwestrowicz, T.; Younes, Z.; Dryden, G.; Fedorak, R.; Greenbloom, S. Randomized, double-blind, placebo-controlled trial of the oral interleukin-12/23 inhibitor apilimod mesylate for treatment of active Crohn's disease. *Inflamm. Bowel. Dis.* **2010**, *16*, 1209–1218. [CrossRef]

45. LeBlanc, K.; Mosli, M.H.; Parker, C.E.; MacDonald, J.K. The impact of biological interventions for ulcerative colitis on health-related quality of life. *Cochrane Database Syst Rev.* **2015**, *37*, Cd008655. [CrossRef]

46. Schreiber, S.; Rutgeerts, P.; Fedorak, R.N.; Khaliq-Kareemi, M.; Kamm, M.A.; Boivin, M.; Bernstein, C.N.; Staun, M.; Thomsen, O.; Innes, A. A randomized, placebo-controlled trial of certolizumab pegol (CDP870) for treatment of Crohn's disease. *Gastroenterology* **2005**, *129*, 807–818. [CrossRef]

47. Schreiber, S.; Khaliq-Kareemi, M.; Lawrance, I.C.; Thomsen, O.; Hanauer, S.B.; McColm, J.; Bloomfield, R.; Sandborn, W.J. Maintenance therapy with certolizumab pegol for Crohn's disease. *N. Engl. J. Med.* **2007**, *357*, 239–250. [CrossRef] [PubMed]

48. Feagan, B.G.; Sandborn, W.J.; Gasink, C.; Jacobstein, D.; Lang, Y.; Friedman, J.R.; Blank, M.A.; Johanns, J.; Gao, L.L.; Miao, Y.; et al. Ustekinumab as Induction and Maintenance Therapy for Crohn's Disease. *N. Engl. J. Med.* **2016**, *375*, 1946–1960. [CrossRef] [PubMed]

49. Targan, S.R.; Feagan, B.G.; Fedorak, R.N.; Lashner, B.A.; Panaccione, R.; Present, D.H.; Spehlmann, M.E.; Rutgeerts, P.J.; Tulassay, Z.; Volfova, M.; et al. Natalizumab for the treatment of active Crohn's disease: Results of the ENCORE Trial. *Gastroenterology* **2007**, *132*, 1672–1683. [CrossRef] [PubMed]

50. Sandborn, W.J.; Feagan, B.G.; Loftus, E.V.; Peyrin-Biroulet, L.; Van Assche, G.; D'Haens, G.; Schreiber, S.; Colombel, J.F.; Lewis, J.D.; Ghosh, S.; et al. Efficacy and Safety of Upadacitinib in a Randomized Trial of Patients with Crohn's Disease. *Gastroenterology* **2020**, *158*, 2123–2138.e2128. [CrossRef] [PubMed]

51. Farrell, D.; Artom, M.; Czuber-Dochan, W.; Jelsness-Jørgensen, L.P.; Norton, C.; Savage, E. Interventions for fatigue in inflammatory bowel disease. *Cochrane Database Syst Rev.* **2020**, *4*, Cd012005. [CrossRef] [PubMed]

52. Lefebvre, C.; Glanville, J.; Briscoe, S.; Littlewood, A.; Marshall, C.; Metzendorf, M.-I.; Noel-Storr, A.; Rader, T.; Shokraneh, F.; Thomas, J.; et al. Chapter 4: Searching for and selecting studies. In *Cochrane Handbook for Systematic Reviews of Interventions Version 6.2*; Higgins, J.P.T., Thomas, J., Chandler, J., Cumpston, M., Li, T., Page, M.J., Welch, V.A., Eds.; Cochrane: Hoboken, NJ, USA, 2022; (updated February 2021); Available online: https://training.cochrane.org/handbook/archive/v6.2 (accessed on 20 January 2022).

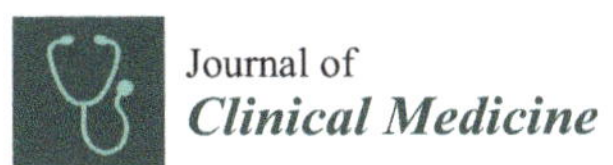

Journal of
Clinical Medicine

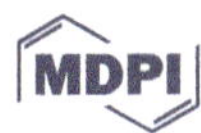

Review

Gastric Cancer Screening in Japan: A Narrative Review

Kazuo Yashima [1,*], **Michiko Shabana** [2], **Hiroki Kurumi** [1], **Koichiro Kawaguchi** [1] and **Hajime Isomoto** [1]

[1] Division of Gastroenterology and Nephrology, Faculty of Medicine, Tottori University, 36-1 Nishicho, Yonago 683-8504, Japan; kurumi_1022_1107@yahoo.co.jp (H.K.); koichiro@tottori-u.ac.jp (K.K.); isomoto@tottori-u.ac.jp (H.I.)

[2] Sanin Rosai Hospital, 1-8-1 Kaikeshinden, Yonago 683-8605, Japan; shabana@saninh.johas.go.jp

[*] Correspondence: yashima@tottori-u.ac.jp; Tel.: +81-859-38-6527; Fax: +81-859-38-6529

Abstract: Gastric cancer is the second leading cause of cancer incidence in Japan, although gastric cancer mortality has decreased over the past few decades. This decrease is attributed to a decline in the prevalence of *H. pylori* infection. Radiographic examination has long been performed as the only method of gastric screening with evidence of reduction in mortality in the past. The revised 2014 Japanese Guidelines for Gastric Cancer Screening approved gastric endoscopy for use in population-based screening, together with radiography. While endoscopic gastric cancer screening has begun, there are some problems associated with its implementation, including endoscopic capacity, equal access, and cost-effectiveness. As *H. pylori* infection and atrophic gastritis are well-known risk factors for gastric cancer, a different screening method might be considered, depending on its association with the individual's background and gastric cancer risk. In this review, we summarize the current status and problems of gastric cancer screening in Japan. We also introduce and discuss the results of gastric cancer screening using *H. pylori* infection status in Hoki-cho, Tottori prefecture. Further, we review risk stratification as a system for improving gastric cancer screening in the future.

Keywords: gastric cancer; gastric cancer screening; endoscopy; *H. pylori*; eradication therapy

Citation: Yashima, K.; Shabana, M.; Kurumi, H.; Kawaguchi, K.; Isomoto, H. Gastric Cancer Screening in Japan: A Narrative Review. *J. Clin. Med.* **2022**, *11*, 4337. https://doi.org/10.3390/jcm11154337

Academic Editor: Sun-Young Lee

Received: 27 June 2022
Accepted: 24 July 2022
Published: 26 July 2022

Publisher's Note: MDPI stays neutral with regard to jurisdictional claims in published maps and institutional affiliations.

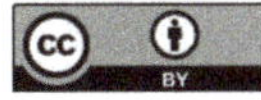

1. Introduction

Gastric cancer is the fifth most common cancer and the fourth leading cause of cancer-related deaths worldwide [1]. *Helicobacter pylori* (*H. pylori*) infection is considered the main cause of gastric cancer [2,3]. In Japan, the adjusted incidence and mortality rates of gastric cancer have decreased over the past few decades [4]. This decrease is mainly attributed to the reduction in *H. pylori* infection rates and the preventative effects of the *H. pylori* eradication therapy [5–10]. Despite this reduction, the number of gastric cancer cases ranks second and the number of deaths caused by gastric cancer ranks third in Japan [11], making it a critical public health problem.

In Japan, radiographic examination has been conducted since the 1960s as a secondary preventive measure for gastric cancer [12]. The revised 2014 Japanese Guidelines for Gastric Cancer Screening approved gastric endoscopy for use in population-based screening, together with radiography [13]. Currently, the government of Japan recommends either radiography or gastroscopic examination for gastric cancer screening [14]. However, there are some barriers, such as participation rate, endoscopic capacity, equal access, and cost-effectiveness [15–18].

Over 99% of gastric cancers in Japan are predisposed by a current or past *H. pylori* infection [19,20]. Furthermore, the background of gastric cancer risk has changed compared to the past due to the rapid decrease in the infection rate of *H. pylori* [5–10]. It has become necessary for efficient gastric cancer screening to classify patients as *H. pylori*-infected [8,21,22].

In recent years, image-enhanced endoscopy (IEE) [23], as well as artificial intelligence (AI), have been introduced in endoscopic diagnostics [24–26]. In this review, the present status and problems of gastric cancer screening in Japan are summarized. We present the results of gastric cancer screening using *H. pylori* infection status in Hoki-cho, Tottori prefecture. Further, we introduce risk stratification as a system for improving gastric cancer screening in the future.

2. Gastric Cancer in Japan

2.1. Epidemiology of Gastric Cancer

In Japan, gastric cancer accounted for almost half of all cancer deaths in the 1960s, but the proportion continues to decline. According to the 2021 cancer statistics forecast of the National Cancer Center Cancer-Information Service, "Cancer Registration and Statistics", gastric cancer ranked third in the number of deaths after lung cancer and colorectal cancer. The total number of cancer deaths was 11.1% (42,000 people) [11]. The number of gastric cancer deaths has remained at 50,000 per year for the past few decades, and since 2011, it has been declining. However, more than 40,000 people lose their lives to stomach cancer every year. Gastric cancer has the second highest incidence rate at 12.9% (130,500 people), following colorectal cancer. As for the annual transition of gastric cancer, the age-standardized incidence and mortality are steadily decreasing, the number of cases is increasing, and the number of deaths tends to plateau due to an increase in the incidence and deaths caused by gastric cancer in the elderly population.

2.2. H. pylori and Gastric Cancer

The International Agency for Research on Cancer designated *H. pylori* as a clear gastric cancer carcinogenic factor (group 1) in 1994 [27] and recommended prevention by eradication in 2014 [28]. The presence of *H. pylori* infection is determined by histologic examination, the rapid urease test, serum antibody test, stool antigen test, or 13C-urea breath test. The effectiveness of the eradication treatment on gastric cancer prevention has been shown in a randomized controlled trial [29], and this primary preventive effect of the eradication of gastric cancer has been reported in recent meta-analyses [30–32]. Eradication of *H. pylori* reduces the risk of gastric cancer and mortality [33–36], but the risk still remains in the second decade after eradication [37]. Moreover, the pathogenicity and carcinogenicity of *H. pylori* depend on its strain. The East Asian type of *H. pylori*, which is popular in Japan, is more carcinogenic than the European-type *H. pylori* [38,39]. In addition, the presence of *H. pylori* with a positive babA2 gene may contribute to an increased risk of GC, especially in the Asian population [39,40]. In Japan, the eradication treatment for gastric and duodenal ulcers was covered by the National Health Insurance in 2000, and *H. pylori*-infected gastritis was added as an indication in 2013 [41]. According to recent reports in Japan, the risk of cumulative incidence of gastric cancer was 17.0% in men and 7.7% in women in the *H. pylori*-infected population, and <1% in the non-infected population [42]. More than 99% of gastric cancers in Japan are associated with *H. pylori*-infection gastritis [19,20]. Histopathological diagnosis of gastric cancer is performed according to the Japanese Classification of Gastric Carcinoma and the Vienna classification system [43,44]. Although gastric cancer that is not associated with *H. pylori* infection is extremely rare, gastric is cancer associated with autoimmune gastritis, gastric cancer due to *CDH1* gene mutation, fundic gland-type cancer, signet ring cell carcinoma, and cardia cancer are known [45]. Cardia cancer is often discovered at an advanced stage; thus, particular attention should be paid to it [46]. Moreover, the main risk factors of cardia cancer, which include gastroesophageal reflux disease and obesity, are different from those of gastric cancer associated with *H. pylori* [47].

As mentioned above, in Japan, the age-standardized incidence and mortality rate of gastric cancer has decreased over the past few decades due to a decrease in the incidence of *H. pylori* infection [4–15]. *H. pylori* infection rates in the 1960s, 1970s, and 1980s or later were 30%, 20%, and <10%, respectively [7]. A meta-analysis of the Japanese population shows that *H. pylori* infection rate is high in patients born in the 1940s; however, the infection rate decreased in patients who were born later, in the 1950s [9]. Although the morbidity rate of gastric cancer has continued to decrease due to the reduced *H. pylori* infection rates and the preventative effect of the *H. pylori* eradication therapy, the prevalence of *H. pylori* eradication has increased remarkably in recent years [8]. In the midst of dynamic changes in the incidence of *H. pylori* infection, it is considered to be important to pay attention to the high-risk groups in gastric cancer screening.

3. Gastric Cancer Screening Methods Used in Japan

3.1. Current Status and Problems of Upper Gastrointestinal Series

Annual radiographic screening for everyone >40 years of age in Japan was implemented in the 1960s as a secondary preventive measure for gastric cancer [12,14]. Gastric cancer screening using radiographic examination has proven to reduce mortality. It has an excellent mass-processing ability, and good accuracy, and is safe and cost-effective [48,49]. Furthermore, in recent case-control studies in Japan and South Korea, the effect of radiographic screening on mortality reduction was limited [50,51]. The Japan Society of Gastroenterological Cancer Screening formulated a revised version of the new gastric radiography guidelines (2011) [52]. The ability to view lesions by gastric radiographic examination has been greatly improved with the use of high-concentration, low-viscosity barium preparations and the advent of digital X ray devices. Consequently, the rate of early detection of gastric cancer has exceeded 70% [53]. In addition, gastric cancer screening has been performed using imaging and AI to detect *H. pylori*-infected gastritis and gastric mucosal atrophy [54]. However, due to aging and immobilization of patients, radiation exposure, and lack of reading physicians and aging facilities, the rate of participation has been sluggish. Although endoscopic examinations have been approved by the revised 2014 Japanese Guidelines for Gastric Cancer Screening [13], it is impossible to replace all conventional radiography with endoscopic examinations due to problems relating to the capacity of endoscopy, budget, and access to examinees [14,15]. In population-based gastric cancer screening, it will be necessary to continue to utilize radiographic examinations with high processing capacity as a safety net.

3.2. Current Status and Problems of Upper Gastrointestinal Endoscopy

Radiographic examination is a screening method limited to Japan, but there is a growing international interest in endoscopic screening [55]. In Korea, in response to the results of domestic research, gastric cancer screening has been limited to endoscopic examinations [55,56].

In 2013, a case-control study was conducted in Japan and Korea. The research conducted in Japan involved a study on the population of Goto Islands in Nagasaki Prefecture [57] and a study on the population of Tottori Prefecture and Niigata City [58]. Although the sample size is small in the Nagasaki study, the mortality rate of gastric cancer was significantly decreased by 79% in participants of endoscopic screening (odds ratio [OR]: 0.206, 95% confidence interval [CI]: 0.044–0.965) [57]. In 2013, a case-control study that was conducted in Niigata City and four cities in Tottori Prefecture reported that the mortality rate was significantly lower by approximately 30% in people who underwent endoscopy 36 months before the date of gastric cancer diagnosis (OR: 0.695, 95% CI: 0.489–0.986) [58]. The studies that were conducted in Korea were large-scale research based on national databases. When the gastroscopic examination was performed even once in the past, the effect of reducing the gastric cancer mortality rate was confirmed to be 47% in individuals aged 40–74 years old (OR: 0.53, 95% CI: 0.51–0.56) [56]. Based on these results, a gastroscopy was recommended as a population-based screening method according to the revised 2014 Japanese Guidelines for Gastric Cancer Screening [13]. At the same time, it has changed from once a year for individuals aged > 40 to once every 2 years for individuals aged > 50 years, reflecting the recent decline in gastric cancer mortality by age group. In 2015, a study of Tottori Prefecture showed that endoscopic screening reduced the gastric cancer mortality rate by 67% compared with radiographic screening [50]. Zhang et al. conducted a meta-analysis that included 342,013 individuals in the six-cohorts and four-case-control studies that were previously published. This analysis demonstrated that endoscopic examination showed a 40% reduction in gastric cancer mortality rate (relative risk: 0.60, 95% CI: 0.49–0.73) [59].

According to reports from the area where endoscopic examinations were introduced, the gastric cancer detection rate was 0.05–0.32% for gastric X-ray examination and 0.30–0.87% for gastroscopic examinations [8,60]. Further, the gastric cancer detection rate of endoscopy was reported to have been approximately three times higher than that of X-ray examination. In Japanese studies, the proportion of early-stage cancer was approximately 70% in the radiographic screening group and >80% in the endoscopic screening group. Similarly, Hosokawa et al. previously reported that the detection rate of early cancer was higher in the endoscopic screening group than in the radiographic screening group [61]. However, the effectiveness of gastric cancer screening should be evaluated by the mortality reduction, and not by the detection rate.

Endoscopy can diagnose early-stage cancers that can be treated by endoscopic surgical dissection. Endoscopic surgical dissection has been performed for approximately half of early-stage cancers detected by endoscopic screening [62]. It seems to contribute to the maintenance of the quality of life after treatment. Moreover, recent development and widespread use of IEE and magnifying endoscopy have improved the endoscopic diagnosis of gastric cancer [23]. IEE is useful for diagnosing gastric cancer after eradication, which is usually difficult to detect [63]. In a recent study, we showed that photodynamic endoscopic diagnosis—based on the fluorescence of photosensitizers that accumulate in tumors—may be useful in the diagnosis of early gastric cancer regardless of the endoscopist's experience and is useful for tumor detection; however, its usefulness has not been established because no prospective studies evaluating its usefulness have been performed [64].

As the participation rate in gastric cancer screening has decreased, its impact on mortality reduction has become limited. Although the participation rate in radiographic screening for gastric cancer has sunk below 10% [65], it is possible to improve the participation rate by introducing endoscopic screening as a method of gastric cancer screening. Notably, the participation rate is approximately 25% in municipalities that have already undergone endoscopic screening [66,67]. Thus, endoscopy is now the first choice for gastrointestinal tract examination instead of X-ray examination.

4. Risk Stratification for Gastric Cancer Screening

4.1. Risk Factors for Gastric Cancer

Risk factors for gastric cancer include *H. pylori* infection and accompanying gastric mucosal atrophy, smoking, and hereditary diseases, such as Lynch syndrome and familial adenomatous coli [23]. In addition, diet, lifestyle preferences, and Epstein-Barr virus infection have been reported as possible risk factors. Recently, it has been reported that approximately one-fifth of diffuse-type gastric cancers in Japan were attributable to the combination of alcohol intake and defective *ALDH2* allele or *CDH1* variants [68]. The most important method of obtaining information about these risk factors before endoscopic screening is a medical questionnaire. In addition, during the endoscopic examination, individuals can be stratified by gastric cancer risk based on *H. pylori* infection status and relevant findings suggestive of gastric cancer risk, as described in the endoscopy-based Kyoto classification of gastritis [69–71]. Endoscopic findings related to the risk of gastric cancer include moderate-to-severe gastric atrophy, enlarged gastric folds, nodular gastritis, xanthoma [72,73], and map-like redness [70]. As a result of examining the accuracy of *H. pylori* infection diagnosis by the "Kyoto classification of gastritis", the sensitivity and specificity of detecting uninfected, existing infection, and current infection were 88.3% and 92.9%, 78.8% and 90.0%, and 67.1% and 91.4%, respectively. Moreover, risk classification by endoscopic examination was confirmed to have very high accuracy. However, to avoid false-negative results, an *H. pylori* antibody test was recommended [74].

4.2. Tests Used for Risk Stratification

According to the 2019 Basic Survey on National Life, 54.2% of men and 45.1% of women aged 40–69 years had undergone gastric cancer screening [75], approaching the target value of 50% of the 3rd Basic Plan for Cancer Countermeasures in Japan. However, in recent years, the number of *H. pylori*-negative people has increased, and the gastric cancer-adjusted mortality rate has naturally decreased [5–11]; following this, there has been a problem with cost-effectiveness in the strategy of simply increasing the participation rate. In the future, it may be necessary to stratify individuals according to gastric cancer risk by determining risk factors—such as a history of *H. pylori* infection and gastric mucosal atrophy—and reflect them in the selection of endoscopy and the determination of the screening interval.

The "ABC method", a combined assay for serum anti-*H. pylori* IgG antibody and serum pepsinogen (PG) levels, is generally used in Japan as a gastric cancer risk classification system [76]. Itoh et al. reported a strong correlation between the ABC classification system and radiological findings in relation to the risk of gastric cancer [77]. However, the revised 2014 Japanese Guidelines for Gastric Cancer Screening do not recommend this method due to insufficient scientific evidence regarding its effectiveness in gastric cancer screening [13]. The risk of gastric cancer can be stratified based on factors, such as the presence of *H. pylori* infection and the extent and severity of gastric atrophy. The serum anti-*H. pylori* IgG antibody titer can predict an individual's *H. pylori* infection status, whereas its titers vary greatly depending on the test kit used.Serum PG levels reflect the status of gastric mucosal inflammation and serve as a marker for atrophic gastritis. Individuals with PG I levels of ≤70 ng/ml and PG I/II ratio of <3 are classified as PG test positive, and people with a history of *H. pylori* eradication, treatment of proton pump inhibitors, previous gastric resection and impairment of renal function are excluded to ensure correct stratification. This method classifies individuals into the following four groups according to their serological status: (1) group A, anti-*H. pylori* IgG antibody (−)PG (−); (2) group B, anti-*H. pylori* IgG antibody (+)/PG (−); (3) group C, anti-*H. pylori* IgG antibody (+)/PG (+); and (4) group D, anti-*H. pylori* IgG antibody (−)/PG (+), which also included those with autoimmune gastritis (type A gastritis) [76]. Notably, a meta-analysis conducted by Terasawa et al. demonstrated that groups A, B, and C + D were significantly different in their respective gastric cancer risk [78]; thus, this stratification is expected to serve as a mass screening system for this disease.

As the development of gastric cancer in patients not infected with *H. pylori* is extremely rare in Japan, it may be expected that the *H. pylori*-uninfected population could be excluded from the mass screening system for gastric cancer. However, group A included patients with a high risk of developing gastric cancer and could not be regarded as truly *H. pylori*-negative [79,80]. The presence of *H. pylori*-infected individuals in group A is a crucial problem because the individuals are wrongly considered to have an extremely low risk for gastric cancer, similar to healthy, *H. pylori*-uninfected individuals. The endoscopic grade of atrophy is an accurate predictive marker for gastric cancer [81,82]. To exclude individuals who are truly *H. pylori*-negative, an endoscopic evaluation of the gastric mucosa should be performed [83,84]. It is inefficient to perform endoscopy in all patients as this is expensive and requires high manpower of endoscopists.

According to a report by the Kanazawa City Medical Association [84], gastric cancer may develop at an annual rate of 0.31% in a state with advanced atrophy (O-3) classified by Kimura and Takemoto [85], and it is possible to stratify the risk of gastric cancer using endoscopic diagnosis. Therefore, endoscopic diagnosis of atrophy may be more effective than the ABC classification system for predicting the risk of gastric cancer.

Several cost-effectiveness analyses demonstrated that endoscopic surveillance is a cost-effective method to reduce gastric cancer mortality. A comprehensive systematic review showed that endoscopic screening is cost-effective in high-incidence countries, and that targeted endoscopic screening of high-risk populations is also generally cost-effective in low-intermediate incidence countries [86]. Recently, Kowada et al. demonstrated that biennial endoscopy for patients with mild-to-moderate gastric mucosal atrophy and annual endoscopy for patients with severe gastric mucosal atrophy were the most cost-effective measures after *H. pylori* eradication [87].

4.3. Gastric Cancer Screening Tests Performed at Hoki-cho, Tottori Prefecture

Since 2000, patients in Tottori Prefecture were able to select between endoscopic and radiographic examinations. The rate of gastric cancer screening by endoscopic or radiographic examination in Hoki-cho, Tottori Prefecture has remained around 20%, which is not sufficient, as the national target is 50%. With the aim of accelerating endoscopic screening and eradication therapy for *H. pylori* infection, Hoki-cho in Tottori Prefecture has implemented a risk evaluation system for gastric cancer for 5 years since 2014 by testing the serum for *H. pylori* antibodies [88]. Target populations included individuals aged 20 and 35–70 years in each year, and who underwent at least one examination through the evaluation system during this period (Figure 1).

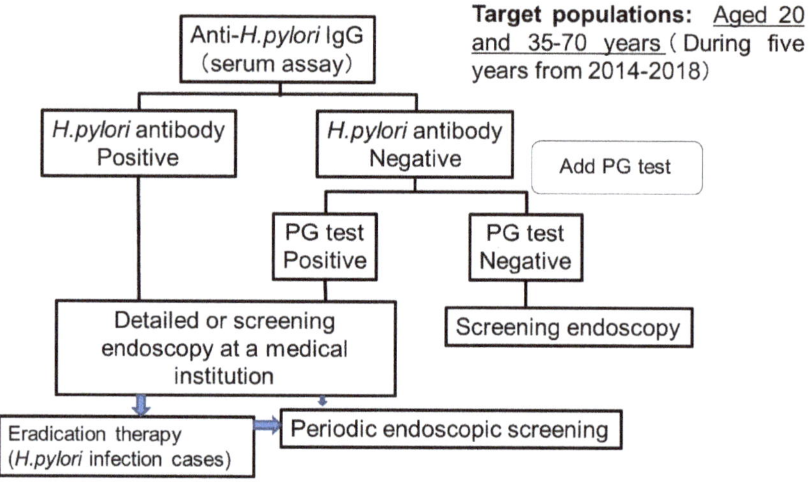

Figure 1. Flow chart of *H. pylori* antibody test project in Hoki-cho, Tottori prefecture. Individuals with PG I levels of ≤70 ng/mL and PG I/II ratio of <3 are classified as PG test positive, which is equal to gastric atrophy. PG, pepsinogen.

In cases with negative results for *H. pylori* diagnosis, we incorporated the serum PG method. During the 5 years from 2014 to 2018, there were a total of 6191 target individuals, of whom 2464 were screened (participation rate: 39.8%). The total number of *H. pylori*-positive cases was 753 (30.6%), and that of cases negative for *H. pylori* antibody and positive for the PG method was 58 (2.4%). The frequency of *H. pylori* positivity was 9.2% in individuals aged 20 years and <40% in individuals aged 60–70 years. This gradually increased with advancing age (Figure 2). The rate was highest (38.4%) among patients aged 60–70 years of age.

Consequently, during the 5-year study period, 71.3% of the examinees underwent a detailed endoscopic examination (Table 1), and two patients with early gastric cancer were detected. Eradication therapy was implemented in 97.6% of cases that had a positive result for *H. pylori* infection after undergoing a detailed endoscopic examination. On the other hand, only 33.7% and 22.8% of individuals with positive screening results in 2014 and 2015, respectively, had received a periodic endoscopic screening at least once during the three years after the following year. Therefore, it is important to increase the participation rate of this project and the rate of detailed endoscopic examinations to further increase in the detection of the risk of gastric cancer and implement periodic endoscopic screening.

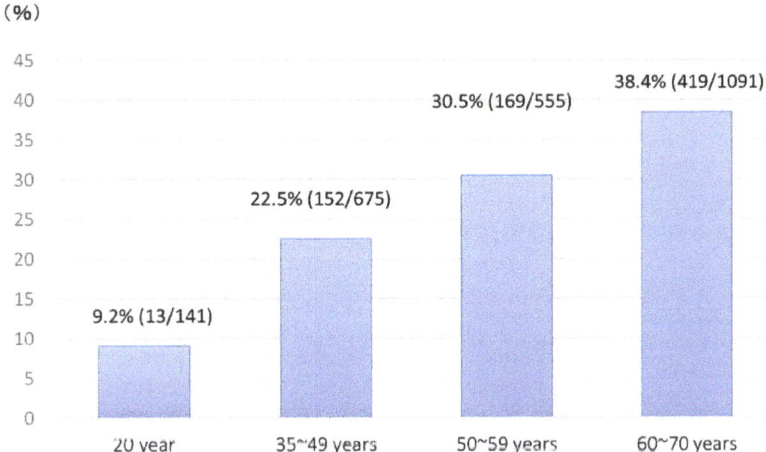

Figure 2. The frequency of *H. pylori* positivity according to age (2014~2018).

Table 1. Results of *H. pylori* antibody test project in Hoki-cho, Tottori Prefecture.

Year	2014	2015	2016	2017, 2018	Total
Examinees (*n*)	910	776	311	467	2464
Cases requiring detailed endoscopy (*n*)	323	259	109	121	811
Examination required rate (%)	35.4	33.4	35.0	25.9	32.9
Cases undergone screeningendoscopy (*n*)	258	181	61	78	578
Examination rate (%)	79.9	69.9	56.0	64.5	71.3

The rate of population-based gastric cancer screening in Hoki-cho was 20.6% in 2013; however, after the introduction of the *H. pylori* infection screening, it increased to 26.2% in 2015, 22.8% in 2016, 23.2% in 2017, and 24.3% in 2018. In 2018, 657 (63.4%) of the 1036 patients had opted for endoscopic examination (26.1% in 2013, 35.3% in 2014, 52.9% in 2015, 50.7% in 2016, and 57.0% in 2017), contributing to the steady increase in the use of endoscopy (Table 2).

Table 2. Annual trends in the rate of participation for population-based gastric cancer screening in Hoki-cho, Tottori Prefecture.

Year	2013	2014	2015	2016	2017	2018	2019
Target population (*n*)	4533	4533	4533	4257	4257	4257	4257
Examinees (*n*)	934	963	1188	970	986	1036	1039
Participation rate (%)	20.6	21.2	26.2	22.8	23.2	24.3	24.4
Proportion of endoscopy among gastric cancer screening tests (%)	26.1	35.3	52.9	50.7	57.0	63.4	65.9

The data were obtained from "Cancer Screening Report in Tottori Prefecture".

This implies that screening using the *H. pylori* antibody test is useful for improving the rate of participation and efficient gastric cancer endoscopy. In the future, it will be necessary to verify the effect of reducing gastric cancer mortality by combining *H. pylori* antibody testing and endoscopic examination and to implement the optimal screening interval for each *H. pylori*-infected and uninfected person. In addition, it is important to improve the true rate of participation by recommending endoscopic examination to those who require it.

5. Future Directions for Gastric Cancer Screening

5.1. Optimal Age and Intervals for Screening

According to Japan's national screening program, the recommended age for gastric cancer screening was changed to >50 years due to a decrease in the incidence of gastric cancer in 40-year-olds [13]. Similarly, the British Society of Gastroenterology guidelines suggested endoscopy screening be considered in individuals aged > 50 years with multiple risk factors for gastric adenocarcinoma (male, smokers, and pernicious anemia) [89]. In Korea, gastric cancer screening is conducted for populations aged 40–74 years [55]. A study in Japan based on nationwide data showed that the endoscopic screening program would be cost-effective when implemented for populations aged 50–75 years [90]. A nationwide study in Singapore revealed that gastric cancer screening was cost-effective when used among Chinese men aged 50–70 years [91].

A different screening interval might be defined and considered depending on its relationship to the individual's background and gastric cancer risk. The incidence of gastric cancer differs according to individual risks and is mainly defined by *H. pylori* infection status and atrophic gastritis. In Korea, an interval of 2 years is recommended [92]. The British Society of Gastroenterology recommends that endoscopic follow-up should be performed every 3 years for individuals with severe chronic atrophic gastritis or intestinal metaplasia, and within one-year intervals for low-grade intraepithelial neoplasia—similar to the management of epithelial precancerous conditions and lesions in the stomach (MAPS II) guideline [93]. In Japan, high-grade intraepithelial neoplasia should be treated clinically. The national program in Japan recommends repeated gastric cancer screening every 2–3 years [14]. However, high-quality prospective research is required to determine the optimal follow-up interval for endoscopic screening in Japan. If individuals with a low risk of gastric cancer could be identified and adopted in the screening programs, their screening interval could be expanded. Hamashima et al. introduced infection atrophy diagnosis using endoscopy and serological testing or risk stratification and conducted a nationwide prospective study to set the interval between risk-specific screenings [17]. It is expected that the results of this research will reduce the burden on patients by appropriately classifying the risk of gastric cancer and extending the interval between screenings for low-risk patients. The research also aims to establish a system that enables the target population to access endoscopic screening fairly by effectively utilizing limited medical resources.

5.2. AI as a New Screening Method

In gastric cancer screening, both radiographic and endoscopic examinations may be eluded by gastric cancer [56,94,95]. In population-based screening, the specialist is required to carry out a double check, the labor is intensive, and the evaluation of the accuracy is difficult. Recently, diagnosis of *H. pylori* infection and detection of gastric cancer using AI have been reported. The sensitivity and specificity of endoscopic *H. pylori* infection diagnosis were 81.9% and 83.4% using AI, 79.0% and 83.2% by an average endoscopist, and 85.2% and 89.3% by an endoscopic specialist, respectively [96]. On the other hand, when AI detection was conducted in three groups. That is, *H. pylori*-positive, *H. pylori*-negative, and eradicated *H. pylori*, the rate of correct diagnosis decreased to 77% [97]; hence, there is room for further improvement in diagnosis using AI, including that of cases following *H. pylori* eradication. AI has a high sensitivity for gastric cancer, but its positive predictive value is low [24–26]. However, this has rapidly improved [98]. In addition to its accuracy, AI diagnostic imaging is expected to reduce the burden of double-checking and effectively extract patients who need follow-up endoscopy [98]. It is expected that intervention of gastric cancer screening using AI may reduce gastric cancer deaths more efficiently than the conventional methods of screening.

6. Conclusions

While endoscopic gastric cancer screening has been initiated nationwide in Japan, the incidence of *H. pylori* infection has decreased and the number of cases following *H. pylori* eradication has increased. Moreover, the importance of ABC classification reflecting *H. pylori* infection status and gastric atrophy before endoscopic screening is being increasingly recognized. Considering its cost-effectiveness, spreading the use of endoscopic screening is desirable to establish a new medical examination provision system that conducts examinations at appropriate screening intervals, according to the individual's background and risks.

Author Contributions: Writing—original draft preparation, K.Y.; writing—review and editing, M.S. and H.I.; supervision, M.S., H.K., K.K. and H.I. All authors have read and agreed to the published version of the manuscript.

Funding: This research received no external funding.

Institutional Review Board Statement: This study was approved by the institutional ethics committee of complies with "The Treaty of Helsinki". The study was conducted in accordance with the Declaration of Helsinki and approved by the Institutional Ethics Committee of Tottori University (1511A080).

Informed Consent Statement: Informed consent was obtained from all subjects involved in the study.

Data Availability Statement: Data will be available from the corresponding author upon reasonable request.

Acknowledgments: The study of *H. pylori* antibody project was supported by Hoki-cho, Tottori prefecture.

Conflicts of Interest: The authors declare no conflict of interest.

References

1. Sung, H.; Ferlay, J.; Siegel, R.L.; Laversanne, M.; Soerjomataram, I.; Jemal, A.; Bray, F. Global cancer statistics 2020: GLOBOCAN estimates of incidence and mortality worldwide for 36 cancers in 185 countries. *CA Cancer J. Clin.* **2021**, *71*, 209–249. [CrossRef] [PubMed]
2. Schistosomes, liver flukes and Helicobacter pylori. International Agency for Research on Cancer monographs on the evaluation of carcinogenesis risks to humans. *IARC Monogr. Eval. Carcinog. Risks Hum.* **1994**, *61*, 208–220.
3. Uemura, N.; Okamoto, S.; Yamamoto, S.; Matsumura, N.; Yamaguchi, S.; Yamakido, M.; Taniyama, K.; Sasaki, N.; Schlemper, R.J. Helicobacter pylori infection and the development of gastric cancer. *N. Engl. J. Med.* **2001**, *345*, 784–789. [CrossRef] [PubMed]
4. Katanoda, K.; Hori, M.; Saito, E.; Shibata, A.; Ito, Y.; Minami, T.; Ikeda, S.; Suzuki, T.; Matsuda, T. Updated trends in cancer in Japan: Incidence in 1985–2015 and mortality in 1958–2018—A sign of decrease in cancer incidence. *J. Epidemiol.* **2021**, *31*, 426–450. [CrossRef]
5. Kobayashi, T.; Kikuchi, S.; Lin, Y.; Yagyu, K.; Obata, Y.; Ogihara, A.; Hasegawa, A.; Miki, K.; Kaneko, E.; Mizukoshi, H.; et al. Trends in the incidence of gastric cancer in Japan and their associations with Helicobacter pylori infection and gastric mucosal atrophy. *Gastric Cancer* **2004**, *7*, 233–239. [CrossRef]
6. Ueda, J.; Gosho, M.; Inui, Y.; Matsuda, T.; Sakakibara, M.; Mabe, K.; Nakajima, S.; Shimoyama, T.; Yasuda, M.; Kawai, T.; et al. Prevalence of Helicobacter pylori infection by birth year and geographic area in Japan. *Helicobacter* **2014**, *19*, 105–110. [CrossRef]
7. Kamada, T.; Haruma, K.; Ito, M.; Inoue, K.; Manabe, N.; Matsumoto, H.; Kusunoki, H.; Hata, J.; Yoshihara, M.; Sumii, K.; et al. Time trends in Helicobacter pylori infection and atrophic gastritis over 40 years in Japan. *Helicobacter* **2015**, *20*, 192–198. [CrossRef]
8. Sugano, K. Screening of gastric cancer in Asia. *Best Pract. Res. Clin. Gastroenterol.* **2015**, *29*, 895–905. [CrossRef]
9. Wang, C.; Nishiyama, T.; Kikuchi, S.; Inoue, M.; Sawada, N.; Tsugane, S.; Lin, Y. Changing trends in the prevalence of H. pylori infection in Japan (1908–2003): A systematic review and meta-regression analysis of 170,752 individuals. *Sci. Rep.* **2017**, *7*, 15491. [CrossRef]
10. Lin, Y.; Kawai, S.; Sasakabe, T.; Nagata, C.; Naito, M.; Tanaka, K.; Sugawara, Y.; Mizoue, T.; Sawada, N.; Matsuo, K. Effects of Helicobacter pylori eradication on gastric cancer incidence in the Japanese population: A systematic evidence review. *Jpn. J. Clin. Oncol.* **2021**, *51*, 1158–1170. [CrossRef]
11. National Cancer Center. Center for Cancer Control and Information Services. 2021. Available online: https://ganjoho.jp/public/index.html (accessed on 1 January 2022).
12. Oshima, A. A critical review of cancer screening programs in Japan. *Int. J. Technol. Assess. Health Care* **1994**, *10*, 346–358. [CrossRef]
13. Hamashima, C. Systematic review group and guideline development group for gastric cancer screening guidelines. Update version of the Japanese Guidelines for Gastric Cancer Screening. *Jpn. J. Clin. Oncol.* **2018**, *48*, 673–683. [CrossRef]

14. Hamashima, C. Cancer screening guidelines and policy making: 15 years of experience in cancer screening guideline development in Japan. *Jpn. J. Clin. Oncol.* **2018**, *48*, 278–286. [CrossRef]
15. Hamashima, C.; Goto, R. Potential capacity of endoscopic screening for gastric cancer in Japan. *Cancer Sci.* **2017**, *108*, 101–107. [CrossRef]
16. Hamashima, C. Overdiagnosis of gastric cancer by endoscopic screening. *World J. Gastrointest. Endosc.* **2017**, *9*, 55–60. [CrossRef]
17. Hamashima, C.; Yoshimura, K.; Fukao, A. A study protocol for expanding the screening interval of endoscopic screening for gastric cancer based on individual risks: Prospective cohort study of gastric cancer screening. *Ann. Transl. Med.* **2020**, *8*, 1604. [CrossRef]
18. Mabe, K.; Inoue, K.; Kamada, T.; Kato, K.; Kato, M.; Haruma, K. Endoscopic screening for gastric cancer in Japan: Current status and future perspectives. *Dig. Endosc.* **2022**, *34*, 412–419. [CrossRef]
19. Matsuo, T.; Ito, M.; Takata, S.; Tanaka, S.; Yoshihara, M.; Chayama, K. Low prevalence of Helicobacter pylori-negative gastric cancer among Japanese. *Helicobacter* **2011**, *16*, 415–419. [CrossRef]
20. Ono, S.; Kato, M.; Suzuki, M.; Ishigaki, S.; Takahashi, M.; Haneda, M.; Mabe, K.; Shimizu, Y. Frequency of Helicobacter pylori-negative gastric cancer and gastric mucosal atrophy in a Japanese endoscopic submucosal dissection series including histological, endoscopic and serological atrophy. *Digestion* **2012**, *86*, 59–65. [CrossRef]
21. Mizota, Y.; Yamamoto, S. How long should we continue gastric cancer screening? From an epidemiological point of view. *Gastric Cancer* **2019**, *22*, 456–462. [CrossRef]
22. Kishikawa, H. The clinical benefits, limitations, and perspectives of the ABC method. *Intern. Med.* **2020**, *59*, 1471–1472. [CrossRef]
23. Yao, K.; Uedo, T.; Kamada, T.; Hirasawa, T.; Nagahama, T.; Yoshinaga, S.; Oka, M.; Inoue, K.; Mabe, K.; Yao, T.; et al. Guidelines for endoscopic diagnosis of early gastric cancer. *Dig. Endosc.* **2020**, *32*, 663–698. [CrossRef]
24. Hirasawa, T.; Aoyama, K.; Tanimoto, T.; Ishihara, S.; Shichijo, S.; Ozawa, T.; Ohnishi, T.; Fujishiro, M.; Matsuo, K.; Fujisaki, J.; et al. Application of artificial intelligence using a convolutional neural network for detecting gastric cancer in endoscopic images. *Gastric Cancer* **2018**, *21*, 653–660. [CrossRef]
25. Ishioka, M.; Hirasawa, T.; Tada, T. Detecting gastric cancer from video images using convolutional neural networks. *Dig. Endosc.* **2019**, *31*, e34–e35. [CrossRef]
26. Ikenoyama, Y.; Hirasawa, T.; Ishioka, M.; Namikawa, K.; Yoshimizu, S.; Horiuchi, Y.; Ishiyama, A.; Yoshio, T.; Tsuchida, T.; Takeuchi, Y.; et al. Detecting early gastric cancer: Comparison between the diagnostic ability of convolutional neural networks and endoscopists. *Dig. Endosc.* **2021**, *33*, 141–150. [CrossRef]
27. Park, J.Y.; Greenberg, E.R.; Parsonnnet, J.; Wild, C.P.; Forman, D.; Herrero, R. *Summary of IARC Working Group Meeting on Helicobacter pylori Eradication as a Strategy for Preventing Gastric Cancer*; IARC Working Group Report 8; International Agency for Research on Cancer: Lyon, France, 2014; pp. 1–4.
28. Greenberg, E.R.; Park, J.Y. Effectiveness of *Helicobacter pylori* eradication. In *Helicobacter pylori Eradication as a Strategy for Preventing Gastric Cancer*; IARC Working Group Report 8; International Agency for Research on Cancer: Lyon, France, 2014; pp. 64–71.
29. Li, W.Q.; Ma, J.L.; Zhang, L.; Brown, L.M.; Li, J.Y.; Shen, L.; Pan, K.F.; Liu, W.D.; Hu, Y.; Han, Z.X.; et al. Effects of *Helicobacter pylori* treatment on gastric cancer incidence and mortality in subgroups. *J. Natl. Cancer Inst.* **2014**, *106*, dju116. [CrossRef]
30. Lee, Y.C.; Chiang, T.H.; Chou, C.K.; Tu, Y.K.; Liao, W.C.; Wu, M.S.; Graham, D.Y. Association between *Helicobacter pylori* eradication and gastric cancer incidence: A systematic review and meta-analysis. *Gastroenterology* **2016**, *150*, 1113–1124.e5. [CrossRef]
31. Sugano, K. Effect of helicobacter pylori eradication on the incidence of gastric cancer: A systematic review and meta-analysis. *Gastric Cancer* **2019**, *22*, 435–445. [CrossRef]
32. Ford, A.C.; Yuan, Y.; Moayyedi, P. Helicobacter pylori eradication therapy to prevent gastric cancer: Systematic review and metaanalysis. *Gut* **2020**, *69*, 2113–2121. [CrossRef]
33. Fukase, K.; Kato, M.; Kikuchi, S.; Inoue, K.; Uemura, N.; Okamoto, S.; Terao, S.; Amagai, K.; Hayashi, S.; Asaka, M.; et al. Effect of eradication of Helicobacter pylori on incidence of metachronous gastric carcinoma after endoscopic resection of early gastric cancer: An openlabel, randomised controlled trial. *Lancet* **2008**, *372*, 392–397. [CrossRef]
34. Li, W.Q.; Zhang, J.Y.; Ma, J.L.; Li, Z.X.; Zhang, L.; Zhang, Y.; Guo, Y.; Zhou, T.; Li, J.Y.; Shen, L.; et al. Effects of helicobacter pylori treatment and vitamin and garlic supplementation on gastric cancer incidence and mortality: Follow-up of a randomized intervention trial. *BMJ* **2019**, *366*, l5016. [CrossRef] [PubMed]
35. Choi, I.J.; Kim, C.G.; Lee, J.Y.; Kim, Y.I.; Kook, M.C.; Park, B.; Joo, J. Family History of Gastric Cancer and Helicobacter pylori Treatment. *N. Engl. J. Med.* **2020**, *382*, 427–436. [CrossRef] [PubMed]
36. Chiang, T.; Chang, W.; Chen, S.L.; Yen, A.M.; Fann, J.C.; Chiu, S.Y.; Chen, Y.R.; Chuang, S.L.; Shieh, C.F.; Liu, C.Y.; et al. Mass eradication of *Helicobacter pylori* to reduce gastric cancer incidence and mortality: A long-term cohort study on Matsu Islands. *Gut* **2021**, *70*, 243–250. [CrossRef] [PubMed]
37. Take, S.; Mizuno, M.; Ishiki, K.; Kusumoto, C.; Imada, T.; Hamada, F.; Yoshida, T.; Yokota, K.; Mitsuhashi, T.; Okada, H. Risk of gastric cancer in the second decade of follow-up after helicobacter pylori eradication. *J. Gastroenterol.* **2020**, *55*, 281–288. [CrossRef]
38. Satomi, S.; Yamakawa, A.; Matsunaga, S.; Masaki, R.; Inagaki, T.; Okuda, T.; Suto, H.; Ito, Y.; Yamazaki, Y.; Kuriyama, M.; et al. Relationship between the diversity of the cagA gene of Helicobacter pylori and gastric cancer in Okinawa, Japan. *J. Gastroenterol.* **2006**, *41*, 668–673. [CrossRef]
39. Yamaoka, Y.; Kato, M.; Asaka, M. Geographic differences in gastric cancer incidence can be explained by differences between Helicobacter pylori strains. *Intern. Med.* **2008**, *47*, 1077–1083. [CrossRef]

40. Kpoghomou, M.A.; Wang, J.; Wang, T.; Jin, G. Association of *Helicobacter pylori* babA2 gene and gastric cancer risk: A meta-analysis. *BMC Cancer* **2020**, *20*, 465. [CrossRef]

41. Asaka, M.; Mabe, K. Strategies for eliminating death from gastric cancer in Japan. *Proc. Jpn. Acad. Ser. B Phys. Biol. Sci.* **2014**, *90*, 251–258. [CrossRef]

42. Kawai, S.; Wang, C.; Lin, Y.; Sasakabe, T.; Okuda, M.; Kikuchi, S. Lifetime incidence risk for gastric cancer in the Helicobacter pylori-infected and uninfected population in Japan: A Monte Carlo simulation study. *Int. J. Cancer* **2022**, *150*, 18–27. [CrossRef]

43. Japanese Gastric Cancer Association. Japanese classification of gastric carcinoma-3rd English edition. *Gastric Cancer* **2011**, *14*, 101–112. [CrossRef]

44. Schlemper, R.J.; Riddell, R.H.; Kato, Y.; Borchard, F.; Cooper, H.S.; Dawsey, S.M.; Dixon, M.F.; Fenoglio-Preiser, C.M.; Fléjou, J.F.; Geboes, K.; et al. The Vienna classification of gastrointestinal epithelial neoplasia. *Gut* **2000**, *47*, 251–255. [CrossRef]

45. Yamamoto, Y.; Fujisaki, J.; Omae, M.; Hirasawa, T.; Igarashi, M. Helicobacter pylori-negative gastric cancer: Characteristics and endoscopic findings. *Dig. Endosc.* **2015**, *27*, 551–561. [CrossRef]

46. Imamura, Y.; Watanabe, M.; Oki, E.; Morita, M.; Baba, H. Esophagogastric junction adenocarcinoma shares characteristics with gastric adenocarcinoma: Literature review and retrospective multicenter cohort study. *Ann. Gastroenterol. Surg.* **2020**, *5*, 46–59. [CrossRef]

47. Crew, K.D.; Neugut, A.I. Epidemiology of gastric cancer. *World J. Gastroenterol.* **2006**, *12*, 354–362. [CrossRef]

48. Ohshima, A.; Hirata, N.; Ubukata, T.; Umeda, K.; Fujimoto, I. Evaluation of a mass screening program for stomach with a case control study design. *Int. J. Cancer* **1986**, *38*, 829–833. [CrossRef]

49. Fukao, A.; Tsubono, Y.; Tsuji, I.; Hisamichi, S.; Sugahara, N.; Takano, A. The evaluation of screening for gastric cancer in Miyagi Prefecture, Japan: A population-based case-control study. *Int. J. Cancer* **1995**, *60*, 45–48. [CrossRef]

50. Hamashima, C.; Shabana, M.; Okada, K.; Okamoto, M.; Osaki, Y. Mortality reduction from gastric cancer by endoscopic and radiographic screening. *Cancer Sci.* **2015**, *106*, 1744–1749. [CrossRef]

51. Jun, J.K.; Choi, K.S.; Lee, H.Y.; Suh, M.; Park, B.; Song, S.H.; Jung, K.W.; Lee, C.W.; Choi, I.J.; Park, E.C.; et al. Effectiveness of the Korean National Cancer Screening Program in Reducing Gastric Cancer Mortality. *Gastroenterology* **2017**, *152*, 1319–1328.e7. [CrossRef]

52. The Japanese Society of Gastrointestinal Cancer Screening. New Guidelines of Radiography for Gastric Cancer Screening. 2011. Available online: https://www.jsgcs.or.jp (accessed on 14 December 2020).

53. The Japanese Society of Gastrointestinal Cancer Screening. Annual Report of Gastrointestinal Cancer Screening 2014. Available online: https://www.jsgcs.or.jp (accessed on 14 December 2020).

54. Togo, R.; Yamamichi, N.; Mabe, K.; Takahashi, Y.; Takeuchi, C.; Kato, M.; Sakamoto, N.; Ishihara, K.; Ogawa, T.; Haseyama, M. Detection of gastritis by a deep convolutional neural network from double-contrast upper gastrointestinal barium x-ray radiography. *J. Gastroenterol.* **2019**, *54*, 321–329. [CrossRef]

55. Choi, K.S.; Jun, J.K.; Suh, M.; Park, B.; Noh, D.K.; Song, S.H.; Jung, K.W.; Lee, H.Y.; Choi, I.J.; Park, E.C. Effect of endoscopy screening on stage at gastric cancer diagnosis: Results of the National Cancer Screening Programme in Korea. *Br. J. Cancer* **2015**, *112*, 608–612. [CrossRef]

56. Choi, K.S.; Jun, J.K.; Park, E.C.; Park, S.; Jung, K.W.; Han, M.A.; Choi, I.J.; Lee, H.Y. Performance of different gastric cancer screening methods in Korea: A population-based study. *PLoS ONE* **2012**, *7*, e50041. [CrossRef] [PubMed]

57. Matsumoto, S.; Yoshida, Y. Efficacy of endoscopic screening in an isolated island: A case-control study. *Indian J. Gastroenterol.* **2014**, *33*, 46–49. [CrossRef]

58. Hamashima, C.; Ogoshi, K.; Okamoto, M.; Shabana, M.; Kishimoto, T.; Fukao, A. A community-based, case-control study evaluating mortality reduction from gastric cancer by endoscopic screening in Japan. *PLoS ONE* **2013**, *8*, e79088. [CrossRef]

59. Zhang, X.; Li, M.; Chen, S.; Hu, J.; Guo, Q.; Liu, R.; Zheng, H.; Jin, Z.; Yuan, Y.; Xi, Y.; et al. Endoscopic Screening in Asian Countries Is Associated With Reduced Gastric Cancer Mortality: A Meta-analysis and Systematic Review. *Gastroenterology* **2018**, *155*, 347–354.e9. [CrossRef] [PubMed]

60. The Japanese Society of Gastrointestinal Cancer Screening. Quality Assurance Manual of Endoscopic Screening for Gastric Cancer in Japanese Communities. *Jpn. J. Clin. Oncol.* **2016**, *46*, 1053–1061. (In Japanese) [CrossRef] [PubMed]

61. Hosokawa, O.; Shinbo, T.; Matsuda, K.; Miyanaga, T. Impact of opportunistic endoscopic screening on the decrease of mortality from gastric cancer. *J. Gatsroenterol. Cancer Screen* **2011**, *49*, 401–409. (In Japanese)

62. Ogoshi, K.; Narisawa, R.; Kato, T.; Saito, S.; Funagoshi, K.; Kinameri, K. Evaluation of endoscopic screening for gastric cancer in Niigata City: The reduction of the mortality rate. *J. Gatsroenterol. Cancer Screen* **2009**, *47*, 531–541. (In Japanese)

63. Shichijo, S.; Uedo, N.; Michida, T. Detection of Early Gastric Cancer after Helicobacter pylori Eradication. *Digestion* **2021**, *2*, 54–61. [CrossRef]

64. Kurumi, H.; Kanda, T.; Ikebuchi, Y.; Yoshida, A.; Kawaguchi, K.; Yashima, K.; Isomoto, H. Current Status of Photodynamic Diagnosis for Gastric Tumors. *Diagnostics* **2021**, *11*, 1967. [CrossRef]

65. Ministry of Health, Labour and Welfare. The Report of Health Promotion and Community Health 2013. Available online: http://www.e-stat.go.jp/SG1/estat/GL08020101.do?_-toGL08020101_&tstatCode=000001030884&requestSender=dsearch (accessed on 1 September 2015).

66. Shabana, M.; Hamashima, C.; Nishida, M.; Miura, K.; Kishimoto, T. Current status and evaluation of endoscopic screening for gastric cancer. *Jpn. J. Cancer Det. Diagn.* **2010**, *17*, 229–235. (In Japanese)

67. Kitagawa, S.; Miyagawa, K.; Iriguchi, Y. The report of gastroenterological screening in 2012. *J. Gastroenterol. Cancer Screen* **2015**, *53*, 60–86. (In Japanese)

68. Suzuki, A.; Katoh, H.; Komura, D.; Kakiuchi, M.; Tagashira, A.; Yamamoto, S.; Tatsuno, K.; Ueda, H.; Nagae, G.; Fukuda, S.; et al. Defined lifestyle and germline factors predispose Asian populations to gastric cancer. *Sci. Adv.* **2020**, *6*, eaav9778. [CrossRef]

69. Sugano, K.; Tack, J.; Kuipers, E.J.; Graham, D.Y.; El-Omar, E.M.; Miura, S.; Haruma, K.; Asaka, M.; Uemura, N.; Malfertheiner, P. Kyoto global consensus report on *Helicobacter pylori* gastritis. *Gut* **2015**, *64*, 1353–1367. [CrossRef]

70. Haruma, K.; Kato, M.; Inoue, K.; Murakami, K.; Kamada, T. *Kyoto Classification of Gastritis*; Nihon Medical Center: Tokyo, Japan, 2017.

71. Yoshii, S.; Mabe, K.; Watano, K.; Ohno, M.; Matsumoto, M.; Ono, S.; Kudo, T.; Nojima, M.; Kato, M.; Sakamoto, N. Validity of endoscopic features for the diagnosis of helicobacter pylori infection status based on the Kyoto classification of gastritis. *Dig. Endosc.* **2020**, *32*, 74–83. [CrossRef]

72. Isomoto, H.; Mizuta, Y.; Inoue, K.; Matsuo, T.; Hayakawa, T.; Miyazaki, M.; Onita, K.; Takeshima, F.; Murase, K.; Shimokawa, I.; et al. A close relationship between Helicobacter pylori infection and gastric xanthoma. *Scand J. Gastroenterol.* **1999**, *34*, 346–352. [CrossRef]

73. Sekikawa, A.; Fukui, H.; Sada, R.; Fukuhara, M.; Marui, S.; Tanke, G.; Endo, M.; Ohara, Y.; Matsuda, F.; Nakajima, J.; et al. Gastric atrophy and xanthelasma are markers for predicting the development of early gastric cancer. *J. Gastroenterol.* **2016**, *51*, 35–42. [CrossRef]

74. Hirai, R.; Hirai, M.; Shimodate, Y.; Minami, M.; Ishikawa, S.; Kanadani, T.; Takezawa, R.; Doi, A.; Nishimura, N.; Mouri, H.; et al. Feasibility of endoscopic evaluation of Helicobacter pylori infection status by using the Kyoto classification of gastritis in the population-based gastric cancer screening program: A prospective cohort study. *Health Sci. Rep.* **2021**, *4*, e325. [CrossRef]

75. Overview of the 2019 Basic Survey on National Life. Available online: https://www.mhlw.go.jp/toukei/saikin/hw/k-tyosa/k-tyosa19/index.html (accessed on 27 June 2022).

76. Miki, K. Gastric cancer screening by combined assay for serum anti-Helicobacter pylori IgG antibody and serum pepsinogen levels "ABC method". *Proc. Jpn. Acad. Ser. B Phys. Biol. Sci.* **2011**, *87*, 405–414. [CrossRef]

77. Itoh, T.; Saito, M.; Marugami, N.; Hirai, T.; Marugami, A.; Takahama, J.; Tanaka, T.; Kichikawa, K. Correlation between the ABC classification and radiological findings for assessing gastric cancer risk. *Jpn. J. Radiol.* **2015**, *33*, 636–644. [CrossRef]

78. Terasawa, T.; Nishida, H.; Kato, K.; Miyashiro, I.; Yoshikawa, T.; Takaku, R.; Hamashima, C. Prediction of gastric cancer development by serum pepsinogen test and Helicobacter pylori seropositivity in Eastern Asians: A systematic review and meta-analysis. *PLoS ONE* **2014**, *9*, e109783. [CrossRef]

79. Kiso, M.; Yoshihara, M.; Ito, M.; Inoue, K.; Kato, K.; Nakajima, S.; Mabe, K.; Kobayashi, M.; Uemura, N.; Yada, T.; et al. Characteristics of gastric cancer in negative test of serum anti-Helicobacter pylori antibody and pepsinogen test: A multicenter study. *Gastric Cancer* **2017**, *20*, 764–771. [CrossRef]

80. Kishino, T.; Oyama, T.; Tomori, A.; Takahashi, A.; Shinohara, T. Usefulness and limitations of a serum screening system to predict the risk of gastric cancer. *Intern. Med.* **2020**, *59*, 1473–1480. [CrossRef]

81. Masuyama, H.; Yoshitake, N.; Sasai, T.; Nakamura, T.; Masuyama, A.; Zuiki, T.; Kurashina, K.; Mieda, M.; Sunada, K.; Yamamoto, H.; et al. Relationship between the degree of endoscopic atrophy of the gastric mucosa and carcinogenic risk. *Digestion* **2015**, *91*, 30–36. [CrossRef]

82. Spence, A.D.; Cardwell, C.R.; McMenamin, U.C.; Hicks, B.M.; Johnston, B.T.; Murray, L.J.; Coleman, H.G. Adenocarcinoma risk in gastric atrophy and intestinal metaplasia: A systematic review. *BMC Gastroenterol.* **2017**, *17*, 157. [CrossRef]

83. Kotachi, T.; Ito, M.; Yoshihara, M.; Boda, T.; Kiso, M.; Masuda, K.; Matsuo, T.; Tanaka, S.; Chayama, K. Serological evaluation of gastric cancer risk based on pepsinogen and helicobacter pylori antibody: Relationship to endoscopic findings. *Digestion* **2017**, *95*, 314–318. [CrossRef]

84. Kaji, K.; Hashiba, A.; Uotani, C.; Yamaguchi, Y.; Ueno, T.; Ohno, K.; Takabatake, I.; Wakabayashi, T.; Doyama, H.; Ninomiya, I.; et al. Grading of atrophic gastritis is useful for risk stratification in endoscopic screening for gastric cancer. *Am. J. Gastroenterol.* **2019**, *114*, 71–79. [CrossRef]

85. Kimura, K.; Takemoto, T. An endoscopic recognition for the atrophic border and its significance in chronic gastritis. *Endoscopy* **1969**, *1*, 87–97. [CrossRef]

86. Canakis, A.; Pani, E.; Saumoy, M.; Shah, S.C. Decision model analyses of upper endoscopy for gastric cancer screening and preneoplasia surveillance: A systematic review. *Therap. Adv. Gastroenterol.* **2020**, *13*, 1756284820941662. [CrossRef] [PubMed]

87. Kowada, A. Endoscopy Is Cost-effective for gastric cancer screening after successful Helicobacter pylori eradication. *Dig. Dis. Sci.* **2021**, *66*, 4220–4226. [CrossRef] [PubMed]

88. Yashima, K.; Hasegawa, R.; Shabana, M.; Kawaguchi, G.; Isomoto, H. Mass screening considering *Helicobacter pylori* infection status for gastric cancer in Hoki-cho, Tottori prefecture. *J. Gatsroenterol. Cancer Screen* **2019**, *57*, 561–570. (In Japanese)

89. Banks, M.; Graham, D.; Jansen, M.; Gotoda, T.; Coda, S.; di Pietro, M.; Uedo, N.; Bhandari, P.; Pritchard, D.M.; Kuipers, E.J.; et al. British Society of Gastroenterology guidelines on the diagnosis and management of patients at risk of gastric adenocarcinoma. *Gut* **2019**, *68*, 1545–1575. [CrossRef]

90. Huang, H.L.; Leung, C.Y.; Saito, E.; Katanoda, K.; Hur, C.; Kong, C.Y.; Nomura, S.; Shibuya, K. Effect and cost-effectiveness of national gastric cancer screening in Japan: A microsimulation modeling study. *BMC Med.* **2020**, *18*, 257. [CrossRef]

91. Dan, Y.Y.; So, J.B.; Yeoh, K.G. Endoscopic screening for gastric cancer. *Clin. Gastroenterol. Hepatol.* **2006**, *4*, 709–716. [CrossRef]

92. Suh, Y.S.; Lee, J.; Woo, H.; Shin, D.; Kong, S.H.; Lee, H.J.; Shin, A.; Yang, H.K. National cancer screening program for gastric cancer in Korea: Nationwide treatment benefit and cost. *Cancer* **2020**, *126*, 1929–1939. [CrossRef]

93. Pimentel-Nunes, P.; Libânio, D.; Marcos-Pinto, R.; Areia, M.; Leja, M.; Esposito, G.; Garrido, M.; Kikuste, I.; Megraud, F.; Matysiak-Budnik, T.; et al. Management of epithelial precancerous conditions and lesions in the stomach (MAPS II): European Society of Gastrointestinal Endoscopy (ESGE), European *Helicobacter* and Microbiota96. Study Group (EHMSG), European Society of Pathology (ESP), and Sociedade Portuguesa de Endoscopia Digestiva (SPED) guideline update 2019. *Endoscopy* **2019**, *51*, 365–388. [CrossRef]

94. Hosokawa, O.; Tsuda, S.; Kidani, E.; Watanabe, K.; Tanigawa, Y.; Shirasaki, S.; Hayashi, H.; Hinoshita, T. Diagnosis of gastric cancer up to three years after negative upper gastrointestinal endoscopy. *Endoscopy* **1998**, *30*, 669–674. [CrossRef]

95. Pimentaelo, A.R.; Monteirooares, M.; Libanio, D.; Dinisibeiro, M. Missing rate for gastric cancer during upper gastrointestinal endoscopy: A systematic review and meta-analysis. *Eur. J. Gastroenterol. Hepatol.* **2016**, *28*, 1041–1049. [CrossRef]

96. Shichijo, S.; Nomura, S.; Aoyama, K.; Nishikawa, Y.; Miura, M.; Shinagawa, T.; Takiyama, H.; Tanimoto, T.; Ishihara, S.; Matsuo, K.; et al. Application of Convolutional Neural Networks in the Diagnosis of Helicobacter pylori Infection Based on Endoscopic Images. *EBioMedicine* **2017**, *25*, 106–111. [CrossRef]

97. Shichijo, S.; Endo, Y.; Aoyama, K.; Takeuchi, Y.; Ozawa, T.; Takiyama, H.; Matsuo, K.; Fujishiro, M.; Ishihara, S.; Ishihara, R.; et al. Application of convolutional neural networks for evaluating Helicobacter pylori infection status on the basis of endoscopic images. *Scand J. Gastroenterol.* **2019**, *54*, 158–163. [CrossRef]

98. Oura, H.; Matsumura, T.; Fujie, M.; Ishikawa, T.; Nagashima, A.; Shiratori, W.; Tokunaga, M.; Kaneko, T.; Imai, Y.; Oike, T.; et al. Development and evaluation of a double-check support system using artificial intelligence in endoscopic screening for gastric cancer. *Gastric Cancer* **2022**, *25*, 392–400. [CrossRef]

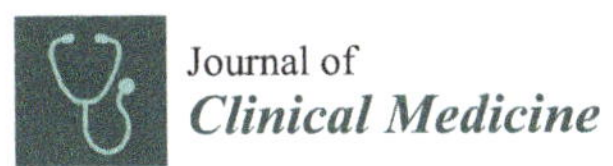

Journal of
Clinical Medicine

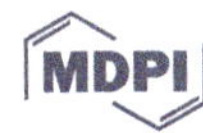

Article

Efficacy of AI-Assisted Personalized Microbiome Modulation by Diet in Functional Constipation: A Randomized Controlled Trial

Naciye Çiğdem Arslan [1], Aycan Gündoğdu [2], Varol Tunali [3,4,*], Oğuzhan Hakan Topgül [1], Damla Beyazgül [5] and Özkan Ufuk Nalbantoğlu [6]

[1] Department of General Surgery, School of Medicine, Medipol University, Istanbul 34214, Turkey
[2] Department of Microbiology and Clinical Microbiology, Faculty of Medicine, Erciyes University, Kayseri 38280, Turkey
[3] Department of Emergency Medicine, Eşrefpaşa Municipality Hospital, Izmir 35170, Turkey
[4] Department of Parasitology, Faculty of Medicine, Celal Bayar University, Manisa 45040, Turkey
[5] Enbiosis Biotechnology, Istanbul 34398, Turkey
[6] Department of Computer Engineering, Faculty of Engineering, Erciyes University, Kayseri 38280, Turkey
* Correspondence: varoltunali@gmail.com

Abstract: Background: Currently, medications and behavioral modifications have limited success in the treatment of functional constipation (FC). An individualized diet based on microbiome analysis may improve symptoms in FC. In the present study, we aimed to investigate the impacts of microbiome modulation on chronic constipation. Methods: Between December 2020–December 2021, 50 patients fulfilling the Rome IV criteria for functional constipation were randomized into two groups. The control group received sodium picosulfate plus conventional treatments (i.e., laxatives, enemas, increased fiber, and fluid intake). The study group underwent microbiome analysis and received an individualized diet with the assistance of a soft computing system (Enbiosis Biotechnology®, Sariyer, Istanbul). Differences in patient assessment constipation–quality of life (PAC-QoL) scores and complete bowel movements per week (CBMpW) were compared between groups after 6-weeks of intervention. Results: The mean age of the overall cohort ($n = 45$) was 31.5 ± 10.2 years, with 88.9% female predominance. The customized diet developed for subjects in the study arm resulted in a 2.5-fold increase in CBMpW after 6-weeks (1.7 vs. 4.3). The proportion of the study group patients with CBMpW > 3 was 83% at the end of the study, and the satisfaction score was increased 4-fold from the baseline (3.1 to 10.7 points). More than 50% improvement in PAC-QoL scores was observed in 88% of the study cohort compared to 40% in the control group ($p = 0.001$). Conclusion: The AI-assisted customized diet based on individual microbiome analysis performed significantly better compared to conventional therapy based on patient-reported outcomes in the treatment of functional constipation.

Keywords: functional bowel disorders; gut microbiota; personalized diet; machine learning; personalized medicine; Turkey

Citation: Arslan, N.Ç.; Gündoğdu, A.; Tunali, V.; Topgül, O.H.; Beyazgül, D.; Nalbantoğlu, Ö.U. Efficacy of AI-Assisted Personalized Microbiome Modulation by Diet in Functional Constipation: A Randomized Controlled Trial. *J. Clin. Med.* **2022**, *11*, 6612. https://doi.org/10.3390/jcm11226612

Academic Editor: Hidekazu Suzuki

Received: 6 October 2022
Accepted: 7 November 2022
Published: 8 November 2022

Publisher's Note: MDPI stays neutral with regard to jurisdictional claims in published maps and institutional affiliations.

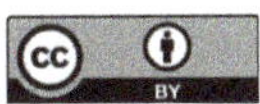

1. Introduction

Constipation is a common gastrointestinal disorder with an estimated global prevalence of 14% [1] and represents a heavy burden for ambulatory healthcare systems [2]. Chronic constipation is defined as difficult and/or infrequent bowel movements and is divided into four subgroups: functional constipation (FC), irritable bowel syndrome (IBS) with constipation, opioid-induced constipation, and functional defecation disorders [3]. Among these, FC has been the least understood and the most desperate group, as only one-third to half of the patients benefit from available treatments [4,5]. Similarly to some common comorbidities, quality of life (QoL) is impaired [6]. The impact of FC is estimated to cause a mean loss of 2.4 active days in a month [7]. Moreover, both direct and indirect healthcare costs are determined by approximately 2.5 million visits and 92,000 hospitalizations per year, with more than 7 billion USD for diagnostic assessments [8,9].

The current guidelines on the diagnosis and management of constipation in adults recommend the symptomatic approach as the initial step [10]. First-line treatments include changes in lifestyle and diet, cessation of medications causing constipation, fiber and/or bulk-forming agents, increased fluid intake, and exercise. The second step includes laxatives, and the third step is the introduction of stimulant laxatives, enemas, as well as prokinetic drugs [10]. In a recent meta-analysis, the results of 33 studies involving 17,214 patients, revealed that almost all medications were superior to placebo in terms of achieving three or more complete bowel movements per week (CBMpW) and the diphenylmethane laxatives (prucalopride and sodium picosulfate) ranked as the most effective [4]. As most of the studies in the literature report results after 4–12 weeks, the long-term effects of the medications and the sustainability of the treatments have been a main topic of debate [4,5,11]. Besides, the main reasons for dissatisfaction with medications are low efficacy and the fact that half of the patients have reported concerns about adverse effects with long-term use [12]. The 'symptomatic approach' rationale of available options and the lack of any radical treatments justify these concerns.

In recent studies, it has been observed that the intestinal microbiota in patients with FC is different from that of healthy individuals [13]. Although the role of the microbiome in CC pathophysiology is not yet fully understood, it is suggested that gut microbiota may have modulating effects on gastrointestinal motility or metabolites, and fermentation products may cause increased gas formation [13]. Animal studies revealed that colonization of germ-free mice with microbiota increased the encoding of several proteins (L-glutamate transporter, L-glutamate decarboxylase, g-aminobutyric acid, vesicle-associated protein 33, enteric g-actin, and cysteine-rich protein 2) which have neuromodulator effects on the enteric nervous system [12]. Human studies have also indicated the crucial role of the microbiome in gastrointestinal motility. An increased proportion of *Actinobacteria*, *Bacteroides*, *Lactococcus*, and *Roseburia* are associated with faster gut transit time, whereas Faecalibacterium correlates with slower motility [12]. The present study aimed to investigate the impact of an AI-assisted microbiome-based personalized diet compared with sodium picosulfate plus conventional therapy (i.e., laxatives, enemas, increased fiber, and fluid intake) on FC patients.

2. Materials and Methods

The study was approved by the Institutional Ethics Committee (Approval no. 10840098-772.02-E.47859) and conducted in line with the Declaration of Helsinki. The patients were thoroughly informed about the protocol, and written consent was obtained. Patients fulfilling the Rome IV criteria for FC and aged between 20–65 years were included in the study. All the patients underwent detailed physical and rectal examinations by a European board-certified coloproctologist (NCA). Patients who had a colonoscopy performed within the last 5 years were included. Colonic transit time and magnetic resonance defecography were obtained from all patients. Exclusion criteria were: the use of antibiotics, probiotics, and/or prebiotics within the last four weeks; gastrointestinal endoscopy within the last four weeks; a history of major gastrointestinal surgery (total/segmental gastrectomy, small bowel resection, and/or colonic resection); cholecystectomy; inflammatory bowel diseases; and celiac disease. Any etiology of chronic constipation other than FC (irritable bowel syndrome, rectocele, dyssynergic defecation, and opioid use) was excluded. Patients with endocrine, metabolic, or neurologic disorders causing constipation (hypothyroidism, Parkinson's disease, and paraplegia) were also excluded from the study.

2.1. Study Design and Groups

This was a single-center, prospective, randomized study. Patients were those who consulted with the Istanbul Medipol University Hospital General Surgery Clinic with constipation. Patients fulfilling inclusion criteria were divided into two groups using block randomization at a 1:1 ratio. The coloproctologist (NCA) was not blinded to randomization as she obtained the fecal samples from the patients in the study group and managed the treatments of the control group. Baseline and post-treatment questionnaires were collected by another surgeon blinded to the randomization (OHT).

After randomization, both groups were recommended to continue their regular diets with increased fluid and fiber intake and informed about the exclusion criteria. The control group received 5 mg of sodium picosulfate (Dulcolax® 2.5 mg, Sanofi, Turkey) daily for ten weeks. In the study group, after fecal samples were taken, patients were suggested to continue their regular diet for four weeks until the microbiome analysis was completed. During the subsequent six weeks, patients in the study group received the personalized microbiome modulatory diet, and those in the control group received 5 mg of sodium picosulfate plus the conventional treatments (i.e., laxatives, enemas, increased fiber, and fluid intake) for FC. The two groups were compared in terms of bowel movements and quality of life.

The primary endpoint was the proportion of patients with a mean of three or more complete bowel movements per week (CBMpW) at ten weeks. The secondary endpoint was a more than 50% improvement in the total Patient Assessment Constipation Quality of Life (PAC-QoL) score.

2.2. Fecal Sampling and 16S Ribosomal RNA Gene Sequencing

Fecal samples were collected using BBL culture swabs (Becton, Dickinson and Company, Sparks, MD, USA) and transported to the laboratory in a DNA/RNA shield buffer medium. DNA extraction was carried out directly from the stool samples using a Qiagen Power Soil DNA Extraction Kit (Qiagen, Hilden, Germany). A NanoDrop (Shimadzu, Japan) device was used to measure the final concentrations of extracted DNA. dsDNA quantification was done using the Qubit dsDNA HS Assay Kit and a Qubit 2.0 Fluorimeter (Thermo Fisher Scientific, Waltham, MA, USA).

The sequencing of 16S rRNA was performed using the Illumina MiSeq (Illumina, San Diego, CA, USA) device according to the manufacturer's protocol.

All amplified products were then checked with 2% agarose gel electrophoresis. Amplicons were purified using the AMPure XP PCR Purification Kit (Beckman Coulter Genomics, Danvers, MA, USA) and quantified using the Qubit dsDNA HS Assay Kit and a Qubit 2.0 Fluorimeter (Thermo Fisher Scientific, Waltham, MA, USA). Approximately 15% of the PhiX Control library (v3) (Illumina, San Diego, CA, USA) was combined with the final sequencing library. The libraries were processed for cluster generation. Sequencing on 250PE MiSeq runs was performed, generating at least 50,000 reads per sample.

Sequencing data were analyzed using the QIIME pipeline [14] after filtering and trimming the reads for a PHRED quality score of 30 via the Trimmomatic tool [15]. Operational taxonomic units were determined using the Uclust method, and the units were assigned to taxonomic clades via PyNAST using the Green Genes database [16] with an open reference procedure. Alpha- and beta-diversity statistics were assessed accordingly by QIIME pipeline scripts. The graph-based visualization of the microbiota profiles was performed using the tmap topological data analysis framework with the Bray-Curtis distance metric.

2.3. The AI-Based Personalized Nutrition Model

The AI-based nutritional recommendations system is based mainly on the eating rates of the individual in a certain period to ensure the homeostasis of the microbiome and increase microbial diversity.

After the analysis reports are released, a detailed health-disease life history is taken, and a six week diet service is provided to the individual with lifestyle-specific diet lists in accordance with his/her comorbidities. Diet lists are updated according to the individual's feedback, recovery level, and wishes during weekly meetings.

While designing an individual's diet list, the modules in the Microbiome Analysis Report provide detailed data and help design results-oriented diet lists. In this study, foods containing "fiber" were prioritized in the AI-based recommended food scores specific to constipated individuals and integrated into the diet list in accordance with the individual's lifestyle. The Enbiosis personalized nutrition model estimates the optimal micronutrient compositions for a required microbiome modulation. The present study computed the microbiome modulation needed for a constipated patient based on the "constipation" indices generated by the machine learning models as described previously [17]. While designing the diet lists, care was taken not to give calories below the basal metabolic rate.

2.4. Assessments and Follow-Up

Demographic and clinical characteristics, as well as the number of CBMpW and PAC-QoL scores of eligible patients, were recorded at baseline. The PAC-QOL questionnaire was previously validated in the Turkish population and assesses constipation-related symptoms on four subscales (physical discomfort, psychosocial discomfort, worries and concerns, and satisfaction) that are scored on a 5-point Likert-type scale (0, none/not at all; 4, extremely/all the time) and are inversely proportional with symptom relief [18]. All the patients were asked to record daily defecation diaries, which include the frequency of bowel movements, presence of straining and/or feeling of incomplete evacuation, and/or use of any rescue enema. The diaries were collected, and PAC- QOL questionnaire was repeated at 10 weeks. The absence of more than 2 weeks of diary records was defined as 'non-responders'. For less than 2 weeks of absent data, the information from last week was copied for the missing weeks.

According to the microbiome test results, patients in the study group received AI-assisted, personally customized diets (Enbiosis Biotechnology®, Sariyer, Istanbul, Turkey) with weekly online dietitian support for six weeks.

2.5. Statistical Analysis

A successful treatment and patient satisfaction rate of 30% was estimated with conventional treatments of FC [19]. With the hypothesis that soft-computed microbiome treatment would increase CBMpW to ≥ 3 in 80% of the patients, the sample size was calculated as 19 patients in each group with $\alpha = 0.05$ and 90% power. Considering a drop-out rate of 25%, a total of 50 patients were recruited for the study. Power and sample size analyses were performed by a web-based software (Raosoft Inc., Seattle, WA, USA) [20].

Continuous variables were expressed as means and standard deviation, and categorical variables as frequency and percentages. The distribution of continuous variables was determined by histograms, skewness, and Kurtosis analyses. The association between parametric variables was tested by an independent samples *t*-test. The association between non-parametric variables was determined by Mann-Whitney-U. Differences in mean CBMpW and PAC-QoL scores before and after treatments were tested by a paired-samples *t*-test. The difference between categorical variables was tested by a *chi*-square test. Statistical significance was defined as $p < 0.05$. Statistical analyses were performed using SPSS 21.0 (IBM, Chicago, IL, USA).

3. Results

Between December 2020 and December 2021, 74 patients with constipation were assessed for eligibility, and 50 were randomized into control ($n = 25$) and study ($n = 25$) groups, yet 5 patients in the control group were excluded for various reasons. The flow diagram is given in Figure 1. The mean age was 31.5 ± 10.2, and 40 (88.9%) patients were female. The mean age in the control group was 34.5 ± 11.4, which higher than the study group mean age (29.1 ± 8.6), but this difference was not statistically significant ($p = 0.076$). Four (8.9%) of the patients had comorbidities including type 2 diabetes ($n = 2$), asthma ($n = 1$), and hypertension ($n = 1$); 10 (22.2%) had proctologic diseases (3 anal fissures and hemorrhoids). The mean duration of constipation was 88.8 ± 66.9 months. The baseline CBMpW was ≥ 3 in 6 (13.3%) of the patients, with a mean value of 1.9 ± 1.92. There was no difference between the groups in terms of gender, body mass index, duration of constipation, or stool frequency (Table 1). The mean baseline PAC-QoL score was 55.3 ± 14.6

and was similar between the groups ($p = 0.101$), except for psychosocial discomfort. The mean scores of PAC-QoL subscales were not different between groups at baseline (Table 1).

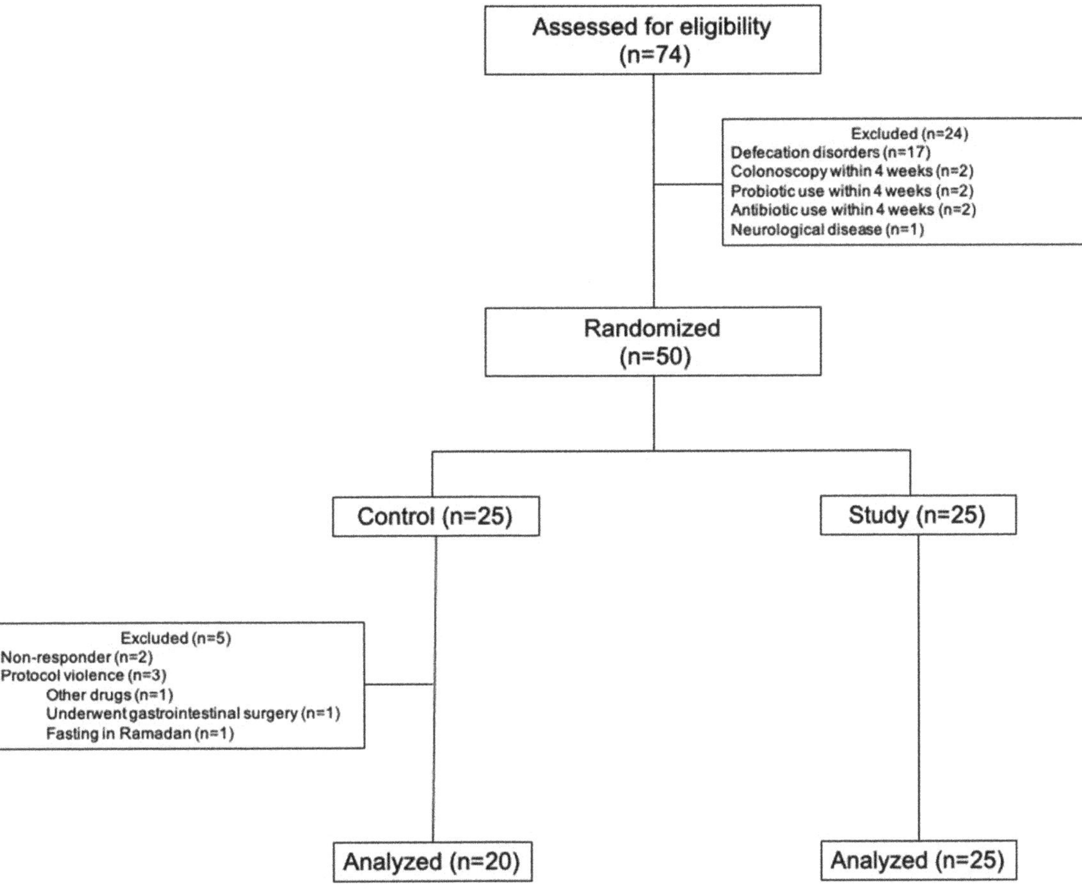

Figure 1. Flow diagram of the study.

Table 1. Demographic and clinical characteristics of the patients, baseline stool frequency, and quality of life scores.

Variables	Total ($n = 45$)	Control Group ($n = 20$)	Study Group ($n = 25$)	p
Age (years, mean ± SD)	31.5 ± 10.2	34.5 ± 11.4	29.1 ± 8.6	0.76 *
Gender				0.608 **
Male	5 (11.1)	2 (10)	3 (12)	
Female	40 (88.9)	18 (90)	22 (88)	
BMI (kg/m^2 mean ± SD)	26.3 ± 5.1	26.1 ± 5	26.5 ± 5.3	0.786 *
Constipation duration (months, mean ± SD)	88.8 ± 66.9	91.9 ± 75.9	86.2 ± 60.2	0.778 *

Table 1. *Cont.*

Variables	Total (n = 45)	Control Group (n = 20)	Study Group (n = 25)	p
CBMpW (n, mean ± SD)	1.9 ± 1.92	2.1 ± 2.2	1.7 ± 1.6	0.374 ***
CBMpW ≥ 3 (n, %)	6 (13.3)	4 (20)	2 (8)	0.383 *
PAC-QoL subscales (points, mean ± SD)				
Physical discomfort	10.33 ± 2.5	10 ± 2.4	10.5 ± 2.5	0.494 *
Psychosocial discomfort	17.33 ± 5.3	20.3 ± 4	15 ± 5.1	0.001 *
Worries and discomfort	30.8 ± 9.4	32.3 ± 5.8	29.6 ± 11.4	0.314 ***
Satisfaction	3.2 ± 2.1	3.3 ± 2.2	3.1 ± 2.1	0.736 *
Total PAC-QoL score (points, mean ± SD)	55.3 ± 14.6	59.3 ± 10.4	52.1 ± 16.9	0.101 *

SD: Standard deviation, BMI: Body mass index, CBMpW: Complete bowel movement per week, PAC-QoL: Patient Assessment Constipation–Quality of Life, *: Student's *t* test, **: Pearson chi-square test, ***: Mann-Whitney-U test.

After 10 weeks, the mean CBMpW improved from 2.1 ± 2.2 to 2.8 ± 2 in the control group (p = 0.003) and from 1.7 ± 1.6 to 4.3 ± 1.8 in the study group (p > 0.001). The mean total PAC-QoL scores improved in both groups. There was a slight but significant improvement in the control group (59.3 ± 10.4 to 55 ± 8.5, p = 0.005)) and an approximately 3.5-fold significant improvement in the study group (52.1 ± 16.9 to 15.9 ± 16, p = 0.001). Among PAC-QoL subscales, only worries and discomfort scores improved after treatment in the control group, whereas the study group has significantly improved scores in every measure (Table 2).

Table 2. Effect of treatments on stool frequency and quality of life at baseline and post-treatment.

	Control Group				Study Group			
	Baseline	After 10 Weeks	T	p *	Baseline	After 10 Weeks	T	p *
CBMpW (n, mean ± SD)	2.1 ± 2.2	2.8 ± 2	−3.462	**0.003**	1.7 ± 1.6	4.3 ± 1.8	−10.718	**<0.001**
PAC-QoL (points, mean ± SD)								
Physical discomfort	10.1 ± 2.4	9.8 ± 2.3	0.677	0.506	10.6 ± 2.5	5 ± 3.9	6.551	**<0.001**
Psychosocial discomfort	20.3 ± 4	19.4 ± 3.5	1.294	0.211	15 ± 5.1	6.5 ± 5.3	6.987	**<0.001**
Worries and discomfort	32.3 ± 5.9	29.8 ± 5.7	2.708	**0.014**	29.6 ± 11.5	15.2 ± 8.1	6.982	**<0.001**
Satisfaction	3.3 ± 2.2	3.9 ± 2.3	−1.332	0.199	3.1 ± 2.1	10.7 ± 3.5	−9.553	**<0.001**
Total PAC-QoL score (points, mean ± SD)	59.3 ± 10.4	55 ± 8.5	3.155	**0.005**	52.1 ± 16.9	15.9 ± 16	9.317	**<0.001**

CBMpW: Complete bowel movement per week, SD: Standard deviation, PAC-QoL: Patient Assessment Constipation Quality of Life, *: Paired samples *t*-test. Bold characters were used for statistically meaningful *p* values.

The mean post-treatment CBMpW was lower than 3 and significantly lower in the control group compared to the study group (2.8 ± 2 vs. 4.3 ± 1.8, p = 0.013). In every measure of PAC-QoL, the study group had significantly better scores than the control group (Table 3). At the end of the trial, 30 (66.7%) of the patients had at least a 50% improvement in their total PAC-QoL score (8 from the control group and 22 from the study group; p = 0.001) and 29 (64.4%) had reported ≥3 CBMpW. In the study group, 84% (n = 21) of the patients had CBMpW ≥ 3 compared to 40% (n = 8) in the control group (p = 0.003).

Table 3. Comparison between groups in terms of post-treatment stool frequency and quality of life measures.

Variables	Total (*n* = 45)	Control Group (*n* = 20)	Study Group (*n* = 25)	*p*
CBMpW (*n*, mean ± SD)	3.6 ± 2	2.8 ± 2	4.3 ± 1.8	0.013 *
PAC-QoL (points, mean ± SD)				
Physical discomfort	7.1 ± 4.1	9.8 ± 2.3	5 ± 3.9	<0.001 *
Psychosocial discomfort	12.2 ± 7.9	19.3 ± 3.5	6.5 ± 5.4	<0.001 **
Worries and discomfort	21.7 ± 10.2	29.9 ± 5.6	15.2 ± 8.1	<0.001 *
Satisfaction	7.7 ± 4.5	3.9 ± 2.3	10.7 ± 3.5	<0.001 **
Total PAC-QoL score (points, mean ± SD)	33.3 ± 23.6	55.1 ± 8.5	15.9 ± 16	<0.001 **
50% improvement in total score (*n*, %)	30 (66.7)	8 (40)	22 (88)	0.001 ***
CBMpW ≥ 3 (*n*, %)	29 (64.4)	8 (40)	21 (84)	0.003 ***

CBMpW: Complete bowel movement per week, SD: Standard deviation, PAC-QoL: Patient Assessment Constipation–Quality of Life. *: Student's *t* test, **: Mann-Whitney-U test, ***: Pearson chi-square test.

4. Discussion

Gut microbiota are affected by changes in the diet. Consuming more fiber in the diet results in higher quantities of *Provotella* spp. in the colon, whereas more protein and fat consumption cause *Bacteroides* spp. to reproduce, causing maladjustment of the gut microbiota, which leads to changes in nutrient absorption, immune response, and tolerance to symbiotic bacteria [21,22].

In a non-randomized controlled study evaluating features of fecal flora in FC patients, it was determined that *Bifidobacterium* and *Bacteroides* species were significantly low in stool samples of patients with FC [23]. The mean Bristol Stool Scores and CBMpW were significantly improved after a 2-week probiotic treatment. In another pivotal cross-sectional study conducted on children with constipation using 16S rRNA gene pyrosequencing, it was determined that *Prevotella* was abundant with several genera of *Firmicutes* in constipated patients compared to controls [24]. It was interpreted that the changes in the microbiome were due to a low-fiber diet, and bacterial fermentation end-products, such as increased butyrate production, might lead to constipation.

Increased fiber intake is a key principle in FC therapy. The physicochemical properties of fiber have a significant effect on the gut microbiota. The type of dietary fiber consumed affects the gut microbiota because not all types of bacteria have the capacity to produce the enzymes necessary for their digestion [25]. In the guidelines, soluble fibers are recommended for the treatment of constipation because there may be tolerance problems with insoluble fibers (e.g., fiber in wheat brans and whole grains) in some patients [26]. Insoluble fibers may lead to or increase abdominal pain, distention, and flatulence. Fruit fiber (e.g., prunes) or mixed soluble fibers are shown to be more effective in the short term than psyllium. Also, oligofructose-probiotic combinations are shown to have significant effects on chronic constipation [22]. In this study, patients on the study arm have achieved significant improvement in 6-week treatment with the personalized diet. Most of the patients on the customized diet were satisfied with the treatment approach, and both the number of CBMpW and the ratio of patients with more than 50% improvement in defecation frequency increased.

Considering the fact that nutrition alters the gut microbiota significantly, it is important to prepare a proper diet for patients with FC according to their needs. In our study, we have determined that personalized microbiome modulation by dietary intervention based on AI-assisted fecal microbiome profiling resulted in improvements in the symptoms of FC patients as well as their quality of life.

There are some limitations to the study. As a single-center pilot study, the results cannot be generalized to the whole patient population with FC. Also, there was no follow-up period after six weeks, so the waxing of symptoms, if any, has not been recorded.

Lastly, due to financial limitations, microbiome tests have only been applied to study group patients instead of all the patients in the study.

In conclusion, customization of a diet based on individual microbiome tests provides better outcomes both clinically and socially in FC patients. Considering the significant social impact and healthcare costs related to FC, effective non-pharmacological therapies should be preferred for these patients. To our knowledge, this is the first study to utilize personalized dietary modulation intervention based on individual microbiome profiles of the FC patient population in Turkey and the literature.

Author Contributions: Conceptualization, N.Ç.A., A.G. and Ö.U.N.; methodology, N.Ç.A., O.H.T. and A.G.; software, Ö.U.N.; validation, V.T., A.G. and Ö.U.N.; formal analysis, D.B.; investigation, N.Ç.A., O.H.T., A.G. and D.B.; resources, D.B. and Ö.U.N.; data curation, V.T.; writing—original draft preparation, V.T.; writing—review and editing, N.Ç.A. and A.G.; visualization, V.T.; supervision, N.Ç.A., Ö.U.N. and V.T.; project administration, Ö.U.N.; funding acquisition, A.G. All authors have read and agreed to the published version of the manuscript.

Funding: This research received no external funding but the microbiome analysis was carried out by ENBIOSIS Biotechnology.

Institutional Review Board Statement: The study was conducted in accordance with the Declaration of Helsinki and approved by the Institutional Review Board of Istanbul Medipol University (Approval No. 10840098-772.02-E.47859 Approval date: 17 September 2020).

Informed Consent Statement: Informed consent was obtained from all subjects involved in the study.

Data Availability Statement: The data presented in this study are available on request from the corresponding author. The data are not publicly available due to privacy reasons.

Conflicts of Interest: D.B. was a dietitian working for Enbiosis Biotechnologies at the time of the study. She was responsible for the administration of personalized dietary interventions for the study group. She did not have access to the results of the study, nor did she have any part in writing the manuscript. She is not currently employed by Enbiosis Biotechnologies. Other authors declare no conflict of interest.

References

1. Ford, A.C.; Suares, N.C. Effect of Laxatives and Pharmacological Therapies in Chronic Idiopathic Constipation: Systematic Review and Meta-Analysis. *Gut* **2011**, *60*, 209–218. [CrossRef] [PubMed]
2. Neri, L.; Basilisco, G.; Corazziari, E.; Stanghellini, V.; Bassotti, G.; Bellini, M.; Perelli, I.; Cuomo, R. Constipation Severity Is Associated with Productivity Losses and Healthcare Utilization in Patients with Chronic Constipation. *United Eur. Gastroenterol. J.* **2014**, *2*, 138–147. [CrossRef] [PubMed]
3. Lacy, B.E.; Mearin, F.; Chang, L.; Chey, W.D.; Lembo, A.J.; Simren, M.; Spiller, R. Bowel Disorders. *Gastroenterology* **2016**, *150*, 1393–1407.e5. [CrossRef] [PubMed]
4. Luthra, P.; Camilleri, M.; Burr, N.E.; Quigley, E.M.M.; Black, C.J.; Ford, A.C. Efficacy of Drugs in Chronic Idiopathic Constipation: A Systematic Review and Network Meta-Analysis. *Lancet Gastroenterol. Hepatol.* **2019**, *4*, 831–844. [CrossRef]
5. Aziz, I.; Whitehead, W.E.; Palsson, O.S.; Törnblom, H.; Simrén, M. An Approach to the Diagnosis and Management of Rome IV Functional Disorders of Chronic Constipation. *Expert Rev. Gastroenterol. Hepatol.* **2020**, *14*, 39–46. [CrossRef]
6. Belsey, J.; Greenfield, S.; Candy, D.; Geraint, M. Systematic Review: Impact of Constipation on Quality of Life in Adults and Children. *Aliment. Pharmacol. Ther.* **2010**, *31*, 938–949. [CrossRef]
7. Johanson, J.F.; Kralstein, J. Chronic Constipation: A Survey of the Patient Perspective. *Aliment. Pharmacol. Ther.* **2007**, *25*, 599–608. [CrossRef]
8. Sun, S.X.; Dibonaventura, M.; Purayidathil, F.W.; Wagner, J.S.; Dabbous, O.; Mody, R. Impact of Chronic Constipation on Health-Related Quality of Life, Work Productivity, and Healthcare Resource Use: An Analysis of the National Health and Wellness Survey. *Dig. Dis. Sci.* **2011**, *56*, 2688–2695. [CrossRef]
9. Dennison, C.; Prasad, M.; Lloyd, A.; Bhattacharyya, S.K.; Dhawan, R.; Coyne, K. The Health-Related Quality of Life and Economic Burden of Constipation. *Pharmacoeconomics* **2005**, *23*, 461–476. [CrossRef]
10. Lindberg, G.; Hamid, S.S.; Malfertheiner, P.; Thomsen, O.O.; Fernandez, L.B.; Garisch, J.; Thomson, A.; Goh, K.-L.; Tandon, R.; Fedail, S.; et al. World Gastroenterology Organisation Global Guideline: Constipation—A Global Perspective. *J. Clin. Gastroenterol.* **2011**, *45*, 483–487. [CrossRef]
11. Bassotti, G.; Usai-Satta, P.; Bellini, M. Linaclotide for the Treatment of Chronic Constipation. *Expert Opin. Pharmacother.* **2018**, *19*, 1261–1266. [CrossRef] [PubMed]

12. Dimidi, E.; Christodoulides, S.; Scott, S.M.; Whelan, K. Mechanisms of Action of Probiotics and the Gastrointestinal Microbiota on Gut Motility and Constipation. *Adv. Nutr.* **2017**, *8*, 484–494. [CrossRef] [PubMed]
13. Vriesman, M.H.; Koppen, I.J.N.; Camilleri, M.; di Lorenzo, C.; Benninga, M.A. Management of Functional Constipation in Children and Adults. *Nat. Rev. Gastroenterol. Hepatol.* **2020**, *17*, 21–39. [CrossRef]
14. Caporaso, J.G.; Kuczynski, J.; Stombaugh, J.; Bittinger, K.; Bushman, F.D.; Costello, E.K.; Fierer, N.; Pēa, A.G.; Goodrich, J.K.; Gordon, J.I.; et al. QIIME Allows Analysis of High-Throughput Community Sequencing Data. *Nat. Methods* **2010**, *7*, 335–336. [CrossRef] [PubMed]
15. Bolger, A.M.; Lohse, M.; Usadel, B. Trimmomatic: A Flexible Trimmer for Illumina Sequence Data. *Bioinformatics* **2014**, *30*, 2114–2120. [CrossRef] [PubMed]
16. McDonald, D.; Price, M.N.; Goodrich, J.; Nawrocki, E.P.; Desantis, T.Z.; Probst, A.; Andersen, G.L.; Knight, R.; Hugenholtz, P. An Improved Greengenes Taxonomy with Explicit Ranks for Ecological and Evolutionary Analyses of Bacteria and Archaea. *ISME J.* **2011**, *6*, 610–618. [CrossRef]
17. Karakan, T.; Gundogdu, A.; Alagözlü, H.; Ekmen, N.; Ozgul, S.; Tunali, V.; Hora, M.; Beyazgul, D.; Nalbantoglu, O.U. Artificial Intelligence-Based Personalized Diet: A Pilot Clinical Study for Irritable Bowel Syndrome. *Gut Microbes* **2022**, *14*, 2138672. [CrossRef]
18. Bengi, G.; Yalçın, M.; Akpınar, H.; Keskinoğlu, P.; Ellidokuz, H. Validity and reliability of the patient assessment of constipation quality of life questionnaire for the Turkish population. *Turk. J. Gastroenterol.* **2015**, *26*, 309–314. [CrossRef]
19. Forootan, M.; Bagheri, N.; Darvishi, M. Chronic Constipation: A Review of Literature. *Medicine* **2018**, *97*, e10631. [CrossRef]
20. Sample Size Calculator by Raosoft, Inc. Available online: http://www.raosoft.com/samplesize.html (accessed on 5 October 2022).
21. Marietta, E.; Horwath, I.; Taneja, V. Microbiome, Immunomodulation, and the Neuronal System. *Neurotherapeutics* **2018**, *15*, 23–30. [CrossRef]
22. Meng, X.; Zhang, G.; Cao, H.; Yu, D.; Fang, X.; de Vos, W.M.; Wu, H. Gut Dysbacteriosis and Intestinal Disease: Mechanism and Treatment. *J. Appl. Microbiol.* **2020**, *129*, 787–805. [CrossRef] [PubMed]
23. Kim, S.E.; Choi, S.C.; Park, K.S.; Park, M.I.; Shin, J.E.; Lee, T.H.; Jung, K.W.; Koo, H.S.; Myung, S.J. Change of Fecal Flora and Effectiveness of the Short-Term VSL#3 Probiotic Treatment in Patients with Functional Constipation. *J. Neurogastroenterol. Motil.* **2015**, *21*, 111–120. [CrossRef] [PubMed]
24. Zhu, L.; Liu, W.; Alkhouri, R.; Baker, R.D.; Bard, J.E.; Quigley, E.M.; Baker, S.S. Structural Changes in the Gut Microbiome of Constipated Patients. *Physiol. Genom.* **2014**, *46*, 679–686. [CrossRef] [PubMed]
25. Abreu, A.T.A.; Milke-García, M.P.; Argüello-Arévalo, G.A.; de la Barca, A.M.C.; Carmona-Sánchez, R.I.; Consuelo-Sánchez, A.; Coss-Adame, E.; García-Cedillo, M.F.; Hernández-Rosiles, V.; Icaza-Chávez, M.E.; et al. Dietary Fiber and the Microbiota: A Narrative Review by a Group of Experts from the Asociación Mexicana de Gastroenterología. *Rev. Gastroenterol. Mex.* **2021**, *86*, 287–304. [CrossRef] [PubMed]
26. Mearin, F.; Ciriza, C.; Mínguez, M.; Rey, E.; Mascort, J.J.; Peña, E.; Cañones, P.; Júdez, J. Clinical Practice Guideline: Irritable Bowel Syndrome with Constipation and Functional Constipation in the Adult. *Rev. Esp. Enferm. Dig.* **2016**, *108*, 332–363. [CrossRef]

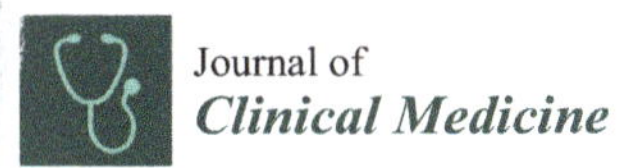

Journal of
Clinical Medicine

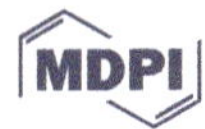

Systematic Review

A Meta-Analysis and Systematic Review of Normothermic and Hypothermic Machine Perfusion in Liver Transplantation

Joseph Mugaanyi [1,2], **Lei Dai** [1], **Changjiang Lu** [1], **Shuqi Mao** [1], **Jing Huang** [1,*] and **Caide Lu** [1,*]

[1]   Department of Hepato-Pancreato-Biliary Surgery, Ningbo Medical Center Li Huili Hospital, The Affiliated Hospital of Ningbo University, Ningbo 315040, China
[2]   School of Medicine, Ningbo University, Ningbo 315211, China
*   Correspondence: huangjingonline@163.com (J.H.); lucaide@nbu.edu.cn (C.L.)

Abstract: Background: The gap between the demand and supply of donor livers is still a considerable challenge. Since static cold storage is not sufficient in marginal livers, machine perfusion is being explored as an alternative. The objective of this study was to assess (dual) hypothermic oxygenated machine perfusion (HOPE/D-HOPE) and normothermic machine perfusion (NMP) in contrast to static cold storage (SCS). Methods: Three databases were searched to identify studies about machine perfusion. Graft and patient survival and postoperative complications were evaluated using the random effects model. Results: the incidence of biliary complications was lower in HOPE vs. SCS (OR: 0.59, 95% CI: 0.36–0.98, $p = 0.04$, I^2: 0%). There was no significant difference in biliary complications between NMP and SCS (OR: 0.76, 95% CI: 0.41–1.40, $p = 0.38$, I^2: 55%). Graft and patient survival were significantly better in HOPE than in SCS (HR: 0.40, 95% CI: 0.23–0.71, $p = 0.002$, I^2: 0%) and (pooled HR: 0.43, 95% CI: 0.20–0.93, $p = 0.03$, I^2: 0%). Graft and patient survival were not significantly different between NMP and SCS. Conclusion: HOPE/D-HOPE and NMP are promising alternatives to SCS for donor liver preservation. They may help address the widening gap between the demand for and availability of donor livers by enabling the rescue and transplantation of marginal livers.

Keywords: machine perfusion; normothermic; hypothermic; liver transplant; survival

Citation: Mugaanyi, J.; Dai, L.; Lu, C.; Mao, S.; Huang, J.; Lu, C. A Meta-Analysis and Systematic Review of Normothermic and Hypothermic Machine Perfusion in Liver Transplantation. *J. Clin. Med.* **2023**, *12*, 235. https://doi.org/10.3390/jcm12010235

Academic Editor: Hidekazu Suzuki

Received: 4 November 2022
Revised: 2 December 2022
Accepted: 5 December 2022
Published: 28 December 2022

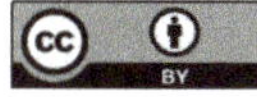

1. Introduction

Although the number of liver transplants performed globally has increased yearly, the availability of donor organs is overshadowed by the demand. More and more centers have optimized and adopted the use of extended criteria donor (ECD) organs to narrow the gap [1,2]. However, ECD organs are more susceptible to ischemia-reperfusion injury and have an increased mortality risk than standard criteria donor organs [3]. Static cold storage (SCS) is the gold-standard method for preserving donor livers. Although SCS has good outcomes for optimal livers, especially donation after brain death (DBD), it has been reported as insufficient in suboptimal livers, with a high risk for complications [4–6]. To address the limitations of SCS, centers worldwide have investigated the use of dynamic preservation of livers using machine perfusion ex situ. Two types of machine perfusion are utilized in the clinical preservation of donor livers: normothermic machine perfusion (NMP) and (dual) hypothermic oxygenated machine perfusion (HOPE/D-HOPE) [7–9]. Normothermic machine perfusion is initiated immediately after standard organ procurement to replace cold storage [10–15]. Unlike NMP, which keeps the liver continuously perfused close to or at normal core temperature, HOPE/D-HOPE involves continuous perfusion of the liver with a cooled, oxygenized perfusate [11,16–19]. HOPE has been associated with improved graft function compared to SCS [18,20–22].

Although numerous studies have explored the dynamic preservation of livers over the past two decades using machine perfusion (NMP or HOPE/D-HOPE) compared to SCS in clinical settings, the majority are small sample-size studies. Based on current literature, it is not very clear which may be comparatively better between HOPE/D-HOPE and NMP when compared with SCS, which is the standard method for preserving donor livers. Ischemia re-perfusion injury is one of the main concerns in SCS. Ischemia re-perfusion injury affects graft survival, which influences patient survival. Machine perfusion aims to address this problem. The occurrence of postoperative complications also has an impact on patient survival. Therefore, in this systematic review and meta-analysis, our primary objective is to assess and compare patient and graft survival in liver transplant patients after ex situ machine perfusion compared to SCS. The secondary objective is to evaluate the occurrence of postoperative complications after liver transplantation.

2. Methods

2.1. Search Strategy

The PubMed, Web of Science and Scopus databases were queried for studies reporting on normothermic and hypothermic machine perfusion in liver transplantation through September 2022. The full search syntax for each database is documented in the Supplementary Materials. Full-text studies reporting on NMP or HOPE with an SCS control group were included. Abstracts, reviews, case reports, editorials and letters and non-English language studies were excluded. First, studies were evaluated for inclusion based on the title and abstract. Studies were subsequently included based on a review of the study's full text. The selection was carried out by two independent reviewers (MJ and DL). The final article inclusion was based on a mutual consensus of the two reviewers. Cross-referencing was performed on the studies to identify any other related studies. Studies comparing either NMP or HOPE to SCS were included; studies that compared NRP, SCS and NMP/HOPE were also included. The most recent study was included if multiple studies reported results from the same source. This manuscript was prepared according to the Cochrane guidelines for interventional system reviews and the PRISMA statement (Preferred Reporting Items for Systematic Reviews and Meta-Analyses) [23,24].

2.2. Quality Assessment

Two independent reviewers performed the quality assessment of all the studies included in the meta-analysis. The evaluation was according to the Downs and Black checklist [25]. We used the modified Downs and Black checklist composed of 5 categories (quality of reporting, external validity, potential for bias, confounding and power analysis). For each study, the maximum possible score is 32 points. Most studies reporting on machine perfusion in liver transplantation have small sample sizes. To address this issue, the last item (study power) was modified from a 5-point scale to assign 5 points if there was adequate study power, 3 if the study power was calculated, and 1 if there was no study power calculation.

2.3. Data Extraction

Data were extracted independently by the two reviewers using standardized forms. Baseline and outcome data were extracted for the research (NMP/HOPE) and control (CSC) groups. Baseline data includes sample size in each group, age, donor type and BMI. Outcome data includes graft survival, patient survival, biliary complications, hospital stay, vascular complications and primary non-function. Data were collected, aggregated and reported. For studies that did not report survival data, the data were extracted from Kaplan–Meier survival curves using methods described by Tierney et al. [26].

2.4. Statistical Analysis

Pooling of available outcome data (biliary complications, vascular complications, graft survival, patient survival, hospital stay and primary non-function) was performed using "Review Manager 5.3" using the random effects model. Study heterogeneity was quantified using the DerSimonian–Laird method. The pooled data were presented with their corresponding 95% confidence intervals (CI). The graft and patient survival between the groups were compared using generic inverse variance described by Tierney et al. [26]. The hazard ratios were reported with the respective 95% CI and corresponding forest plots used for visual reporting. The random effects model was used for biliary complications, vascular complications, hospital stay and primary non-function, and the odds ratios (OR) with 95% CI were reported on forest plots. Study heterogeneity was assessed using the I^2 statistic. *p*-value < 0.05 was considered significant.

3. Results

3.1. Literature Search Results

A text search was performed on 13 September 2022. A PRISMA flow chart of the search process is presented in Figure 1. Upon initial search, 529 results were returned, and 70 articles were selected for full-text assessment. Finally, 10 articles were included in the analysis [7,11,18,20,27–32]. The quality assessment of all the included studies is summarized in Table 1. The studies were of moderately good quality; the median score was 20 out of 32 points (range 17–23). Three studies had DCD and DBD donors in the analyzed [7,11,27]. Dutkowski et al. compared DCD HOPE to DCS SCS and DBD SCS [29]. Gaurav et al. compared SCS, NMP and NRP [30]; only SCS and NMP data were included. Vascular complications were reported in eight studies [11,18,20,28–32], PNF in six [7,11,18,29–31], biliary complications in nine [11,18,20,27–32] and hospital stay in eight [7,11,20,27–31]. Seven studies reported adequate data to compare patient survival [11,18,20,28,30–32], and nine to compare graft survival [7,11,18,20,28–32]. The baseline demographic and clinical data of the included studies are summarized in Table 2. In total, 1104 liver transplant recipients were included (504 machine-perfused livers and 600 static cold-storage livers) in this study. Of the 504 perfused livers, 371 were NMP and 133 were HOPE. In one study, HOPE was combined with NRP [28]. Three studies only reported patient survival rates without sufficient data to extract survival data [7,27,29]. Bral et al. did not provide sufficient data to extract graft survival data [27].

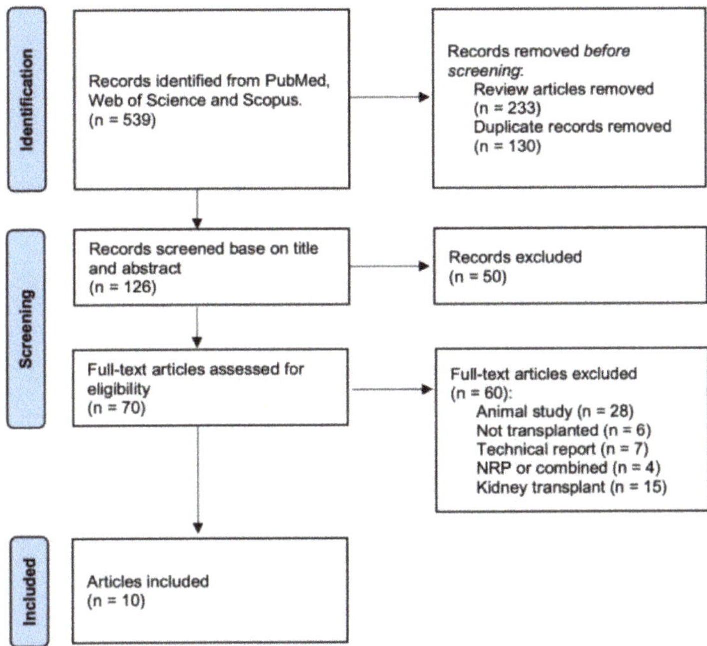

Figure 1. PRISMA flow chart.

Table 1. Quality assessment based on the downs and black checklist.

References	Reporting	External Validity	Internal Validity (Risk of Bias)	Internal Validity (Confounding)	Power	Total Points
Dutkowski et al., 2015	10	3	5	3	1	22
Guarrera et al., 2015	9	2	5	2	1	19
Bral et al., 2017	8	3	6	2	1	20
Van Rijn et al., 2017	8	3	6	4	1	22
Nasralla et al., 2018	9	3	6	4	1	23
Schlegel et al., 2019	8	3	5	4	1	21
Mergental et al., 2020	8	3	5	2	1	19
Riccardo et al., 2021	7	3	5	1	1	17
Gaurav et al., 2022	8	3	5	1	1	18
Markmann et al., 2022	8	3	5	3	1	20
Maximum score	11	3	7	6	5	32

Table 2. Study characteristics.

References	n		Age		MELD		CIT		Perfusion Time
	HOPE	SCS	HOPE	SCS	HOPE	SCS	HOPE	SCS	
Dutkowski et al., 2015	25	50	60 (57–64)	56 (49–59)	13 (9–15)	16 (10–21)	188 (141–264)	395 (349–447)	317 (280–391)
Guarrera et al., 2015 *	31	30	57.5 ± 8	58.4 ± 9.6	19.5 ± 5.9	21.4 ± 6.3	553 ± 96	516 ± 114	228 ± 54
Van Rijn et al., 2017	10	20	57 (54–62)	52 (42–60)	16 (15–22)	22 (17–27)	-	503 (476–526)	126 (123–135)
Schlegel et al., 2019	50	50	58 (56–62)	57 (51–61)	11 (8–14)	11.8(8.5–15.8)	264 (210–312)	282 (258–318)	120 (96–144)
Riccardo et al., 2021	37	37	58 (37–70)	56 (38–66)	9 (6–25)	13 (6–19)	411 (330–660)	390 (240–583)	120 (42–380)

References	n		Age		MELD		CIT		Perfusion Time
	NMP	SCS	NMP	SCS	NMP	SCS	NMP	SCS	
Bral et al., 2017	10	30	53(28–67)	59(43–69)	13 (9–32)	19 (7–34)	167 (95–293)	233 (64–890)	690 (198–1350)
Nasralla et al., 2018	121	101	55(48–62)	55(48–62)	13 (10–18)	14 (9–18)	126 (106.5–143)	465 (375–575)	547.5(372.5–710.5)
Mergental et al., 2020	22	44	56(46–65)	-	12 (9–16)	-	452 (389–600)	-	587 (450–705)
Gaurav et al., 2022	67	97	59(51–63)	56(50–62)	14 (10–18)	16 (13–20)	396 (346–441)	430 (397–474)	460 (330–569)
Markmann et al., 2022 *	151	142	57 ± 10.3	58.4 ± 10.1	28.4 ± 6.9	28 ± 5.7	175. 4 ± 43.5	338.8 ± 91.5	276.6 ± 117.4

MELD: Model For End-Stage Liver Disease. CIT: Cold Ischemia Time. HOPE: Hypothermic oxygenated machine perfusion. SCS: Static Cold Storage; NMP: Normothermic Machine Perfusion. * values were reported as mean ± standard deviation. Elsewhere, values were reported as median (range).

3.2. Complications after Liver Transplant

Biliary and vascular complications and primary non-function are summarized in Table 3. Biliary complications were reported in 269/1038 patients in 10 studies. The incidence of biliary complications was higher in SCS than in MP (Pooled OR: 0.59, 95% CI: 0.44–0.80, $p < 0.001$, I^2: 0%, Figure 2a) [7,11,18,20,27–32]. When comparing HOPE to SCS, biliary complications were higher in SCS (Pooled OR: 0.59, 95% CI: 0.36–0.98, $p = 0.04$, I^2: 0%, Figure 2b) [18,20,28,29,31]. There was no significant difference in biliary complications between NMP and SCS (Pooled OR: 0.76, 95% CI: 0.41–1.40, $p = 0.38$, I^2: 55%, Figure 2c) [7,11,27,30,32]. Vascular complications were reported in 81/1019 patients in 8 studies [11,18,20,28–32]. There was no significant difference in vascular complications between NM and SCS (Pooled OR: 0.79, 95% CI: 0.49–1.28, $p = 0.35$, I^2: 0%, Figure 3a) [11,18,20,28–32]. There was no significant difference in vascular HOPE and SCS (Pooled OR: 0.54 95% CI: 0.2–1.28, $p = 0.16$, I^2: 0%, Figure 3b) [18,20,28,29,31], nor between NMP and SCS (Pooled OR: 0.94, 95% CI: 0.53–1.68, $p = 0.84$, I^2: 0%, Figure 3c) [7,11,27,30,32]. Vascular complications were not reported in two of the studies [7,27]. PNF was reported in 23/579 patients in six studies [7,11,18,29–31]. There was no significant difference in PNF between NM and SCS (Pooled OR: 1.92, 95% CI: 0.46–7.97, $p = 0.37$, I^2: 50%, Figure 4a) [7,11,18,29–31]. PNF was also not significantly different between HOPE and SCS, nor between NMP and SCS; (Pooled OR: 2.82, 95% CI: 0.56–14.18, $p = 0.21$, I^2: 38%, Figure 4b) [18,29,31] and (Pooled OR: 0.58, 95% CI: 0.12–2.77, $p = 0.49$, I^2: 0%, Figure 4c) [7,11,30], respectively.

Table 3. Postoperative complications.

References	Biliary Complications			Vascular Complications			PNF		
	Total	MP	SCS	Total	MP	SCS	Total	MP	SCS
Dutkowski et al., 2015	28	5	23	4	1	3	10	7	3
Guarrera et al., 2015	17	4	13	5	3	2	3	1	2
Bral et al., 2017	4	0	4	-	-	-	-	-	-
Van Rijn et al., 2017	18	5	13	2	0	2	-	-	-
Nasralla et al., 2018	28	13	15	23	13	10	2	2	0
Schlegel et al., 2019	34	16	18	10	4	6	1	1	0
Mergental et al., 2020	-	-	-	-	-	-	1	0	1
Riccardo et al., 2021	19	8	11	9	1	8	-	-	-
Gaurav et al., 2022	61	23	38	12	5	7	6	1	5
Markmann et al., 2022	60	21	39	16	7	9	-	-	-

MP: Machine Perfusion; SCS: Static Cold Storage. PNF: Primary Non-Function.

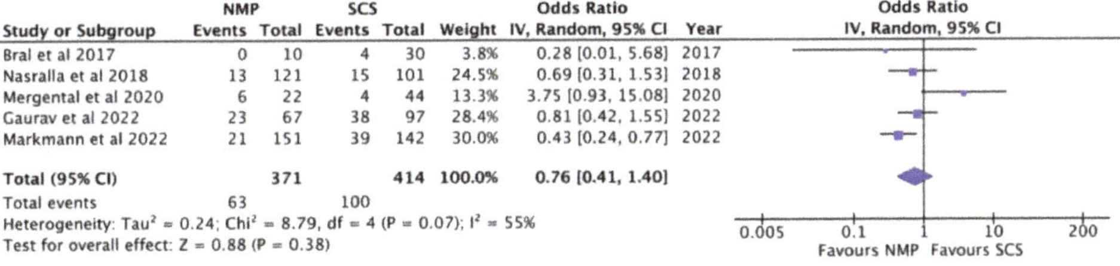

Figure 2. Forest plots for biliary complications. (**a**) Machine perfusion (hypothermic or normothermic) vs. SCS (*P* < 0.001). (**b**) HOPE vs. SCS (*P* = 0.04). (**c**) NMP vs. SCS (*P* = 0.38).

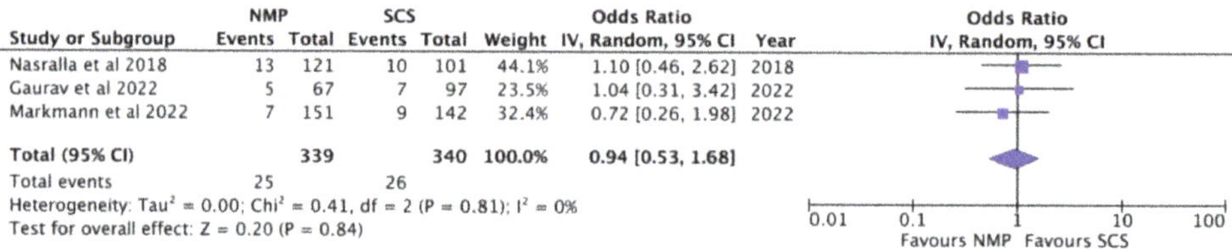

Figure 3. Forest plots for vascular complications. (**a**) Machine perfusion (hypothermic or normothermic) vs. SCS (*P* = 0.35). (**b**) HOPE vs. SCS (*P* = 0.16). (**c**) NMP vs. SCS (*P* = 0.84).

3.3. Graft and Patient Survival after Liver Transplant

The graft and patient survival rates for each of the studies are summarized in Tables 4 and 5. Re-transplantation was reported in 68/566 patients in five studies (Pooled OR: 0.43, 95% CI: 0.23–0.83, *p* = 0.01, I^2: 0%, Figure S1) [11,20,29–31]. Reported 1-year graft survival ranged between 81 and 98% in MP and 69 and 99% in SC. Reported 1-year patient survival ranged between 80 and 100% in the MP and between 80 and 97% in SCS. Graft and patient survival were compared between HOPE and SCS and between NMP and SCS. Graft survival was significantly better in the MP group than SCS (pooled HR: 0.46, 95% CI: 0.23–0.93, *p* = 0.03, I^2: 74%, Figure 5a) [7,11,18,20,28–32]. HOPE was associated with reduced graft loss compared to SCS (pooled HR: 0.40, 95% CI: 0.23–0.71, *p* = 0.002, I^2: 0%, Figure 5b) [18,20,28,29,31]. Graft was slightly favorable in NMP compared to SCS but not statistically significant (pooled HR: 0.60, 95% CI: 0.15–2.37, *p* = 0.47, I^2: 89%, Figure 5c) [7,11,30,32]. There was no significant difference in patient survival between MP and SCS (pooled HR: 0.74, 95% CI: 0.47–1.17, *P* = 0.20, I^2: 4%, Figure 5a) [11,18,20,28,30–32]. Patient survival was significantly better in HOPE than SCS (pooled HR: 0.43, 95% CI: 0.20–0.93, *p* = 0.03, I^2: 0%, Figure 6b) [18,20,28,31]. There was no significant difference in patient survival between NMP and SCS (pooled HR: 0.99, 95% CI: 0.57–1.72, *p* = 0.98, I^2: 0%, Figure 6c) [11,30,32]. Funnel plots for studies included in the various analyzes are provided in the supplement; HOPE vs SCS in Figure S2, NMP vs SCS in Figure S3 and MP vs SCS in Figure S4.

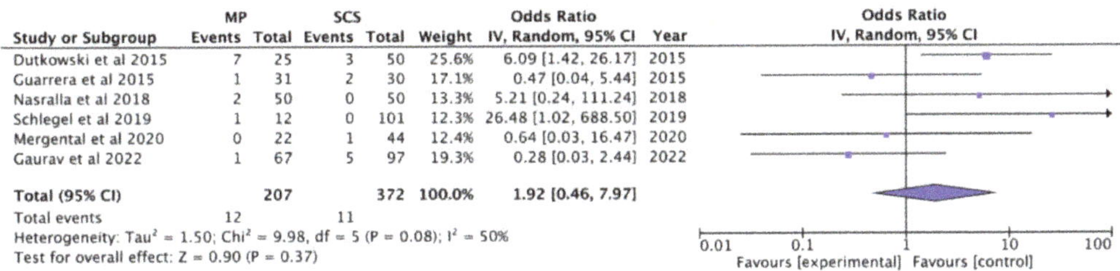

a) Machine perfusion vs SCS

b) HOPE vs SCS

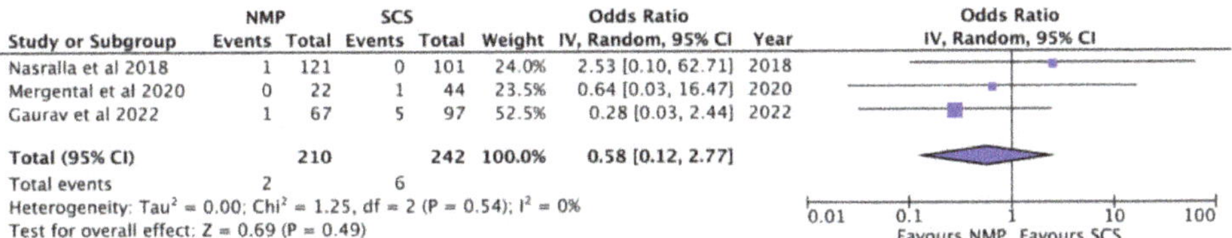

c) NMP vs SCS

Figure 4. Forest plots for primary non-function. (**a**) Machine perfusion (hypothermic or normothermic) vs. SCS (*P* = 0.37). (**b**) HOPE vs. SCS (*P* = 0.21). (**c**) NMP vs. SCS (*P* = 0.49).

Table 4. Graft survival.

References	Proportion (%) Graft Survival			
	6 Months		**1 Year**	
	MP	**SCS**	**MP**	**SCS**
Dutkowski et al., 2015	-	-	90	69
Guarrera et al., 2015	-	-	81	80
Bral et al., 2017	80	100	-	-
Van Rijn et al., 2017	100	80	100	67
Nasralla et al., 2018	-	-	95	96
Schlegel et al., 2019	-	-	90	82
Mergental et al., 2020	-	-	86.4	86.4
Riccardo et al., 2021	-	-	91.8	83.8
Gaurav et al., 2022	90	87	75	83
Markmann et al., 2022	99	99	98	99

Table 5. Patient survival.

References	Proportion (%) Patient Survival	
	1 Year	
	MP	**SCS**
Dutkowski et al., 2015	-	-
Guarrera et al., 2015	84	80
Bral et al., 2017	100	85
Van Rijn et al., 2017	100	67
Nasralla et al., 2018	95	97
Schlegel et al., 2019	98	86
Mergental et al., 2020	100	95.5
Riccardo et al., 2021	100	91.8
Gaurav et al., 2022	80	94
Markmann et al., 2022	94	93.7

a) Machine perfusion vs SCS

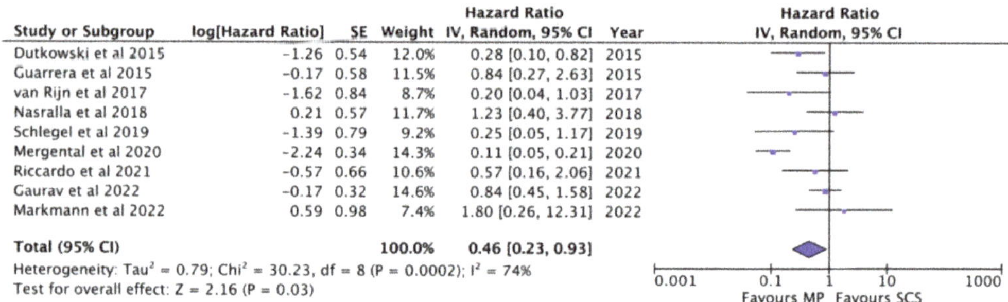

b) HOPE vs SCS

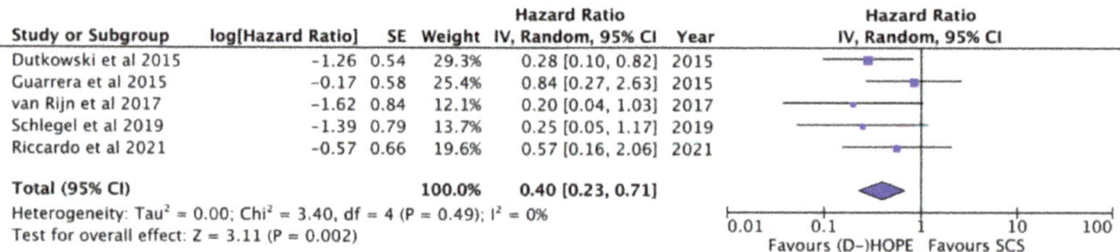

c) NMP vs SCS

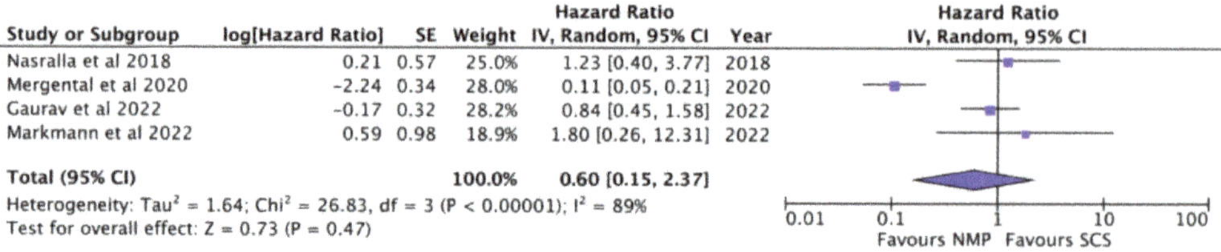

Figure 5. Forest plots for graft survival. (**a**) Machine perfusion (hypothermic or normothermic) vs. SCS (*P* = 0.03). (**b**) HOPE vs. SCS (*P* = 0.02). (**c**) NMP vs. SCS (*P* = 0.47).

a) Machine perfusion vs SCS

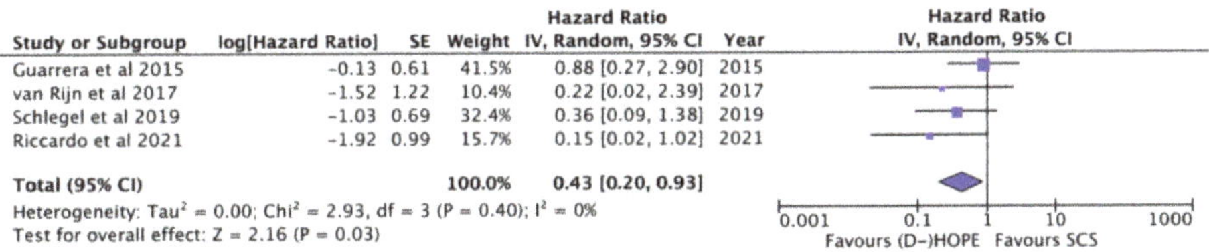

b) HOPE vs SCS

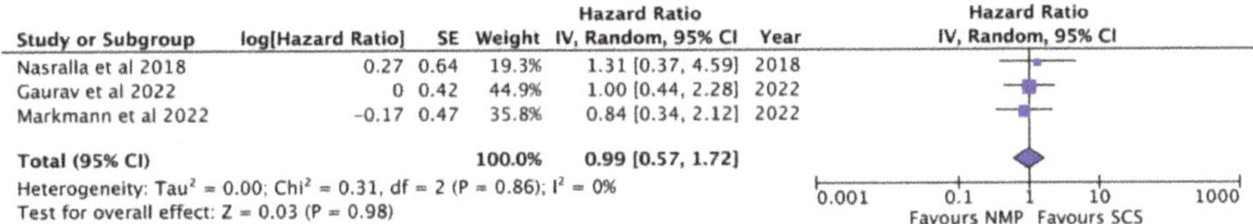

c) NMP vs SCS

Figure 6. Forest plots for patient survival. (**a**) Machine perfusion (hypothermic or normothermic) vs. SCS ($P = 0.20$). (**b**) HOPE vs. SCS ($P = 0.03$). (**c**) NMP vs. SCS ($P = 0.98$).

4. Discussion

Given the increasing demand for donor livers, the gap between supply and demand has kept widening. Several approaches have been taken to try to address this issue. One of which has been the use of ECD organs [33,34]. However, ECD organs are often discarded due to being suboptimal. Secondly, marginal livers are associated with less optimal postoperative outcomes than standard-criteria donor organs. Numerous transplant centers have explored the use of machine perfusion to rescue discarded livers [7,8,35]. The utilization of machine perfusion, however, extends beyond the rescue of discarded organs, and studies have investigated the possibility of replacing SCS with NMP or HOPE/D-HOPE [11,12,18,20,29]. Based on current literature, machine perfusion is associated with more favorable postoperative outcomes. However, there appears to be some difference in the postoperative outcomes of HOPE/D-HOPE vs. SCS and those of NMP vs. SCS.

Both graft and patient survival in liver transplant recipients of grafts that underwent HOPE/D-HOPE instead of SCS were significantly better. The improvement in graft survival may be associated with reduced ischemia-reperfusion injury in grafts that are preserved using HOPE [28,31,36]. The improved patient survival may also be a result of the reduced incidence of postoperative complications and the reduced incidence of graft loss in HOPE compared to SCS. In the HOPE subgroup analysis, graft survival favored the HOPE group in all the studies included. The same was true for patient survival. In both analyses, the studies were homogeneous (I^2: 0%).

However, in the studies that compared NMP to SCS, there was no significant difference in graft and patient survival, although graft survival slightly favored NMP. We do note though that based on I^2-statistic, these studies were heterogenous (I^2: 89%). On further investigation, we found graft survival in Mergental et al. [7] to be the outlier (OR: -2.24, SE: 0.34, in favor of NPM). Without their study included in the subgroup analysis, the studies were homogenous (I^2: 0%). This heterogeneity may be a result of the much smaller sample size in this study compared to the other three studies in the analysis. The NPM and SCS group sample sizes were 22 and 44, respectively, in Mergental et al. [7]; 67 and 97, respectively, in Gaurav et al. [30]; 170 and 164, respectively, in Nasralla et al. [11]; and 142 and 151 in Markmann et al. [32].

Based on these results, HOPE/D-HOPE may provide more favorable graft and patient survival outcomes than NMP. However, we cannot provide concrete backing for this deduction. As such, it should be interpreted as a bird's-eye-view takeaway from the findings, which merit further investigation.

In a pooled analysis of machine perfusion (NMP and HOPE/D-HOPE) vs. SCS, graft survival was significantly better in the machine perfusion group (p = 0.03). However, the studies were significantly heterogeneous (I^2: 74%). The heterogeneity here is most likely a result of the different methods of machine perfusion used in the different studies (HOPE vs. NMP). The patient survival was not significantly better in the machine perfusion group than in SCS, although machine perfusion was slightly favored (p = 0.2). Unlike the graft-survival analysis, in this case, the studies were homogenous (I^2: 4%). The patient outcome was mostly affected by the survival results in the studies that used NMP. This is perhaps expected since HOPE and NMP are considered to be distinct graft-preservation techniques. HOPE has been reported to promote mitochondrial functional recovery, increase adenosine triphosphate levels and reduce the donor liver injuring the rewarming phase [16,37]. NPM, on the other hand, has been reported to enable liver metabolism at physiological temperature. NPM has most been used to assess the viability of suboptimal organs [15,38]. Based on current literature, there appears to be no evidence showing a significant benefit of NPM in improving the quality of suboptimal livers. Furthermore, NPM machines have been reported to be technically challenging and prone to human error. Injury to the liver during NPM has a considerably more negative impact on the organ than under HOPE [39].

Since HOPE and NMP may have distinct benefits, with HOPE seemingly being more beneficial to mitigating reperfusion injury, and NPM to allowing for viability testing, some centers are now investigating the combination of HOPE and NPM [40], while some are looking at sub-normothermic machine perfusion [12,14]. We are yet to see whether the sequential use of HOPE followed by NMP can yield much more positive postoperative outcomes coupled with the potential for rescuing marginal and suboptimal organs than may have otherwise been discarded.

We found a similar situation with respect to biliary complications. HOPE had a significantly lower incidence of biliary complications than SCS (p = 0.04, I^2: 0%). However, the difference was not significant for NPM vs. SCS, and yet again, the studies were heterogeneous (I^2: 55%). As with graft survival in the studies that compared NPM to SCS, Mergental et al. [7] seems to be the source of the heterogeneity. Analysis without this study included is homogenous with I^2 of 0%. We did, however, find biliary complications to be lower in machine perfusion as a whole vs. SCS (p < 0.001, I^2: 0%). For the other postoperative outcomes we analyzed (PNF and vascular complications), there were no significant differences between HOPE and SCS, nor between NMP and SCS.

We could not conduct a detailed analysis of the potential mediating and confounding factors that may have impacted graft and patient survival in the included studies due to patient data availability limitations. However, this is an important aspect of survival analysis. Graft survival in liver transplant patients may be affected by male recipient–female donor sex mismatch, recipient blood group, number of transplantations, advanced donor age, pre-existing portal vein thrombosis and prolonged cold ischemia time [41–43]. Patient survival may be influenced by the need for re-transplantation, graft rejection, advanced donor age and prolonged cold ischemia time [42]. To the best of our knowledge, at the time of writing, there is no published study directly comparing HOPE/D-HOPE to NMP. We believe that a standardized multi-center, large sample-size study comparing the two methods and analyzing the potential mediating and confounding factors would be of considerable significance to our understanding of these approaches to donor liver preservation.

The limitations of this study include relatively small sample sizes in some of the studies included. However, since the transplantation of machine-perfused livers is currently being investigated at a limited number of centers, the sample size limitation is still unavoidable. This will undoubtedly change as more liver transplantation centers adopt machine perfusion. Heterogeneity may also have had some impact on the results, especially in the NMP subgroup. In either case, the source of the heterogeneity was a single study whose sample size was much smaller compared to the other studies in the analysis. There may also be limitations due to the inclusion or exclusion bias. There may also be differences in surgical experience at different centers and protocols for HOPE and NMP in the different studies. For all the studies, survival data and hazard ratios were extracted and calculated using the method described by Tierney et al. [26] in their paper. The process of extracting this data may introduce some inaccuracy; however, we think this is mostly negligible since almost all studies tended to favor the research group. The survival rates reported were short-term survival; therefore, for long-term graft and patient survival, further studies are needed.

5. Conclusions

Machine perfusion is gaining more interest in donor liver preservation and viability testing for marginal/suboptimal organs. In reported studies, HOPE/D-HOPE has been associated with improved graft and patient survival and reduced biliary complications. NMP has been reported to be helpful in the viability evaluation and rescue of marginal livers. Therefore, HOPE/D-HOPE and NMP are promising alternatives to SCS for donor liver preservation. They may help address the widening gap between the demand for and availability of donor livers by enabling the rescue and transplantation of marginal livers.

Supplementary Materials: The following are available online at https://www.mdpi.com/article/10.3390/10.3390/jcm12010235/s1, Figure S1: Forest plots for re-transplantation in Machine Perfusion vs. Static Cold Storage, Figure S2: Funnel plots for HOPE vs. Static Cold Storage, Figure S3: Funnel plots for Normothermic Machine Perfusion vs. Static Cold Storage, Figure S4: Funnel plots for Machine Perfusion vs. Static Cold Storage

Author Contributions: Conceptualization, J.M. and J.H.; writing-original draft preparation, J.M.; writing-review and editing, C.L. (Changjiang Lu) and J.M.; supervision, C.L. (Caide Lu); resources, J.H. and C.L. (Caide Lu); data curation: L.D., J.M. and S.M.; Methodology, J.M., C.L. (Changjiang Lu) and L.D.; formal analysis, J.M. and S.M. All authors have read and agreed to the published version of the manuscript.

Funding: The authors have declared no funding.

Institutional Review Board Statement: Not applicable.

Informed Consent Statement: Not applicable.

Data Availability Statement: Not applicable.

Conflicts of Interest: The authors have no conflicts of interest to declare.

References

1. Durand, F.; Renz, J.F.; Alkofer, B.; Burra, P.; Clavien, P.A.; Porte, R.J.; Freeman, R.B.; Belghiti, J. Report of the Paris consensus meeting on expanded criteria donors in liver transplantation. *Liver Transpl.* **2008**, *14*, 1694–1707. [CrossRef]
2. Morrissey, P.E.; Monaco, A.P. Donation after circulatory death: Current practices, ongoing challenges, and potential improvements. *Transplantation* **2014**, *97*, 258–264. [CrossRef] [PubMed]

3. Nemes, B.; Gámán, G.; Polak, W.G.; Gelley, F.; Hara, T.; Ono, S.; Baimakhanov, Z.; Piros, L.; Eguchi, S. Extended-criteria donors in liver transplantation Part II: Reviewing the impact of extended-criteria donors on the complications and outcomes of liver transplantation. *Expert Rev. Gastroenterol. Hepatol.* **2016**, *10*, 841–859. [CrossRef] [PubMed]

4. Callaghan, C.J.; Charman, S.C.; Muiesan, P.; Powell, J.J.; Gimson1, A.E.; van der Meulen, J.H.P. Outcomes of transplantation of livers from donation after circulatory death donors in the UK: A cohort study. *BMJ Open* **2013**, *3*, e003287. [CrossRef] [PubMed]

5. de Vries, Y.; von Meijenfeldt, F.A.; Porte, R.J. Post-transplant cholangiopathy: Classification, pathogenesis, and preventive strategies. *Biochim. Biophys. Acta Mol. Basis Dis.* **2018**, *1864*, 1507–1515. [CrossRef]

6. den Dulk, A.C.; Sebib Korkmaz, K.; de Rooij, B.J.F.; Sutton, M.E.; Braat, A.E.; Inderson, A.; Dubbeld, J.; Verspaget, H.W.; Porte, R.J.; van Hoek, B. High peak alanine aminotransferase determines extra risk for nonanastomotic biliary strictures after liver transplantation with donation after circulatory death. *Transpl. Int.* **2015**, *28*, 492–501. [CrossRef] [PubMed]

7. Mergental, H.; Laing, R.W.; Kirkham, A.J.; Perera, M.T.P.R.; Boteon, Y.L.; Attard, J.; Barton, D.; Curbishley, S.; Wilkhu, M.; Neil, D.A.; et al. Transplantation of discarded livers following viability testing with normothermic machine perfusion. *Nat. Commun.* **2020**, *11*, 2939. [CrossRef] [PubMed]

8. van Leeuwen, O.B.; de Vries, Y.; Fujiyoshi, M.; Nijsten, M.W.; Ubbink, R.; Pelgrim, G.J.; Werner, M.J.; Reyntjens, K.M.; van den Berg, A.P.; de Boer, M.T.; et al. Transplantation of High-risk Donor Livers After Ex Situ Resuscitation and Assessment Using Combined Hypo- and Normothermic Machine Perfusion: A Prospective Clinical Trial. *Ann. Surg.* **2019**, *270*, 906–914. [CrossRef]

9. Schlegel, A.; Kron, P.; Dutkowski, P. Hypothermic machine perfusion in liver transplantation. *Curr. Opin. Organ Transplant.* **2016**, *21*, 308–314. [CrossRef]

10. Detelich, D.; Markmann, J.F. The dawn of liver perfusion machines. *Curr. Opin. Organ Transplant.* **2018**, *23*, 151–161. [CrossRef]

11. Nasralla, D.; Coussios, C.C.; Mergental, H.; Akhtar, M.Z.; Butler, A.J.; Ceresa, C.D.; Chiocchia, V.; Dutton, S.J.; García-Valdecasas, J.C.; Heaton, N.; et al. A randomized trial of normothermic preservation in liver transplantation. *Nature* **2018**, *557*, 50–56. [CrossRef] [PubMed]

12. Bruinsma, B.G.; Yeh, H.; Özer, S.; Martins, P.N.; Farmer, A.; Wu, W.; Saeidi, N.; Op den Dries, S.; Berendsen, T.A.; Smith, R.N.; et al. Subnormothermic machine perfusion for ex vivo preservation and recovery of the human liver for transplantation. *Am. J. Transplant.* **2014**, *14*, 1400–1409. [CrossRef] [PubMed]

13. Bruinsma, B.G.; Berendsen, T.A.; Izamis, M.L.; Yarmush, M.L.; Uygun, K. Determination and extension of the limits to static cold storage using subnormothermic machine perfusion. *Int. J. Artif. Organs* **2013**, *36*, 775–780. [CrossRef] [PubMed]

14. Gringeri, E.; Bonsignore, P.; Bassi, D.; D'Amico, F.E.; Mescoli, C.; Polacco, M.; Buggio, M.; Luisetto, R.; Boetto, R.; Noaro, G.; et al. Subnormothermic machine perfusion for non-heart-beating donor liver grafts preservation in a Swine model: A new strategy to increase the donor pool? *Transplant. Proc.* **2012**, *44*, 2026–2028. [CrossRef]

15. Mergental, H.; Perera, M.T.P.R.; Laing, R.W.; Muiesan, P.; Isaac, J.R.; Smith, A.; Stephenson, B.T.F.; Cilliers, H.; Neil, D.A.H.; Hübscher, S.G.; et al. Transplantation of Declined Liver Allografts Following Normothermic Ex-Situ Evaluation. *Am. J. Transplant.* **2016**, *16*, 3235–3245. [CrossRef] [PubMed]

16. Schlegel, A.; de Rougemont, O.; Graf, R.; Clavien, P.A.; Dutkowski, P. Protective mechanisms of end-ischemic cold machine perfusion in DCD liver grafts. *J. Hepatol.* **2013**, *58*, 278–286. [CrossRef]

17. Patrono, D.; Surra, A.; Catalano, G.; Rizza, G.; Berchialla, P.; Martini, S.; Tandoi, F.; Lupo, F.; Mirabella, S.; Stratta, C.; et al. Hypothermic Oxygenated Machine Perfusion of Liver Grafts from Brain-Dead Donors. *Sci. Rep.* **2019**, *9*, 9337. [CrossRef]

18. Schlegel, A.; Muller, X.; Kalisvaart, M.; Muellhaupt, B.; Perera, M.T.P.; Isaac, J.R.; Clavien, P.A.; Muiesan, P.; Dutkowski, P. Outcomes of DCD liver transplantation using organs treated by hypothermic oxygenated perfusion before implantation. *J. Hepatol.* **2019**, *70*, 50–57. [CrossRef] [PubMed]

19. Burlage, L.C.; Hessels, L.; van Rijn, R.; Matton, A.P.; Fujiyoshi, M.; van den Berg, A.P.; Reyntjens, K.M.; Meyer, P.; de Boer, M.T.; de Kleine, R.H.; et al. Opposite acute potassium and sodium shifts during transplantation of hypothermic machine perfused donor livers. *Am. J. Transplant.* **2019**, *19*, 1061–1071. [CrossRef]

20. van Rijn, R.; Karimian, N.; Matton, A.P.; Burlage, L.C.; Westerkamp, A.C.; van den Berg, A.P.; de Kleine, R.H.; de Boer, M.T.; Lisman, T.; Porte, R.J. Dual hypothermic oxygenated machine perfusion in liver transplants donated after circulatory death. *Br. J. Surg.* **2017**, *104*, 907–917. [CrossRef] [PubMed]

21. van Rijn, R.; Schurink, I.J.; de Vries, Y.; van den Berg, A.P.; Cortes Cerisuelo, M.; Darwish Murad, S.; Erdmann, J.I.; Gilbo, N.; de Haas, R.J.; Heaton, N.; et al. Hypothermic Machine Perfusion in Liver Transplantation—A Randomized Trial. *N. Engl. J. Med.* **2021**, *384*, 1391–1401. [CrossRef] [PubMed]

22. van Rijn, R.; van Leeuwen, O.B.; Matton, A.P.; Burlage, L.C.; Wiersema-Buist, J.; van den Heuvel, M.C.; de Kleine, R.H.; de Boer, M.T.; Gouw, A.S.; Porte, R.J. Hypothermic oxygenated machine perfusion reduces bile duct reperfusion injury after transplantation of donation after circulatory death livers. *Liver Transpl.* **2018**, *24*, 655–664. [CrossRef] [PubMed]

23. Higgins, J.P. *Cochrane Handbook for Systematic Reviews of Interventions Version*; John Wiley & Sons: Chichester, UK, 2022.

24. Moher, D.; Shamseer, L.; Clarke, M.; Ghersi, D.; Liberati, A.; Petticrew, M.; Shekelle, P.; Stewart, L.A. Preferred reporting items for systematic review and meta-analysis protocols (PRISMA-P) 2015 statement. *Syst. Rev.* **2015**, *4*, 1. [CrossRef]

25. Downs, S.H.; Black, N. The feasibility of creating a checklist for the assessment of the methodological quality both of randomised and non-randomised studies of health care interventions. *J. Epidemiol. Community Health* **1998**, *52*, 377–384. [CrossRef]

26. Tierney, J.F.; Stewart, L.A.; Ghersi, D.; Burdett, S.; Sydes, M.R. Practical methods for incorporating summary time-to-event data into meta-analysis. *Trials* **2007**, *8*, 16. [CrossRef] [PubMed]

27. Bral, M.; Gala-Lopez, B.; Bigam, D.; Kneteman, N.; Malcolm, A.; Livingstone, S.; Andres, A.; Emamaullee, J.; Russell, L.; Coussios, C.; et al. Preliminary Single-Center Canadian Experience of Human Normothermic Ex Vivo Liver Perfusion: Results of a Clinical Trial. *Am. J. Transplant.* **2017**, *17*, 1071–1080. [CrossRef]

28. De Carlis, R.; Schlegel, A.; Frassoni, S.; Olivieri, T.; Ravaioli, M.; Camagni, S.; Patrono, D.; Bassi, D.; Pagano, D.; Di Sandro, S.; et al. How to Preserve Liver Grafts from Circulatory Death With Long Warm Ischemia? A Retrospective Italian Cohort Study with Normothermic Regional Perfusion and Hypothermic Oxygenated Perfusion. *Transplantation* **2021**, *105*, 2385–2396. [CrossRef]

29. Dutkowski, P.; Polak, W.G.; Muiesan, P.; Schlegel, A.; Verhoeven, C.J.; Scalera, I.; DeOliveira, M.L.; Kron, P.; Clavien, P.A. First Comparison of Hypothermic Oxygenated PErfusion Versus Static Cold Storage of Human Donation After Cardiac Death Liver Transplants: An International-matched Case Analysis. *Ann. Surg.* **2015**, *262*, 764–770. [CrossRef]

30. Gaurav, R.; Butler, A.J.; Kosmoliaptsis, V.; Mumford, L.; Fear, C.; Swift, L.; Fedotovs, A.; Upponi, S.; Khwaja, S.; Richards, J.; et al. Liver Transplantation Outcomes from Controlled Circulatory Death Donors SCS vs in situ NRP vs ex situ NMP. *Ann. Surg.* **2022**, *275*, 1156–1164. [CrossRef]

31. Guarrera, J.V.; Henry, S.D.; Samstein, B.; Reznik, E.; Musat, C.; Lukose, T.I.; Ratner, L.E.; Brown, R.S., Jr.; Kato, T.; Emond, J.C. Hypothermic machine preservation facilitates successful transplantation of "orphan" extended criteria donor livers. *Am. J. Transplant.* **2015**, *15*, 161–169. [CrossRef]

32. Markmann, J.F.; Abouljoud, M.S.; Ghobrial, R.M.; Bhati, C.S.; Pelletier, S.J.; Lu, A.D.; Ottmann, S.; Klair, T.; Eymard, C.; Roll, G.R.; et al. Impact of Portable Normothermic Blood-Based Machine Perfusion on Outcomes of Liver Transplant The OCS Liver PROTECT Randomized Clinical Trial. *Jama Surg.* **2022**, *157*, 189–198. [CrossRef]

33. Vodkin, I.; Kuo, A. Extended Criteria Donors in Liver Transplantation. *Clin. Liver Dis.* **2017**, *21*, 289–301. [CrossRef] [PubMed]

34. Guorgui, J.; Ito, T.; Younan, S.; Agopian, V.G.; Dinorcia, J., III; Farmer, D.G.; Busuttil, R.W.; Kaldas, F.M. The Utility of Extended Criteria Donor Livers in High Acuity Liver Transplant Recipients. *Am. Surg.* **2021**, *87*, 1684–1689. [CrossRef]

35. Seidita, A.; Longo, R.; Di Francesco, F.; Tropea, A.; Calamia, S.; Panarello, G.; Barbara, M.; Gruttadauria, S. The use of normothermic machine perfusion to rescue liver allografts from expanded criteria donors. *Updates Surg.* **2022**, *74*, 193–202. [CrossRef] [PubMed]

36. Zhou, W.; Zhong, Z.; Lin, D.; Liu, Z.; Zhang, Q.; Xia, H.; Peng, S.; Liu, A.; Lu, Z.; Wang, Y.; et al. Hypothermic oxygenated perfusion inhibits HECTD3-mediated TRAF3 polyubiquitination to alleviate DCD liver ischemia-reperfusion injury. *Cell Death Dis.* **2021**, *12*, 211. [CrossRef]

37. Schlegel, A.; Graf, R.; Clavien, P.A.; Dutkowski, P. Hypothermic oxygenated perfusion (HOPE) protects from biliary injury in a rodent model of DCD liver transplantation. *J. Hepatol.* **2013**, *59*, 984–991. [CrossRef] [PubMed]

38. Watson, C.J.E.; Kosmoliaptsis, V.; Randle, L.V.; Gimson, A.E.; Brais, R.; Klinck, J.R.; Hamed, M.; Tsyben, A.; Butler, A.J. Normothermic Perfusion in the Assessment and Preservation of Declined Livers Before Transplantation: Hyperoxia and Vasoplegia-Important Lessons From the First 12 Cases. *Transplantation* **2017**, *101*, 1084–1098. [CrossRef]

39. Czigany, Z.; Lurje, I.; Tolba, R.H.; Neumann, U.P.; Tacke, F.; Lurje, G. Machine perfusion for liver transplantation in the era of marginal organs-New kids on the block. *Liver Int.* **2019**, *39*, 228–249. [CrossRef]

40. Boteon, Y.L.; Boteon, Y.L.; Laing, R.W.; Schlegel, A.; Wallace, L.; Smith, A.; Attard, J.; Bhogal, R.H.; Neil, D.A.; Hübscher, S.; et al. Combined Hypothermic and Normothermic Machine Perfusion Improves Functional Recovery of Extended Criteria Donor Livers. *Liver Transpl.* **2018**, *24*, 1699–1715. [CrossRef] [PubMed]

41. Matinlauri, I.H.; Nurminen, M.M.; Hockerstedt, K.A.; Isoniemi, H.M. Risk factors predicting survival of liver transplantation. *Transplant. Proc.* **2005**, *37*, 1155–1160. [CrossRef]

42. Moore, D.E.; Feurer, I.D.; Speroff, T.; Gorden, D.L.; Wright, J.K.; Chari, R.S.; Pinson, C.W. Impact of donor, technical, and recipient risk factors on survival and quality of life after liver transplantation. *Arch. Surg.* **2005**, *140*, 273–277. [CrossRef] [PubMed]

43. Bastos-Neves, D.; Salvalaggio, P.R.O.; Almeida, M.D. Risk factors, surgical complications and graft survival in liver transplant recipients with early allograft dysfunction. *Hepatobiliary Pancreat. Dis. Int.* **2019**, *18*, 423–429. [CrossRef] [PubMed]

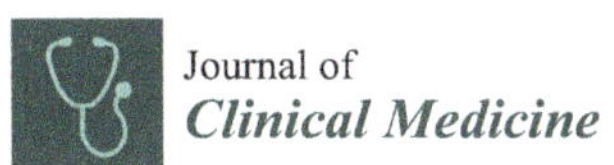

Journal of
Clinical Medicine

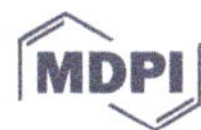

Article

Ustekinumab Promotes Radiological Fistula Healing in Perianal Fistulizing Crohn's Disease: A Retrospective Real-World Analysis

Jiayin Yao [1,†], Heng Zhang [2,†], Tao Su [1,†], Xiang Peng [1], Junzhang Zhao [1], Tao Liu [1], Wei Wang [1], Pinjin Hu [1], Min Zhi [1,*] and Min Zhang [1,*]

[1] Department of Gastroenterology, Guangdong Provincial Key Laboratory of Colorectal and Pelvic Floor Disease, The Sixth Affiliated Hospital, Sun Yat-Sen University, Guangzhou 510655, China
[2] Department of Colorectal Surgery, Guangdong Provincial Key Laboratory of Colorectal and Pelvic Floor Disease, The Sixth Affiliated Hospital, Sun Yat-Sen University, Guangzhou 510655, China
* Correspondence: zhimin@mail.sysu.edu.cn (M.Z.); zhangm72@mail.sysu.edu.cn (M.Z.); Tel.: +86-13710910365 (M.Z.); +86-13825086505 (M.Z.)
† These authors contributed equally to this work.

Abstract: There is insufficient evidence to confirm the efficacy of ustekinumab (UST) in promoting fistula closure in perianal fistulizing Crohn's disease (CD) patients. We aimed to evaluate the efficacy of UST in a real-world setting. The data were retrospectively analyzed. Intestinal clinical and endoscopic changes were evaluated. Fistula radiological outcomes were determined using the Van Assche score. A total of 108 patients were included, 43.5% of whom had complex perianal fistulas. Intestinal clinical and endoscopic remission was achieved in 65.7% and 31.5% of patients, respectively. The fistula clinical remission and response rates were 40.7% and 63.0%, respectively, with a significant reduction in Perianal Crohn's disease Activity Index [5.0(3.0, 8.0) vs. 7.5(5.0, 10.0), $p < 0.001$] and Crohn's Anal Fistula Quality of Life [23.5(9.3, 38.8) vs. 49.0(32.3, 60.0), $p < 0.001$]. Radiological healing, partial response, no change, and deterioration were observed in 44.8%, 31.4%, 13.4%, and 10.4% of patients, respectively. The cut-off UST trough concentration for predicting fistula clinical remission was 2.11 μg/mL with an area under the curve of 0.795, a sensitivity of 93.3%, and a specificity of 67.6%. UST is efficacious in promoting radiological fistula closure in patients with perianal fistulizing CD. A UST trough concentration over 2.11 μg/mL was correlated with a higher likelihood of perianal fistula clinical remission.

Keywords: Crohn's disease; ustekinumab; perianal fistula; radiological fistula remission

Citation: Yao, J.; Zhang, H.; Su, T.; Peng, X.; Zhao, J.; Liu, T.; Wang, W.; Hu, P.; Zhi, M.; Zhang, M. Ustekinumab Promotes Radiological Fistula Healing in Perianal Fistulizing Crohn's Disease: A Retrospective Real-World Analysis. *J. Clin. Med.* **2023**, *12*, 939. https://doi.org/10.3390/jcm12030939

Academic Editor: Hidekazu Suzuki

Received: 31 December 2022
Revised: 17 January 2023
Accepted: 22 January 2023
Published: 25 January 2023

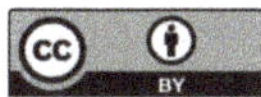

1. Introduction

Perianal fistula is the most common complication of Crohn's disease (CD), affecting approximately 40% of patients [1]. It represents an aggressive phenotype of CD, which is likely to respond poorly to multiple medications, has a high risk of relapse and disease-associated disability, and faces early-onset surgery [2,3]. Patients with perianal fistulizing CD suffer from anal pain, purulent discharge, restricted sexual activity, and abdominal symptoms, which undoubtedly result in a lower quality of life. Therefore, management and monitoring of perianal fistulizing CD remains challenging.

A multidisciplinary approach is recommended for the treatment of perianal fistulizing CD because of its complexity [4]. According to the global consensus established by Gecse in 2014 [5], for patients with perianal abscesses and active draining fistula, seton or fistulotomy should be performed, followed by aggressive medical therapies. Monoclonal antibodies against tumor necrosis factor (anti-TNF) agents, including infliximab and adalimumab, are effective in perianal fistulizing CD, as shown by the results of the ACCENT II [6] and CHARM [7] trials. However, it should not be ignored that a proportion of patients are primary non-responders to anti-TNF agents, and some have to switch to other biologics targeting different inflammatory pathways due to loss of response or development of severe adverse effects.

Ustekinumab (UST), an antibody targeting the p40 subunit shared by interleukin 12 and 23, effectively induces disease remission, as supported by the UNITI-1 and UNITI-2 clinical trials [8,9]. Our recently published study demonstrated that clinical and endoscopic remission rates were 84.2% and 73.7%, respectively, at week 16/20 after UST initiation, which adds evidence to the effectiveness of UST in refractory CD [10]. However, there is still no strong evidence supporting the efficacy of UST in treating perianal fistulizing CD, despite a series of post hoc or subgroup analyses [11,12].

We aimed to assess the short-term efficacy of UST in treating perianal fistulizing CD, especially in promoting radiological fistula healing, and to evaluate the UST trough concentration for predicting clinical fistula remission.

2. Methods

2.1. Study Design

This was a retrospective cohort study based on the data of patients with perianal fistulizing CD from 1 March 2020 to 31 October 2022 at the Sixth Affiliated Hospital of Sun Yat-Sen University (Guangzhou, China). This study was approved by the Ethics Committee of Sun Yat-Sen University (2021ZSLYEC-066) and the Clinical Trial Registry (NCT04923100). Consent from the patients was waived because all the data we used were anonymous. All procedures were performed in accordance with the principles of the Declaration of Helsinki.

2.2. Patients

Consecutive patients meeting the following inclusion criteria were included: First, patients underwent comprehensive screening and diagnosis for CD according to internationally accepted criteria [13,14] with supportive clinical, endoscopic, radiological, and histopathological findings. Second, active perianal fistula was confirmed by clinical symptoms and baseline magnetic resonance imaging (MRI). Third, patients were administered UST therapy and followed up until the third infusion at weeks 16 or 20, with a drug interval of q8w or q12w, respectively. Patients with incomplete data, development of severe adverse events, and discontinuation of UST therapy within 16 weeks were excluded.

All patients were first infused with intravenous UST (260 mg for those weighing <55 kg, 520 mg for those weighing >85 kg, and 390 mg for those weighing between 55–85 kg) and subcutaneous UST (90 mg every 8 or 12 weeks) afterward [15]. Perianal surgeries were performed if needed before the initiation of UST infusion. The indications for surgery include the following: (1) acute abscess formation; (2) marked purulent external orifice, which worsens the quality of life; (3) an active fistula revealed by MRI scan with the characteristics including lesion range larger than 1 cm, deep ramification, or multiple ramification formation. The protocols for prior surgery include abscess incision, partial extra-sphinteric fistulotomy or fistulectomy, and loose seton drainage. Concomitant oral antibiotics including metronidazole and ciprofloxacin were prescribed for 4 weeks after surgery. As for the patients with loose seton, a second definite surgical repair or seton removal was evaluated at week 16/20 after UST initiation. The UST trough concentration and antidrug antibodies were detected before the third infusion of UST. Data on patient characteristics, serologic biomarkers (including C-reactive protein [CRP], erythrocyte sedimentation rate, platelets, hemoglobin, and albumin, and imaging were extracted from hospital digital records.

2.3. Definition

CD was classified using the widely accepted Montreal classification system [16]. Crohn's disease activity index (CDAI) [17], perianal Crohn's disease activity index (PDAI) [18], and Crohn's anal fistula quality of life (CAF-QoL) [19] were evaluated at baseline and at week 16/20. Intestinal clinical remission was defined as a CDAI < 150, and intestinal clinical response was defined as a >70 reduction in CDAI and/or CDAI < 150 [17]. Fistula clinical remission was defined as the absence of any draining fistula, and fistula clinical response was defined as a decrease of >50% in the number of draining fistulas according to the fistula drainage assessment index (FDA) [1]. Rutgeerts [20] scores and simple endoscopic score for Crohn's disease (SES-CD) [21] were used to evaluate the changes in endoscopic findings in patients with or without colectomy, respectively. Endoscopic remission was defined as a Rutgeerts score ≤i1 or SES-CD ≤2 [20,21]. Endoscopic response was defined as a reduction of one grade from baseline in Rutgeerts score or a reduction of >50% in SES-CD [20,21]. C-reactive protein (CRP) normalization was defined as a CRP level of <4 mg/L.

MRI was performed to evaluate the fistula status. The number of fistulas, anatomical-classification, hyperintensity on the fat-saturated T2 sequence, and track thickness and volume were recorded. A simple fistula was defined as a superficial/inter-sphincteric/trans-sphincteric fistula with only one track, without extension or abscess. Complex fistulas were defined as inter-sphincteric/trans-sphincteric fistulas with more than one track, or supra-sphincteric/extra-sphincteric/rectovaginal fistula [1]. Four MRI-based radiological outcomes were described, including healing, improvement, no change, and deterioration. Radiological fistula healing was defined as the absence of a high signal track on fat satu rated T2 sequences. Improvement was defined as a reduction in the number and volume of fistula, and >10% decrease in the MRI signal. No change was defined as the same in the number of fistulas and the volume of inflammation. Deterioration was defined as an increase in the size and number of fistula tracks [22]. Van Assche scores [23] ranging from 0 to 22 reflected fistula activity, including fistula number, location, extension, hyperintensity on T2, collections, and rectal wall involvement. Two specialists from the Colorectal Department (HZ and BH) diagnosed perianal fistulizing CD and assessed the improvement of perianal fistula based on gentle compression, examination under anesthesia, and MRI scans. Two experienced radiologists (WTC and WRL) read the MRI scans, evaluated the radiological outcomes, and recorded the Van Assche scores. Clinical, endoscopic, and radiological evaluations were recommended at week 16/20.

2.4. Statistical Analysis

Continuous data were presented as mean ± standard error (S.D.E) or median with interquartile range (IQR), while categorical data were presented as percentages. Student's *t*-test or Wilcoxon test was performed to compare indicators before and after UST treatment. A receiver operating characteristic (ROC) curve was established to figure out the cut-off value of UST trough concentration for predicting clinical fistula remission with the area under the curve (AUC), sensitivity, and specificity calculated. All analyses were conducted using SPSS 22.0. A statistically significant *p*-value was defined as a two-sided *p*-value < 0.05.

3. Results

3.1. Patients' Characteristics

A total of 308 patients diagnosed with CD and receiving scheduled UST treatment were enrolled. Of these, 137 patients were excluded due to the absence of perianal fistula based on clinical symptoms and MRI scans, 51 for insufficient follow-up duration, and 12 for incomplete data (Figure 1). A total of 108 eligible patients were finally included, 74.1% of whom were male, with a mean age of 29.2 ± 1.0 years at diagnosis and a mean disease duration of 4.3 ± 0.4 years. As for the Montreal classification, 61.1% of the patients were assigned to B1 (non-stricturing, non-penetrating) and 71.3% to L3 (ileocolonic) phenotypes. Most fistulas were inter-sphincteric (63.9%), followed by superficial (18.5%), trans-sphincteric (15.7%), and supra-sphincteric (1.9%). Of the fistulas, 43.5% were complex fistulas, with a median baseline Van Assche score of 9.0 (7.0,14.0), as determined by MRI scans. Of the patients, 29.6% had perianal abscesses and 57.4% had proctitis. Among them, 14 patients underwent fistulotomy before UST therapy, 2 of whom received additional ileostomy due to the severe proximal intestinal lesion. The baseline characteristics are listed in Table 1.

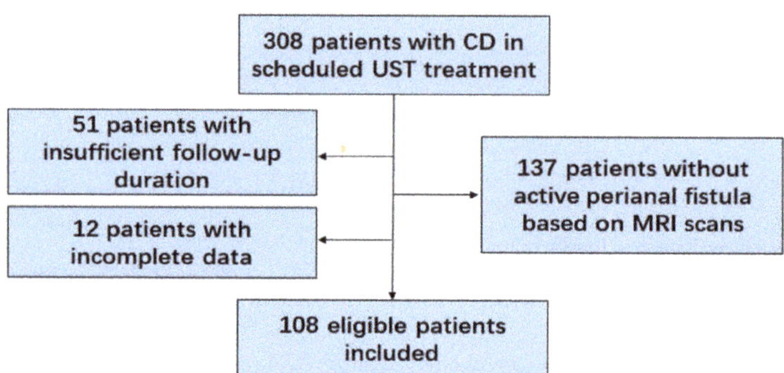

Figure 1. Flow chart of the study (CD, Crohn's disease; UST, ustekinumab; MRI, magnetic resonance imaging).

Table 1. Baseline characteristics of overall patients.

Variables	Total Patients (*n* = 108)
Male, *n* (%)	80 (74.1)
Age at diagnosis, [years, mean ± S.D.E]	29.2 ± 1.0
Disease duration, [years, mean ± S.D.E]	4.3 ± 0.4
Montreal classification	
Age, *n* (%)	
A1 (≤16 years)	8 (7.4)
A2 (17–40 years)	87 (80.6)
A3 (>40 years)	13 (12.0)
Disease behavior, *n* (%)	
B1 (non-stricturing, non-penetrating)	66 (61.1)
B2 (stricturing)	13 (12.0)
B3 (penetrating)	29 (26.9)
Disease location, *n* (%)	
L1 (ileal)	20 (18.5)
L2 (colonic)	11 (10.2)
L3 (ileocolonic)	77 (71.3)
L4 (upper GI)	21 (19.4)
Fistula type, *n* (%)	
Simple	61 (56.5)
Complex	47 (43.5)
Fistula location, *n* (%)	
Superficial	20 (18.5)
Inter-sphincteric	69 (63.9)
Trans-sphincteric	17 (15.7)
Supra-sphincteric	2 (1.9)
Extra-sphincteric	0 (0)
Van Assche at baseline, median (IQR)	9.0 (7.0,14.0)
Proctitis, *n* (%)	62 (57.4)
Perianal abscess, *n* (%)	32 (29.6)
Previous medication, *n* (%)	
Steroids	50 (46.3)
Immunosuppressants [1]	76 (70.4)
Anti-TNF agents [2]	70 (64.8)
Previous intestinal surgery, *n* (%)	27 (25.0)
Extraintestinal manifestation, *n* (%)	8 (7.4)

[1] Immunosuppressants includes thiopurines, methotrexate, cyclophosphane, and thalidomide. [2] Anti-TNF agents refers to infliximab or/and adalimumab. IQR, interquartile range; S.D.E, standard error; GI, gastrointestinal.

3.2. Efficacy of UST on CD

After administration of UST, the patients showed less inflammatory burden manifested by a significant decrease in CRP (14.6 ± 2.4 vs. 24.0 ± 3.2, $p = 0.002$), and improved nutrition manifested by an increase in hemoglobin (129.8 ± 2.1 vs. 119.0 ± 2.1, $p < 0.001$) and Alb (40.2 ± 5.7 vs. 36.9 ± 5.1, $p < 0.001$) (Table 2). Intestinal clinical remission was observed in 65.7% of patients, and intestinal clinical response was observed in 71.3% of patients (Figure 2A). CRP normalization was achieved in 55.6% of patients (Figure 2B). A total of 99 patients had endoscopy reexamination, of whom 22 patients were evaluated by Rutgeerts score and 77 by SES-CD. Endoscopic remission and response were achieved in 31.5% and 45.4% of patients, respectively (Figure 2C).

Table 2. Efficacy of UST on patients with perianal fistulizing CD ($n = 108$).

Variables	Baseline	Week 16/20	p Value
Inflammatory burden (mean $\pm$ S.D.E)			
CRP (mg/L)	24.0 ± 3.2	14.6 ± 2.4	0.002
ESR (mm/h)	22.8 ± 2.3	18.2 ± 1.6	0.051
Platelet ($\times 109$/L)	311.9 ± 9.4	296.4 ± 9.1	0.090
Nutritional state (mean $\pm$ S.D.E)			
Hemoglobin (g/L)	119.0 ± 2.1	129.8 ± 2.1	<0.001
Alb (g/L)	36.9 ± 5.1	40.2 ± 5.7	<0.001
BMI	19.0 ± 2.9	19.3 ± 3.3	0.247
Intestinal clinical evaluation (IQR)			
CDAI	179.5 (117.6, 258.2)	112.2 (71.9, 171.8)	<0.001
Fistula clinical evaluation (IQR)			
PDAI	7.5 (5.0, 10.0)	5.0 (3.0, 8.0)	<0.001
CAF-QoL	49.0 (32.3, 60.0)	23.5 (9.3, 38.8)	<0.001

CRP: c-reactive protein; ESR: erythrocyte sedimentation rate; Alb: albumin; BMI: body mass index; CDAI: Crohn's disease activity index; PDAI: perianal Crohn's disease activity index; CAF-QoL: Crohn's anal fistula quality of life; CD, Crohn's disease; UST, ustekinumab; IQR, interquartile range; S.D.E, standard error.

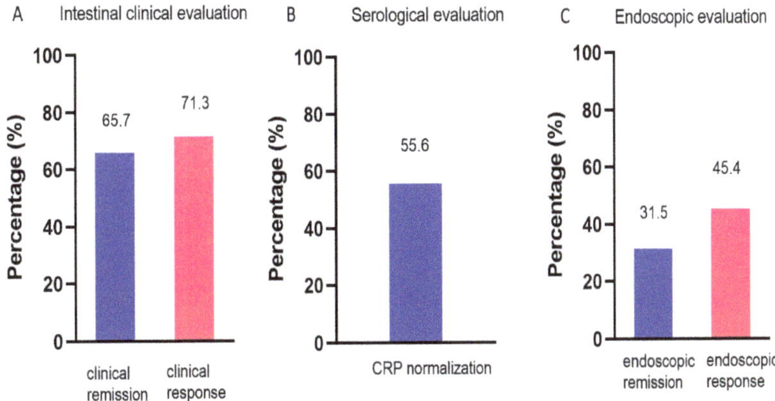

Figure 2. Efficacy of UST on CD. (**A**) Intestinal clinical evaluation using CDAI at week 16/20, $n = 108$. (**B**) Serological evaluation determined by CRP levels, $n = 108$. (**C**) Endoscopic evaluation using Rutgeerts score or SES-CD, $n = 99$. UST: ustekinumab; CDAI: Crohn's disease activity index; CRP: C-reactive protein; SES-CD: simple endoscopic score for Crohn's disease.

3.3. Efficacy of UST on Perianal Fistulas

For all enrolled patients, a marked reduction in PDAI (5.0(3.0, 8.0) vs. 7.5(5.0, 10.0), $p < 0.001$) and CAF-QoL (23.5(9.3, 38.8) vs. 49.0(32.3, 60.0), $p < 0.001$) indicated the mitigation of fistulas (Table 2). Fistula clinical remission was observed in 40.7% and fistula clinical response in 63.0% of patients (Figure 3A). All the patients were required to return at week 16/20 after UST initiation for clinical, endoscopic, and radiological reevaluation. However, a proportion of patients refused MRI reexamination due to disappearance of perianal symptoms, economic burden, or time constraint. Eventually, 62.0% (67/108) of the patients underwent MRI scans. The percentages of patients with fistula healing, partial response, no change, and deterioration were 44.8%, 31.4%, 13.4%, and 10.4%, respectively (Figure 3B). After UST treatment, the Van Assche score significantly decreased (5.5(0.0, 10.0) vs. 9.0(7.0, 14.0), $p < 0.001$), indicating the confirmed amelioration in fistula radiological outcomes (Figure 3C).

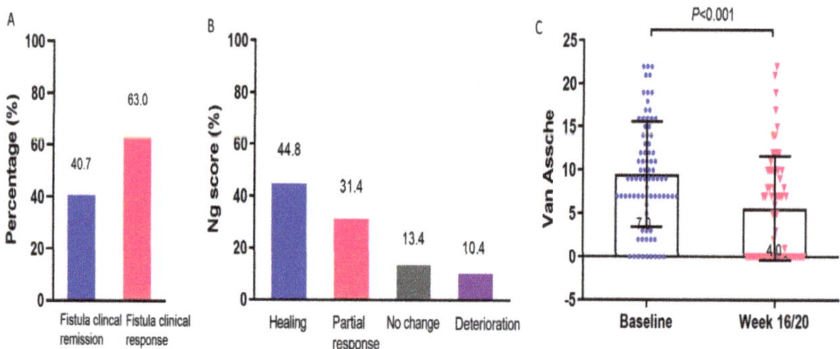

Figure 3. Efficacy of UST on perianal fistula. (**A**) Fistula clinical remission and response rates determined by PDAI, $n = 108$. (**B**) Radiological outcomes evaluated by Ng score, $n = 67$. (**C**) Changes in Van Assche scores before and after UST therapy, $n = 67$. UST: ustekinumab; PDAI: perianal Crohn's disease activity index.

3.4. Efficacy of UST on Anti-TNF Naïve and Exposure Patients

We further evaluated the efficacy of UST on patients who were anti-TNF naïve and those who had anti-TNF exposure. Intestinal clinical remission rate in anti-TNF naïve patients was significantly higher than that in anti-TNF exposure patients (78.9% vs. 58.6%, $p = 0.033$). There was no significant difference in intestinal clinical response, fistula clinical remission and response, endoscopic remission and response, and radiological remission between the two groups (Table 3). Nevertheless, we did observe more favorable remission and response rates in clinical, endoscopic, and radiological evaluations in anti-TNF naïve patients, although not statistically significant, according to the subgroup analysis.

Table 3. Efficacy of UST on patients with anti-TNF exposure and anti-TNF naïve.

Variables	Anti-TNF Naïve [1]	Anti-TNF Exposure	*p* Value
Intestinal clinical remission, n/n (%) ($n = 108$)	30/38 (78.9)	41/70 (58.6)	0.033
Intestinal clinical response, n/n (%) ($n = 108$)	30/38 (78.9)	47/70 (67.1)	0.195
Fistula clinical remission, n/n (%) ($n = 108$)	20/38 (52.6)	24/70 (34.3)	0.064

Table 3. *Cont.*

Variables	Anti-TNF Naïve [1]	Anti-TNF Exposure	*p* Value
Fistula clinical response, *n/n* (%) (*n* = 108)	25/38 (65.8)	42/70 (60.0)	0.554
Endoscopic remission, *n/n* (%) (*n* = 99)	14/35 (40.0)	17/64 (26.6)	0.381
Endoscopic response, *n/n* (%) (*n* = 99)	20/35 (57.1)	25/64 (39.1)	0.260
Radiological remission, *n/n* (%) (*n* = 67)	14/25 (56.0)	16/42 (38.1)	0.154

[1] Anti-TNF agents refers to infliximab or/and adalimumab.

3.5. Relationship of CD Clinical Remission and Clinical Fistula Response

Fistula clinical fistula remission/response was observed in 80.3% of the patients who had achieved intestinal clinical remission, but only 43.2% in those who did not, indicating that intestinal clinical remission positively correlated with fistula clinical remission.

3.6. Exposure–Response Effect of UST on Perianal Fistulizing CD

Overall, 64 patients had UST trough concentration detected at week 16/20 after initiation of UST. The median UST trough concentration at week 16/20 was 2.4 (0.9, 3.5) µg/mL. In a quartile analysis of UST trough concentrations, we demonstrated that fistula clinical remission and response rates correlated with UST trough levels. Higher rates of fistula clinical remission and response were observed in the higher UST trough concentration group (Figure 4A). A significantly higher fistula remission and response rate was found in the higher UST trough concentration quartile. The cut-off UST trough concentration predicting clinical fistula remission was 2.11 µg/mL, with an AUC of 0.795, a sensitivity of 93.3%, and a specificity of 67.6% (Figure 4B). Figure 5 showed a typical case manifesting radiological fistula healing after UST therapy in patients with perianal fistulizing CD.

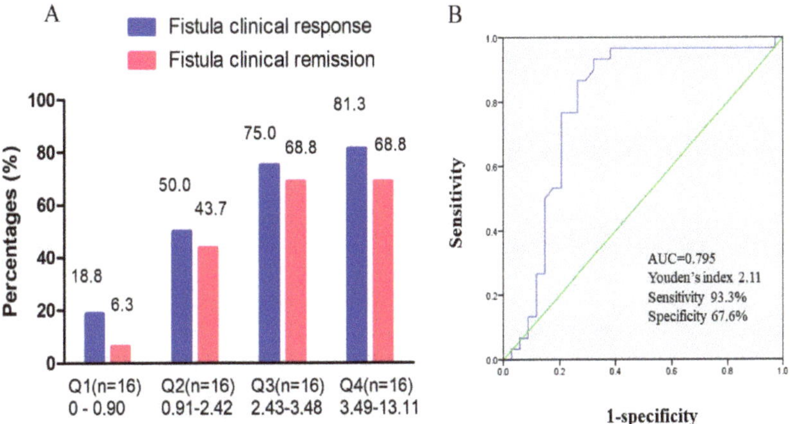

Figure 4. Exposure–response effect of UST on fistula clinical outcome. (**A**) Quartile analysis of UST trough concentration associated with fistula clinical remission and response. (**B**) ROC curve of UST trough concentration at week 16/20 predicting clinical fistula remission. The cut-off UST trough concentration was 2.11 µg/mL, with an AUC of 0.795 [95%CI: 0.675–0.915], a sensitivity of 93.3%, and a specificity of 67.6%. ROC, receiver operating characteristic; UST, ustekinumab; AUC, area under the curve; CI, confidence interval.

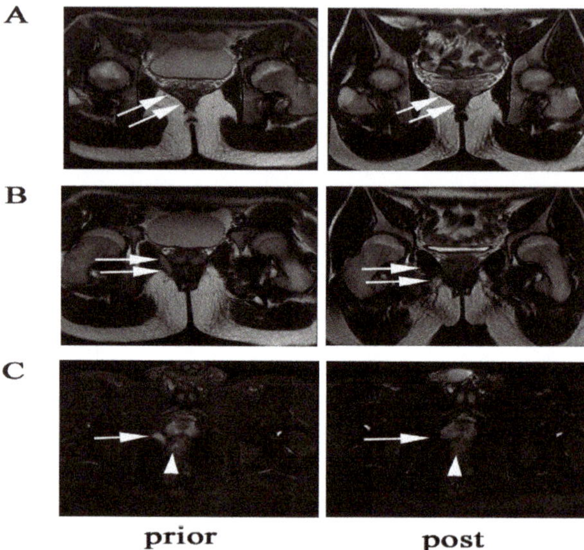

Figure 5. A case showing radiological fistula healing of a supralevator fistula. (**A**) The arrows show the supralevator part of the fistula closure with scarring. (**B**) The arrows show the infralevator part of the fistulas closure with scarring. (**C**) The arrows show vanishment of the supralevator lesion, and the triangle shows improvement of proctitis.

4. Discussion

In this study, approximately 40% of the patients achieved fistula clinical remission after UST initiation. Of note, 44.8% of the patients achieved deep radiological fistula healing according to post-treatment MRI. Our clinical and radiological results verified the acceptable short-term efficacy of UST for perianal fistulizing CD, particularly in promoting radiological fistula closure.

Infliximab was the first proven effective biologic in promoting and maintaining CD-related fistula closure, supported by high-quality randomized controlled trials (RCTs) with fistula closure as the primary endpoint [24]. According to a multicenter, double-blind RCT conducted by Daniel et al. [6], 40% of patients had a complete fistula response at week 54 after scheduled infliximab administration. Adalimumab is effective in treating fistulizing CD, however only with low-grade evidence [25]. Majority of studies reported that 30–50% of patients achieved clinical fistula remission after long-term anti-TNF therapies [6,26,27]. Our results manifested that 40.7% of the patients presented fistula closure after initiation of UST, which was similar to those reported previously. Given that this study focused solely on the short-term efficacy of UST, favorable long-term outcomes may be expected.

UST is the second-line biologic recommended for perianal fistulizing CD. A post hoc analysis of UNITI-1/UNITI-2 reported that 24.7% of patients achieved fistula closure at week 8 and 80% of patients achieved clinical fistula response at week 44 after UST treatment [28]. The BioLAP study [29], including 207 patients with perianal CD, was a retrospective trial with the largest sample size reported to date. Therapeutic success was achieved in 38.5% of patients treated with UST. A prospective observational study in the Netherlands reported that 35.7% (10/28) of patients achieved clinical fistula remission 24 weeks after UST initiation [30]. However, RCTs are still lacking with regards to fistula closure as the primary endpoint to evaluate the efficacy of UST on perianal fistula.

UST was first approved for the treatment of CD in 2016 in America and in 2020 in China. The efficacy of UST on CD has rarely been reported in China, and has never been reported in perianal fistulizing CD. To our knowledge, this is the first real-world study conducted in Chinese population to report the effectiveness of UST in perianal fistulizing CD. The fistula clinical remission rate was 40.7%, similar to that reported previously [31]. We focused more on radiological outcome regarding that radiological fistula healing always lags behind fistula clinical remission and calls for greater efforts to realize it. However, our results showed approximately 45% of patients had achieved radiological fistula healing, which undoubtedly adds our confidence in efficacy of UST in the treatment of perianal fistulizing CD. Moreover, a better performance of UST was seen on patients who were biologic-naïve manifested by the significantly higher rate in intestinal clinical remission according to our subgroup analysis, which was consistent with the well-known SUCCESS trial [32]. Nevertheless, there was no significant difference in the effectiveness of UST in promoting clinical or radiological fistula healing in biologic-naïve and biologic-exposure patients.

Pelvic MRI is a pivotal tool for perianal fistula diagnosis, classification, severity evaluation, and monitoring. Radiological fistula healing continues after clinical fistula closure, for internal tracks may persist despite closure of the external opening, leading to a higher rate of relapse [33]. Patients who achieve radiological fistula remission may maintain fistula resolution, regardless of continuation or discontinuation of anti-TNF therapy [34]. In this study, all eligible patients had a precise diagnosis and classification of perianal fistula based on MRI scans. In addition, 62.0% (67/108) of the patients underwent MRI scans at the post-therapy follow-up. The radiological fistula healing rate was 44.8%, indicating the ideal efficacy of UST for complete fistula closure. Follow-up imaging can assist with disease monitoring and therapeutic management.

Perianal fistulizing CD exerts profound effects on patient's psychosocial state and daily life [35]. To date, limited data have been obtained regarding the effect of perianal fistulas on quality of life. The PDAI is widely used to measure CD-associated perianal disease activity. It is neither specific to perianal fistulas nor patient-centered [36]. CAF-QoL is the first disease-specific and patient-reported outcome index in clinical practice, involving factors such as burden of symptoms and treatment, and negative impact on quality of life [19]. In this study, we combined the PDAI and CAF-QoL to evaluate the impact of perianal fistulas on patients with CD. Favorable changes in both the PDAI and CAF-QoL were observed after UST therapy.

It has been reported that an IFX concentration of 12 µg/mL is associated with fistula remission. Optimizing biologics correlates with a higher response rate in perianal fistulizing CD patients [37,38]. Nevertheless, no studies have yet proposed a cut-off UST trough level associated with fistula healing. Sands et al. concluded that perianal fistula resolution is not associated with a higher UST serum concentration [39]. In contrast, one observational study noted that 50% of patients with UST escalation into q4w or q6w administration intervals achieved a clinical response in perianal disease [40]. In this study, we did manifest the exposure–effect relationship between clinical fistula remission and UST trough levels. The cut-off value of UST we reported was 2.11 µg/mL, which was much higher than 1.12 µg/mL, the cut-off value of UST associated with clinical remission (defined as CDAI < 150) that we reported previously [10]. Undoubtedly, more high-quality studies are needed to further verify the relationship between UST escalation and fistula outcome.

This study had some limitations. First, this was a single-center study with a relatively small sample size. The evidence from this retrospective study should be validated further in a larger sample size from multiple IBD centers nationwide. Moreover, we only manifested the short-term efficacy of UST in perianal fistulizing CD with short-term follow-up; hence, and the long-term efficacy and the safety of UST for perianal fistula was not evaluated. The strengths of this study include strict definitions, radiological evaluation combined with clinical assessment, and emphasis on quality of life.

5. Conclusions

In conclusion, UST is effective in promoting clinical and radiological fistula remission in patients with CD. A trough concentration of UST higher than 2.11 µg/mL was associated with clinical fistula remission at week 16/20. More RCTs with fistula closure as the primary outcome are warranted to evaluate the efficacy of UST in treating perianal fistulizing CD in-depth.

Author Contributions: All authors have made a significant contribution to this research article. J.Y., H.Z. and T.S.: Study concept and design, analysis of data and manuscript drafting. X.P., J.Z., T.L., W.W. and P.H.: Acquisition and analysis of data. M.Z. (Min Zhi) and M.Z. (Min Zhang): Critical revision of the manuscript. M.Z. (Min Zhi) and M.Z. (Min Zhang): Final approval of the version to be submitted. All authors approved the final manuscript as well as the authorship list. All authors have read and agreed to the published version of the manuscript.

Funding: This research was funded by the National Natural Science Foundation of China [81900490 81670477 and 82270544], Project 5010 of Sun Yat-Sen University [2014008], Project 1010 of Sixth Affiliated Hospital of Sun Yat-Sen University [1010PY(2020)-55], Qingfeng Scientific Research Fund of the China Crohn's & Colitis Foundation (CCCF-QF-2022A53-2 and CCCF-QF-2022B43-14) and Young Teacher Foundation of Sun Yat-Sen University [22qntd3604].

Institutional Review Board Statement: This study was approved by the Ethics Committee of Sun Yat-Sen University (2021ZSLYEC-066) and was approved by the Clinical Trial Registry (NCT04923100).

Informed Consent Statement: Due to the retrospective study design, which used anonymous data, written informed consent from the patients was waived.

Data Availability Statement: The data that support the findings of this study are available from the corresponding author upon reasonable request.

Acknowledgments: The authors thank Wuteng Cao and Wenru Li from Department of Radiology, Bang Hu from Department of Colorectal Surgery, Sixth Affiliated Hospital, Sun Yat-Sen University for their assistance in radiological assessment.

Conflicts of Interest: The authors declare no conflict of interest.

References

1. Caron, B.; D'Amico, F.; Danese, S.; Peyrin-Biroulet, L. Endpoints for Perianal Crohn's Disease Trials: Past, Present and Future. *J. Crohns Colitis* **2021**, *15*, 1387–1398. [CrossRef]
2. Shmidt, E.; Ho, E.Y.; Feuerstein, J.D.; Singh, S.; Terdiman, J.P. Spotlight: Medical Management of Moderate to Severe Luminal and Perianal Fistulizing Crohn's Disease. *Gastroenterology* **2021**, *160*, 2511. [CrossRef]
3. Barreiro Dominguez, E.M.; Vazquez-Garcia, I.; Perez-Corbal, L.; Ballinas Miranda, J.R.; Antelo, J.S.; Parajo Calvo, A. Mesenchymal stem cells for the treatment of perianal fistulizing Crohn's disease-A video vignette. *Colorectal Dis.* **2022**, *24*, 1441–1442. [CrossRef]
4. Wiseman, J.; Chawla, T.; Morin, F.; de Buck van Overstraeten, A.; Weizman, A.V. A Multi-Disciplinary Approach to Perianal Fistulizing Crohn's Disease. *Clin. Colon. Rectal Surg.* **2022**, *35*, 51–57. [CrossRef]
5. Gecse, K.B.; Bemelman, W.; Kamm, M.A.; Stoker, J.; Khanna, R.; Ng, S.C.; Panes, J.; van Assche, G.; Liu, Z.; Hart, A.; et al. A global consensus on the classification, diagnosis and multidisciplinary treatment of perianal fistulising Crohn's disease. *Gut* **2014**, *63*, 1381–1392. [CrossRef]
6. Sands, B.E.; Anderson, F.H.; Bernstein, C.N.; Chey, W.Y.; Feagan, B.G.; Fedorak, R.N.; Kamm, M.A.; Korzenik, J.R.; Lashner, B.A.; Onken, J.E.; et al. Infliximab maintenance therapy for fistulizing Crohn's disease. *N. Engl. J. Med.* **2004**, *350*, 876–885. [CrossRef]
7. Colombel, J.F.; Sandborn, W.J.; Rutgeerts, P.; Enns, R.; Hanauer, S.B.; Panaccione, R.; Schreiber, S.; Byczkowski, D.; Li, J.; Kent, J.D.; et al. Adalimumab for maintenance of clinical response and remission in patients with Crohn's disease: The CHARM trial. *Gastroenterology* **2007**, *132*, 52–65. [CrossRef]
8. Adedokun, O.J.; Xu, Z.; Gasink, C.; Jacobstein, D.; Szapary, P.; Johanns, J.; Gao, L.L.; Davis, H.M.; Hanauer, S.B.; Feagan, B.G.; et al. Pharmacokinetics and Exposure Response Relationships of Ustekinumab in Patients with Crohn's Disease. *Gastroenterology* **2018**, *154*, 1660–1671. [CrossRef]
9. Feagan, B.G.; Sandborn, W.J.; Gasink, C.; Jacobstein, D.; Lang, Y.; Friedman, J.R.; Blank, M.A.; Johanns, J.; Gao, L.L.; Miao, Y.; et al. Ustekinumab as Induction and Maintenance Therapy for Crohn's Disease. *N. Engl. J. Med.* **2016**, *375*, 1946–1960. [CrossRef]
10. Yao, J.Y.; Zhang, M.; Wang, W.; Peng, X.; Zhao, J.Z.; Liu, T.; Li, Z.W.; Sun, H.T.; Hu, P.; Zhi, M. Ustekinumab trough concentration affects clinical and endoscopic outcomes in patients with refractory Crohn's disease: A Chinese real-world study. *BMC Gastroenterol.* **2021**, *21*, 380. [CrossRef]
11. Rubin de Celix, C.; Chaparro, M.; Gisbert, J.P. Real-World Evidence of the Effectiveness and Safety of Ustekinumab for the Treatment of Crohn's Disease: Systematic Review and Meta-Analysis of Observational Studies. *J. Clin. Med.* **2022**, *11*, 4202. [CrossRef]
12. Honap, S.; Meade, S.; Ibraheim, H.; Irving, P.M.; Jones, M.P.; Samaan, M.A. Effectiveness and Safety of Ustekinumab in Inflammatory Bowel Disease: A Systematic Review and Meta-Analysis. *Dig. Dis. Sci.* **2022**, *67*, 1018–1035. [CrossRef]
13. Gomollon, F.; Dignass, A.; Annese, V.; Tilg, H.; Van Assche, G.; Lindsay, J.O.; Peyrin-Biroulet, L.; Cullen, G.J.; Daperno, M.; Kucharzik, T.; et al. 3rd European Evidence-based Consensus on the Diagnosis and Management of Crohn's Disease 2016: Part 1: Diagnosis and Medical Management. *J. Crohns Colitis* **2017**, *11*, 3–25. [CrossRef]

14. Inflammatory Bowel Disease Group; Chinese Society of Gastroenterology; Chinese Medical Association. Chinese consensus on diagnosis and treatment in inflammatory bowel disease (2018, Beijing). *J. Dig. Dis.* **2021**, *22*, 298–317. [CrossRef]
15. Kotze, P.G.; Ma, C.; Almutairdi, A.; Panaccione, R. Clinical utility of ustekinumab in Crohn's disease. *J. Inflamm. Res.* **2018**, *11*, 35–47. [CrossRef]
16. Satsangi, J.; Silverberg, M.S.; Vermeire, S.; Colombel, J.F. The Montreal classification of inflammatory bowel disease: Controversies, consensus, and implications. *Gut* **2006**, *55*, 749–753. [CrossRef]
17. Thia, K.; Faubion, W.A., Jr.; Loftus, E.V., Jr.; Persson, T.; Persson, A.; Sandborn, W.J. Short CDAI: Development and validation of a shortened and simplified Crohn's disease activity index. *Inflamm. Bowel Dis.* **2011**, *17*, 105–111. [CrossRef] [PubMed]
18. Irvine, E.J. Usual therapy improves perianal Crohn's disease as measured by a new disease activity index. McMaster IBD Study Group. *J. Clin. Gastroenterol.* **1995**, *20*, 27–32.
19. Adegbola, S.O.; Dibley, L.; Sahnan, K.; Wade, T.; Verjee, A.; Sawyer, R.; Mannick, S.; McCluskey, D.; Bassett, P.; Yassin, N.; et al. Development and initial psychometric validation of a patient-reported outcome measure for Crohn's perianal fistula: The Crohn's Anal Fistula Quality of Life (CAF-QoL) scale. *Gut* **2021**, *70*, 1649–1656. [CrossRef]
20. Rutgeerts, P.; Geboes, K.; Vantrappen, G.; Beyls, J.; Kerremans, R.; Hiele, M. Predictability of the postoperative course of Crohn's disease. *Gastroenterology* **1990**, *99*, 956–963. [CrossRef]
21. Daperno, M.; D'Haens, G.; Van Assche, G.; Baert, F.; Bulois, P.; Maunoury, V.; Sostegni, R.; Rocca, R.; Pera, A.; Gevers, A.; et al. Development and validation of a new, simplified endoscopic activity score for Crohn's disease: The SES-CD. *Gastrointest. Endosc.* **2004**, *60*, 505–512. [CrossRef]
22. Ng, S.C.; Plamondon, S.; Gupta, A.; Burling, D.; Swatton, A.; Vaizey, C.J.; Kamm, M.A. Prospective evaluation of anti-tumor necrosis factor therapy guided by magnetic resonance imaging for Crohn's perineal fistulas. *Am. J. Gastroenterol.* **2009**, *104*, 2973–2986. [CrossRef]
23. Van Assche, G.; Vanbeckevoort, D.; Bielen, D.; Coremans, G.; Aerden, I.; Noman, M.; D'Hoore, A.; Penninckx, F.; Marchal, G.; Cornillie, F.; et al. Magnetic resonance imaging of the effects of infliximab on perianal fistulizing Crohn's disease. *Am. J. Gastroenterol.* **2003**, *98*, 332–339. [CrossRef]
24. Gu, B.; Venkatesh, K.; Williams, A.J.; Ng, W.; Corte, C.; Gholamrezaei, A.; Ghaly, S.; Xuan, W.; Paramsothy, S.; Connor, S. Higher infliximab and adalimumab trough levels are associated with fistula healing in patients with fistulising perianal Crohn's disease. *World J. Gastroenterol.* **2022**, *28*, 2597–2608. [CrossRef]
25. Dunleavy, K.A.; Pardi, D.S. Biologics: How far can they go in Crohn's disease? *Gastroenterol. Rep.* **2022**, *10*, goac049. [CrossRef]
26. Yang, B.L.; Chen, Y.G.; Gu, Y.F.; Chen, H.J.; Sun, G.D.; Zhu, P.; Shao, W.J. Long-term outcome of infliximab combined with surgery for perianal fistulizing Crohn's disease. *World J. Gastroenterol.* **2015**, *21*, 2475–2482. [CrossRef]
27. Papamichael, K.; Vande Casteele, N.; Jeyarajah, J.; Jairath, V.; Osterman, M.T.; Cheifetz, A.S. Higher Postinduction Infliximab Concentrations Are Associated with Improved Clinical Outcomes in Fistulizing Crohn's Disease: An ACCENT-II Post Hoc Analysis. *Am. J. Gastroenterol.* **2021**, *116*, 1007–1014. [CrossRef]
28. Sands, B.E.; Gasink, C.; Jacobstein, D.; Gao, L.L.; Johanns, J.; Colombel, J.F.; de Villiers, W.J.; Sandborn, W.J. Fistula healing in prvotal studies of Ustekinumab in Crohn's disease. *Gastroenterology* **2017**, *152*, S185. [CrossRef]
29. Chapuis-Biron, C.; Kirchgesner, J.; Pariente, B.; Bouhnik, Y.; Amiot, A.; Viennot, S.; Serrero, M.; Fumery, M.; Allez, M.; Siproudhis, L.; et al. Ustekinumab for Perianal Crohn's Disease: The BioLAP Multicenter Study from the GETAID. *Am. J. Gastroenterol.* **2020**, *115*, 1812–1820. [CrossRef]
30. Biemans, V.B.C.; van der Meulen-de Jong, A.E.; van der Woude, C.J.; Lowenberg, M.; Dijkstra, G.; Oldenburg, B.; de Boer, N.K.H.; van der Marel, S.; Bodelier, A.G.L.; Jansen, J.M.; et al. Ustekinumab for Crohn's Disease: Results of the ICC Registry, a Nationwide Prospective Observational Cohort Study. *J. Crohns Colitis* **2020**, *14*, 33–45. [CrossRef]
31. Attauabi, M.; Burisch, J.; Seidelin, J.B. Efficacy of ustekinumab for active perianal fistulizing Crohn's disease: A systematic review and meta-analysis of the current literature. *Scand. J. Gastroenterol.* **2021**, *56*, 53–58. [CrossRef]
32. Johnson, A.M.; Barsky, M.; Ahmed, W.; Zullow, S.; Galati, J.; Jairath, V.; Narula, N.; Peerani, F.; Click, B.H.; Coburn, E.S.; et al. The Real-World Effectiveness and Safety of Ustekinumab in the Treatment of Crohn's Disease: Results from the SUCCESS Consortium. *Am. J. Gastroenterol.* **2022**, in press. [CrossRef] [PubMed]
33. Tao, Y.; Li, H.; Xu, H.; Tang, W.; Fan, G.; Yang, X. Can the simplified magnetic resonance index of activity be used to evaluate the degree of activity in Crohn's disease? *BMC Gastroenterol.* **2021**, *21*, 409. [CrossRef] [PubMed]
34. Karmiris, K.; Bielen, D.; Vanbeckevoort, D.; Vermeire, S.; Coremans, G.; Rutgeerts, P.; Van Assche, G. Long-term monitoring of infliximab therapy for perianal fistulizing Crohn's disease by using magnetic resonance imaging. *Clin. Gastroenterol. Hepatol.* **2011**, *9*, 130–136. [CrossRef]
35. Panes, J.; Rimola, J. Perianal fistulizing Crohn's disease: Pathogenesis, diagnosis and therapy. *Nat. Rev. Gastroenterol. Hepatol.* **2017**, *14*, 652–664. [CrossRef] [PubMed]
36. Hindryckx, P.; Jairath, V.; Zou, G.; Feagan, B.G.; Sandborn, W.J.; Stoker, J.; Khanna, R.; Stitt, L.; van Viegen, T.; Shackelton, L.M.; et al. Development and Validation of a Magnetic Resonance Index for Assessing Fistulas in Patients with Crohn's Disease. *Gastroenterology* **2019**, *157*, 1233–1244.e35. [CrossRef]
37. El-Matary, W.; Walters, T.D.; Huynh, H.Q.; deBruyn, J.; Mack, D.R.; Jacobson, K.; Sherlock, M.E.; Church, P.; Wine, E.; Carroll, M.W.; et al. Higher Postinduction Infliximab Serum trough Levels Are Associated with Healing of Fistulizing Perianal Crohn's Disease in Children. *Inflamm. Bowel Dis.* **2019**, *25*, 150–155. [CrossRef]

38.	Grossberg, L.B.; Cheifetz, A.S.; Papamichael, K. Therapeutic Drug Monitoring of Biologics in Crohn's Disease. *Gastroenterol. Clin. N. Am.* **2022**, *51*, 299–317. [CrossRef]
39.	Sands, B.E.; Kramer, B.C.; Gasink, C.; Jacobstein, D.; Gao, L.L.; Ma, T.; Adedokun, O.J.; Colombel, J.F.; Schwartz, D.A. Association of Ustekinumab Serum Concentrations and Perianal Fistula Resolution inthe Crohn's Disease Uniti Program. *Gastroenterology* **2019**, *156*, S1099–S1100. [CrossRef]
40.	Glass, J.; Alsamman, Y.; Chittajallu, P.; Ahmed, T.; Fudman, D. Ustekinumab Dose Escalation Effective in Real-World Use for Luminal and Perianal Crohn's Disease. *Inflamm. Bowel Dis.* **2020**, *26*, S76. [CrossRef]

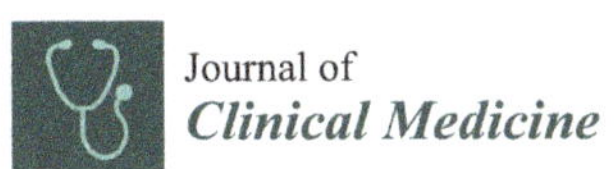

Journal of
Clinical Medicine

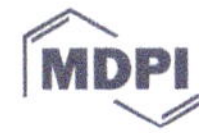

Article

Impact of Sarcopenia on Survival in Patients Treated with FOLFIRINOX in a First-Line Setting for Metastatic Pancreatic Carcinoma

Lisa Lellouche [1], Maxime Barat [2,3,4], Anna Pellat [1,3], Juliette Leroux [1,3], Felix Corre [1,3], Rachel Hallit [1,3], Antoine Assaf [1,3], Catherine Brezault [1], Marion Dhooge [1], Philippe Soyer [2,3,4] and Romain Coriat [1,3,4,*]

[1] Gastroenterology and Digestive Oncology Unit, Cochin Hospital AP-HP, 75014 Paris, France
[2] Department of Radiology, Cochin Hospital AP-HP, 75014 Paris, France
[3] UFR de Médecine, Université Paris Cité, 75006 Paris, France
[4] INSERM U1016, CNRS UMR8104, Institut Cochin, Université Paris Cité, 75006 Paris, France
[*] Correspondence: romain.coriat@aphp.fr; Tel.: +33-(15)-8411901

Abstract: Sarcopenia, defined as decreased muscle mass and strength, can be evaluated by a computed tomography (CT) examination and might be associated with reduced survival in patients with carcinoma. The prognosis of patients with metastatic pancreatic carcinoma is poor. The FOLFIRINOX (a combination of 5-fluorouracil, irinotecan, and oxaliplatin) chemotherapy regimen is a validated first-line treatment option. We investigated the impact of sarcopenia on overall survival (OS) and progression-free survival (PFS) in patients with metastatic pancreatic carcinoma. Clinical data and CT examinations of patients treated with FOLFIRINOX were retrospectively reviewed. Sarcopenia was estimated using baseline CT examinations. Seventy-five patients were included. Forty-three (57.3%) were classified as sarcopenic. The median OS of non-sarcopenic and sarcopenic patients were 15.6 and 14.1 months, respectively ($p = 0.36$). The median PFS was 10.3 in non-sarcopenic patients and 9.3 in sarcopenic patients ($p = 0.83$). No differences in toxicity of FOLFIRINOX were observed. There was a trend towards a higher probability of short-term death (within 4 months of diagnosis) in sarcopenic patients. In this study, the detection of sarcopenia failed to predict a longer OS or PFS in selected patients deemed eligible by a physician for triplet chemotherapy and receiving the FOLFIRINOX regimen in a first-line setting, confirming the major importance of a comprehensive patient assessment by physicians in selecting the best treatment option.

Keywords: metastatic pancreatic carcinoma; FOLFIRINOX; sarcopenia; oxaliplatin

Citation: Lellouche, L.; Barat, M.; Pellat, A.; Leroux, J.; Corre, F.; Hallit, R.; Assaf, A.; Brezault, C.; Dhooge, M.; Soyer, P.; et al. Impact of Sarcopenia on Survival in Patients Treated with FOLFIRINOX in a First-Line Setting for Metastatic Pancreatic Carcinoma. *J. Clin. Med.* **2023**, *12*, 2211. https://doi.org/10.3390/jcm12062211

Academic Editors: Stanley W. Ashley and Rajinder Dawra

Received: 13 January 2023
Revised: 20 February 2023
Accepted: 9 March 2023
Published: 13 March 2023

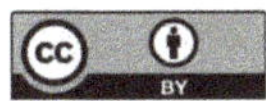

1. Introduction

Pancreatic cancer is expected to become the second leading cause of cancer-related death by 2030 [1]. While surgical resection is the only potentially curative treatment, only 15–20% of patients are candidates for surgery at diagnosis, because the majority of patients are diagnosed at a locally advanced stage of the metastatic stage of the disease [2].

Gemcitabine was first identified as the cornerstone of the treatment of patients with metastatic pancreatic carcinoma [3]. In 2011 and 2013, two large phase 3 trials pinpointed a survival benefit with FOLFIRINOX (5-fluorouracil, irinotecan, and oxaliplatin) and gemcitabine plus nab-paclitaxel in comparison to gemcitabine monotherapy [4,5]. These combinations are now considered as the two validated options in the first-line setting for patients with metastatic pancreatic cancer, pending a good performance status (PS) (i.e., Eastern Co-operative Oncology Group [ECOG] PS 0 or 1). Despite these treatment improvements, the prognosis of patients with metastatic pancreatic adenocarcinoma is still poor [6].

Sarcopenia, defined as the decrease in skeletal muscle mass and strength, is a component of cancer cachexia, which is characterized by a negative protein and energy balance, resulting from multiple factors, such as reduced food intake, inflammation, and excessive catabolism [7,8]. In clinical practice, the most commonly used method for skeletal muscle mass assessment is obtained using cross-sectional imaging at the level of the third lumbar vertebra (L3), using computed tomography (CT) [9,10]. Skeletal muscle index (SMI) cut-offs based on gender and body mass index (BMI) to classify sarcopenia have been published [11,12]. Sarcopenia was significantly associated with a shortened overall survival (OS) ($p < 0.001$) and a reduced cancer-specific survival (CSS) ($p < 0.001$) in a large meta-analysis including 7843 patients with solid tumors [13]. At the time of diagnosis, the prevalence of sarcopenia in patients with solid tumors was estimated to be around 40% [12]. In pancreatic adenocarcinoma, the prevalence of sarcopenia ranges from 19 to 65% [12,14,15]. Recently, a Japanese study identified a shortened OS in sarcopenic patients treated with FOLFIRINOX for advanced pancreatic carcinoma ($p = 0.001$) [16].

The aim of this study was to determine whether sarcopenia was associated with an unfavorable outcome in a Western population of patients with metastatic pancreatic cancer treated with FOLFIRINOX in a first-line setting.

2. Material and Methods

2.1. Study Design and Objectives

We performed a single-center, retrospective study in patients with metastatic pancreatic carcinoma treated with a modified FOLFIRINOX regimen in the first-line treatment, from January 2012 to December 2020 in our tertiary center. The primary endpoint of the study was OS, defined as the time from diagnosis to death (or last news if alive). Secondary endpoint was PFS, defined as the time from diagnosis to radiological progression. Our study received approval from our local institutional review board (AAA-2022-08011).

2.2. Patients and Treatment

Patients were included in the study if they had a histologically proven diagnosis of metastatic pancreatic carcinoma and had received at least one cycle of a triplet chemotherapy with 5-fluorouracil, oxaliplatin, and irinotecan (FOLFIRINOX regimen). All patients received prophylactic growth factors to prevent severe neutropenia.

Patients were excluded if they did not have CT examination within the 30 days before the treatment initiation, if they did not have follow-up with CT examination, or if they had undergone a surgical resection or local treatment of the primary tumor or metastasis after the diagnosis of metastatic pancreatic cancer. Patients presenting with mixed tumors, or neuroendocrine tumors were excluded. Patients with metachronous metastasis were included in the present study.

2.3. Toxicity Assessment

Treatment toxicity was evaluated during medical visit by experienced physicians after four to six cycles of chemotherapy and at progression. All side-effects were graded according to the Common Terminology Criteria for Adverse Events version (CTCAE) version 4 [17].

2.4. Anthropometric Measurement

For each patient, weight and height were measured according to standard methods, and body mass index (BMI) was calculated.

2.5. Image Analysis

Sarcopenia was assessed using CT examination at the time of diagnosis of metastatic pancreatic cancer. A radiologist with 10 years of experience in pancreatic imaging analyzed CT images at the third lumbar vertebra (L3) and identified skeletal muscles according to anatomic features and predefined thresholds of Hounsfield units (-29 to $+150$) (Figure 1) [11]. Skeletal muscle area (cm^2) was normalized by height (m^2), allowing calculation of the skeletal muscle index (SMI) (cm^2/m^2).

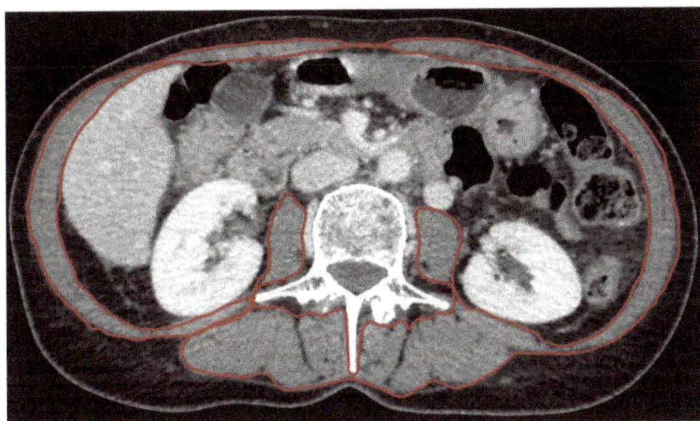

Figure 1. CT image in the axial plane at the level of the third lumbar vertebra in a sarcopenic patient with metastatic pancreatic carcinoma. Regions of interest (ROI) for sarcopenia measurements on axial CT image are indicated inside the red zone.

To define sarcopenia, we used the threshold values previously determined by Martin et al. which were associated with poor survival in patients with solid tumors [11]. Patients were considered sarcopenic when the following values were observed: SMI < 43 cm^2/m^2 for men with BMI < 25 kg/m^2, <53 cm^2/m^2 for men with BMI $\geq$ 25 kg/m^2, and <41 cm^2/m^2 for women, regardless of BMI. Radiologic progression was defined using the Response Evaluation Criteria In Solid Tumors (RECIST 1.1) criteria [18].

2.6. Statistical Analysis

The normality of the distribution of quantitative variables was assessed using Shapiro–Wilk test. Quantitative variables were expressed as means $\pm$ standard deviations (SD) and ranges when normally distributed, or as medians and interquartile ranges (Q1 and Q3) when non-normally distributed [19]. Qualitative variables were expressed as raw numbers, proportions, and percentages. Comparison between patients with sarcopenia and patients without sarcopenia was performed using Student t-test for continuous variables or the Chi2 test for qualitative variables. Survival in patients with sarcopenia and in patients without sarcopenia was analyzed by the Kaplan–Meier method and compared using the log-rank test. A *p*-value < 0.05 was considered to indicate significant differences. Calculations were performed with NCSSC 2007 software (NCSS, Kaysville, UT, USA).

3. Results

3.1. Patients

One hundred and seventy patients with histologically proven metastatic pancreatic carcinoma were initially identified. Among them, 24 were excluded due to the lack of a CT examination at the time of diagnosis, surgical resection of the primary tumor or metastasis (n = 3), or exclusive supportive care (n = 15). One hundred and twenty-eight patients (75.3%) received chemotherapy. Among them, 75 received a FOLFIRINOX regimen (58.7%), 33 received FOLFOX (25.8%), nine received gemcitabine plus nab-paclitaxel (7%), eight received gemcitabine monotherapy (6.2%), and three received FOLFIRI (2.3%). The study flow-chart is displayed in Figure 2.

We included 75 patients who received at least one cycle of FOLFIRINOX. There were 38 women (50.7%) and 37 men (49.3%), with a mean age of 64 $\pm$ 11.2 (SD) years (range: 34–85 years). The patients' baseline characteristics are reported in Table 1. All patients had a pancreatic ductal adenocarcinoma (PDAC) or variants (acinar cell carcinoma, n = 2; adenosquamous carcinoma, n = 1; undifferentiated carcinoma with osteoclast-like giant cells, n = 2). Ten patients had a past history of cephalic duodenopancreatectomy (n = 4) or pancreatosplenectomy (n = 6). Forty-three patients (57.3%) were identified as sarcopenic.

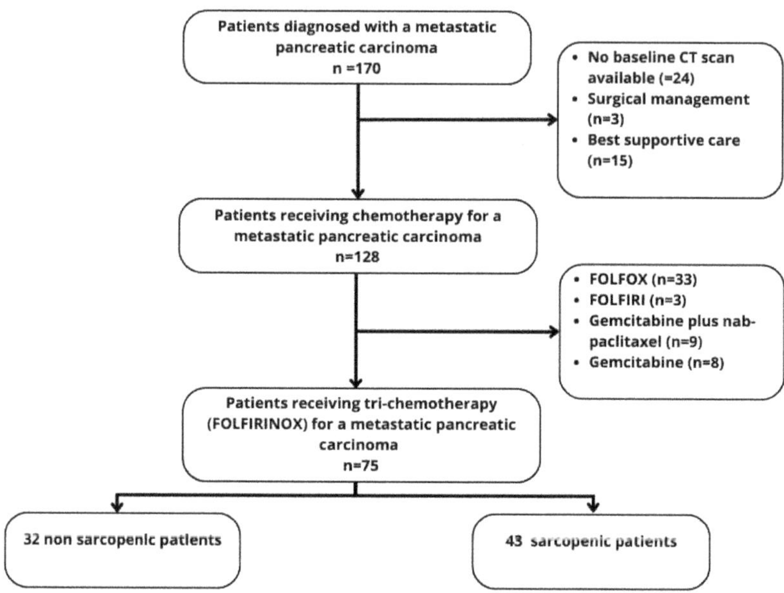

Figure 2. Flow-chart.

Table 1. Patients' characteristics at baseline.

Patients' Characteristics	All Patients	Non-Sarcopenic Patients	Sarcopenic Patients	*p*-Value
Patients, n (%)	75	32 (42.7)	43 (57.3)	
Sex, n (%)				0.98
Women	38 (51)	13 (34.2)	25 (65)	
Men	37 (49.3)	19 (51.3)	18 (48.7)	
Age, mean (SD)	64 (11.2)	63.4 (11.7)	64.4 (11)	0.68
Weight (kg), mean (SD)	67.9 (13,5)	73 (12.4)	64 (13)	0.002
BMI, mean (SD)	23.6 (4.4)	25.3 (5.1)	22.3 (3.3)	0.005
Underweight (BMI < 18.5), n (%)	3 (4)	0 (0)	3 (7)	
Normalweight ($18.5 \leq$ BMI < 25), n (%)	49 (65.3)	18 (56.2)	31 (72)	
Overweight ($25 \leq$ BMI < 30), n (%)	17 (22.7)	10 (31.2)	7 (16.3)	
Obese ($30 \leq$ BMI), n (%)	4 (5.3)	3 (9.4)	1 (2.3)	
Skeletal muscle L3 area (cm^2), mean (SD)	123.3 (31.5)	144.5 (24.5)	107.6 (26.7)	<0.001
SMI (cm^2/m^2) (men), mean (SD)	45.3 (7.5)	49.6 (4.7)	40.8 (7.3)	<0.001
SMI (cm^2/m^2) (women), mean (SD)	39.6 (9.1)	48.9 (8.8)	34.7 (4.3)	<0.001
ECOG PS, n (%)				0.2
0	14 (18.7)	8 (25)	6 (14)	
1	31 (41.3)	16 (50)	15 (34.9)	
2	11 (14.7)	3 (9.4)	8 (18.6)	
3	2 (2.6)	0 (0)	2 (4.6)	
Unknown	17 (22.6)	5 (15.6)	12 (28)	
Site of tumor, n (%)				0.36
Head	40 (53.3)	16 (50)	24 (55.8)	
Body or tail	33 (44)	16 (50)	17 (39.5)	
Unknown	2 (2.6)	0 (0)	2 (4.6)	
Biliary drainage, *n* (%)	19 (25.3)	9 (28)	10 (23.2)	0.6
Liver metastasis, n (%)	54 (72)	23 (71.9)	31 (72)	0.98
Pulmonary metastasis, n (%)	24 (32)	11 (34.4)	13 (30)	0.7
Peritoneum metastasis, n (%)	18 (24)	6 (18.7)	12 (28)	0.35
Previous therapy for localized cancer				
Adjuvant chemotherapy, n (%)	9 (12.0)	6 (18.7)	3 (7)	0.12

Table 1. *Cont.*

Patients' Characteristics	All Patients	Non-Sarcopenic Patients	Sarcopenic Patients	*p*-Value
Pancreatic surgery, n (%)	10 (13.3)	6 (18.7)	4 (9.3)	0.23
CRP (mg/L), median (IQR)	13.6 (3.9–33.9)	13.5 (3.4–32.3)	15.1 (4.9–35.2)	0.8
Ca 19.9 (U/mL), median (IQR)	462.5 (48.9–3910.7)	425 (87.4–5179.5)	500 (39.2–1823)	0.08
CEA (ng/mL), median (IQR)	7 (3.8–29.7)	5.5 (3.3–12.6)	17.1 (6.3–36.6)	0.25
Total bilirubin (umol/L), median (IQR)	8.3 (5.5–16)	9.7 (6–16.5)	7.35 (5.3–15)	0.69
Albumin (g/L), median (IQR)	38.5 (34–41)	39 (36–42)	38 (33–40)	0.22

No differences were observed regarding tumor and metastasis localization, albumin, CRP, bilirubin, and CA 19–9 levels. Significant differences in mean BMI (22.3 kg/m^2 vs. 25.3 kg/m^2, respectively; $p = 0.005$) and mean weight (64 kg vs. 73 kg; $p = 0.002$) were found between sarcopenia and non-sarcopenia patients. Mean skeletal muscle L3 area (107.6 vs. 144.5; $p < 0.0001$) and SMI (34.7 vs. 48.9 for women and 40.8 vs. 49.6 for men; $p < 0.0001$) were significantly different between the two groups.

3.2. Toxicity

In the overall population, 22.7% of patients (n = 17) experienced grade 3/4 hematological adverse events (Table 2). The most common grade 3/4 hematological adverse event was neutropenia or febrile neutropenia (12%) despite prophylactic treatment. Non-hematological grade 3/4 adverse events occurred in 26.7% of patients (n = 20), including diarrhea (n = 10), nausea (n = 5), vomiting (n = 3), and chemotherapy-induced neuropathy (n = 2). There were no significant differences regarding the adverse effects between sarcopenic and non-sarcopenic patients, except for anemia, which was significantly higher in non-sarcopenic patients. Oxaliplatin and irinotecan were discontinued in 44% and 18.7% of patients, respectively (Table 3). No significant differences were found in terms of treatment reduction or discontinuation between the two groups.

Table 2. Toxicity in patients receiving FOLFIRINOX regimen for metastatic pancreatic carcinoma.

	All Patients (n = 75)	Non-Sarcopenic Patients (n = 32)	Sarcopenic Patients (n = 43)	*p*-Value
Neutropenia				
Any grade	14 (18.6)	7 (21.9)	7 (16.3)	0.53
Grade $\geq$ 3	6 (8)	3 (9.4)	3 (7)	1
Febrile neutropenia				
Any grade	NA	NA	NA	
Grade $\geq$ 3	3 (4)	2 (6.2)	1 (2.3)	0.57
Thrombopenia				
Any grade	19 (25.3)	11 (34.4)	8 (18.6)	0.12
Grade $\geq$ 3	3 (4)	2 (6.2)	1 (2.3)	0.57
Anemia				
Any grade	30 (40)	17 (53)	13 (30)	**0.045**
Grade $\geq$ 3	5 (6)	2 (6.2)	3 (7)	1
Diarrhea				
Any grade	42 (56)	19 (59)	23 (53.5)	0.61
Grade $\geq$ 3	10 (13.3)	3 (9.4)	7 (16.3)	0.38
Nausea				
Any grade	34 (45.3)	17 (53)	17 (39.5)	0.24
Grade $\geq$ 3	5 (6.7)	2 (6.2)	3 (6.9)	0.90
Vomiting				
Any grade	21 (28)	9 (28.1)	12 (27.9)	0.98
Grade $\geq$ 3	3 (4)	1 (3.1)	2 (4.7)	1
Peripheral neuropathy				
Any grade	51 (68)	24 (75)	27 (62.8)	0.26
Grade $\geq$ 3	2 (2.6)	2 (6.2)	0 (0)	0.17

NA: Not applicable.

Table 3. Treatment interruption and dose reduction.

	All Patients n = 75	Non-Sarcopenic Patients n = 32	Sarcopenic Patients n = 43	*p*-Value
Oxaliplatin, n (%)				
Dose reduction	38 (50.7)	18 (56.2)	20 (46.5)	0.4
Discontinuation	33 (44)	15 (46.9)	18 (41.9)	0.66
Irinotecan, n (%)				
Dose reduction	29 (38.7)	10 (31.2)	19 (44.2)	0.25
Discontinuation	14 (18.7)	5 (15.6)	9 (20.9)	0.55
5-fluorouracil, n (%)				
Dose reduction	14 (18.7)	5 (15.6)	9 (20.9)	0.55
Discontinuation	0	0	0	NA

3.3. Survival

The median number of cycles of FOLFIRINOX administrated was 10 (range: 1–58) in the entire cohort, with no difference between sarcopenic and non-sarcopenic patients (9 vs. 10, p = 0.83). There were no significant differences in terms of the median OS (15.6 versus 14.1 months; 95% CI, 0.56–1.45; p = 0.36) or median PFS (10.3 vs. 9.3 months; 95% CI, 0.65–1.89; p = 0.83) between the non- and the sarcopenic patients (Figure 3).

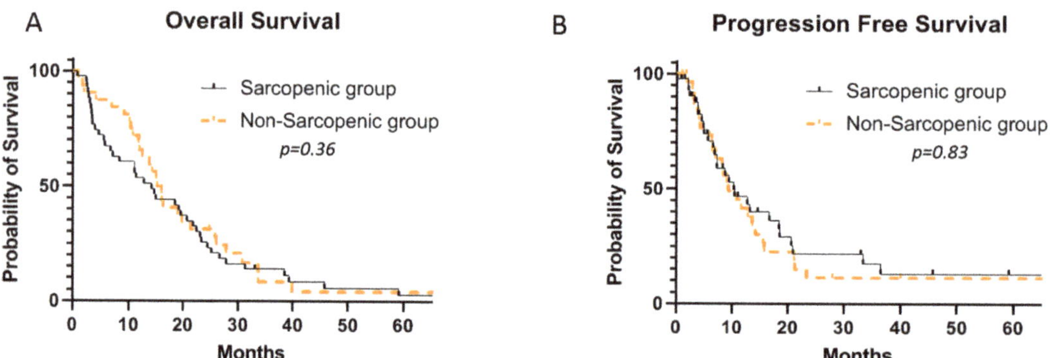

Figure 3. Median OS (**A**) and PFS (**B**) in sarcopenic and non-sarcopenic patients receiving FOLFIRINOX for metastatic pancreatic carcinoma.

There were numerically more patients in the sarcopenic group who had an early death (25.6 versus 9.4%), within 4 months of diagnosis of metastatic pancreatic carcinoma, although this did not reach a statistical significance (p = 0.07) (Table 4). Seventy-two percent of sarcopenic patients who had a short-term death did not have a radiologically proven disease progression. There was no difference between the two groups in the percentage of deaths within 12 months of diagnosis.

At progression, 41.3% (n = 31) of patients received second-line chemotherapy (Table 5), and 58.7% (n = 44) received best supportive care. Sarcopenic patients received significantly less second-line chemotherapy than non-sarcopenic patients (30.2% vs. 56.3%, p = 0.02). The second-line treatment was gemcitabine monotherapy for 11 patients (14.7%) and gemcitabine plus nab-paclitaxel for 20 patients (26.7%). The median second OS (since the start of the second-line chemotherapy) for sarcopenic and non-sarcopenic patients was 12.3 months (5.9–16.6) in the patients receiving gemcitabine plus nab-paclitaxel, and 4.6 months (1.8–9.7) in the patients receiving gemcitabine monotherapy.

Table 4. Early death in patients receiving FOLFIRINOX for metastatic pancreatic carcinoma.

	All Patients (n = 75)	Non-Sarcopenic Patients (n = 32)	Sarcopenic Patients (n = 43)	*p*-Value
Death within 4 months from diagnosis, n (%)				
Death before confirmed radiological progression	10 (13.3)	2 (6.2)	8 (18.6)	0.08
Death before or after confirmed radiological progression	14 (18.6)	3 (9.4)	11 (25.6)	0.07
Death within 12 months from diagnosis, n (%)				
Death before confirmed radiological progression	12 (16)	4 (12.5)	8 (18.6)	0.54
Death before or after radiological progression	32 (42.7)	11 (34)	21 (48)	0.24

Table 5. Treatment at progression after FOLFIRINOX.

	All Patients n = 75	Non-Sarcopenic Patients n = 32	Sarcopenic Patients n = 43	*p*-Value
Best supportive care	44 (58.7)	12 (43.7)	30 (69.8)	**0.02**
Second-line therapy	31 (41.3)	18 (56.3)	13 (30.2)	**0.02**
Gemcitabine monotherapy, n (%)	11 (14.7)	6 (18.7)	5 (11.6)	0.38
Gemcitabine plus nab-paclitaxel, n (%)	20 (26.7)	12 (37.5)	8 (18.6)	0.06

4. Discussion

Our study evaluated the association between sarcopenia at baseline and survival in 75 patients with metastatic pancreatic cancer who received FOLFIRINOX as the first-line therapy. We found no significant association between sarcopenia at baseline and OS or PFS. These findings are inconsistent with previous reports from Kurita et al. [16], who showed that sarcopenia at the time of diagnosis was an independent poor prognosis factor in 82 patients with advanced pancreatic cancer. There might be several explanations for these conflicting results. First, nearly half of the patients included in the study by Kurita et al. had previously received systemic therapy for advanced pancreatic cancer, whereas our study included only chemotherapy-naïve patients. Therefore, patients included in our study might have had a better general condition. Secondly, as the study by Kurita et al. involved an Asian population, the cut-offs used for the diagnosis of sarcopenia (SMI < 45.3 cm^2/m^2 and 37.1 cm^2/m^2 for men and women, respectively) were different than ours (SMI < 43 cm^2/m^2 for males with BMI < 25 kg/m^2, <53 cm^2/m^2 for males with BMI $\geq$ 25 kg/m^2, and <41 cm^2/m^2 for women, regardless of BMI). One difficulty in studying the impact of sarcopenia in clinical practice is the lack of consensus regarding the SMI thresholds for diagnosis. We chose to use those reported by Martin et al. in a large cohort of 1473 patients with lung or gastrointestinal tumors [11], but only 9.9% of the included patients had pancreatic carcinoma, the vast majority of them having a colon or rectum cancer. We might hypothesize that, because patients with pancreatic carcinoma suffer from cachexia more often than those with colon or rectal cancer, the SMI thresholds for the diagnosis of sarcopenia should be different. In another study including only obese patients with a lung or gastrointestinal cancer, Prado et al. found different sex-specific SMI cut-offs associated with mortality (52.4 cm^2/m^2 for men and 38.5 cm^2/m^2 for women) [9]. The narrative review by Bozzetti et al. reported that the cut-offs for defining sarcopenia ranged from 36 to 55 cm^2/m^2 in men [12].

In this study, we chose to include only patients who were treated with FOLFIRI-NOX, which is a validated first-line standard for patients with an ECOG PS of 0 or 1. As FOLFIRINOX is considered an aggressive regimen, it is recommended only for patients in good general condition based on the oncologist's clinical assessment. In our center, of the 170 patients diagnosed with metastatic pancreatic cancer, only 44% ultimately received FOLFIRINOX, with the remaining patients receiving 5-fluorouracil-based bichemotherapy (21.2%), gemcitabine plus nab-paclitaxel (5.3%), gemcitabine monotherapy (4.7%), or exclusive support care (8.9%). Of the 75 patients receiving FOLFIRINOX, 11 (14.7%) and two (2.7%) had a reported ECOG PS of 2 and 3, respectively. These results should be interpreted with caution, as the literature reports conflicting data regarding the reproducibility of the ECOG PS scale [20,21]. In these 75 patients deemed eligible to receive FOLFIRINOX based on the physician global assessment, sarcopenia was not a predictor of reduced PFS of OS.

In our study, sarcopenic patients received significantly less second-line chemotherapy than non-sarcopenic patients, although there was no difference in the median OS between the two groups. In metastatic pancreatic carcinoma, there are no large prospective randomized studies of second-line chemotherapy after FOLFIRINOX failure, as most data are from retrospective studies. In a prospective cohort of 57 patients receiving gemcitabine plus nab-paclitaxel after FOLFIRINOX failure, Portal et al. [22] identified a median second OS (since the start of the second-line chemotherapy) of 8.8 months. In our study, the median second OS in sarcopenic and non-sarcopenic patients treated with gemcitabine plus-paclitaxel was 12.3 months.

While sarcopenia at baseline was not a prognosis factor for OS or PFS in our study, there was a trend toward a higher proportion of early deaths (within 4 months of diagnosis of metastatic pancreatic carcinoma) in sarcopenic patients. This may argue for the early detection of sarcopenia in patients undergoing chemotherapy, to improve the overall management of patients and attempt to reverse skeletal muscle loss and cachexia. Recently, the APACaP trial randomized 313 patients with advanced pancreatic cancer, to chemotherapy or chemotherapy plus adapted physical activity (APA) [23]. In this trial, APA was shown to be feasible in patients with pancreatic carcinoma, and was associated with an improvement in several quality-of-life dimensions. Moreover, there was a tendency for a longer OS and PFS in the patients randomized to the APA arm, although this result did not reach a statistical difference. In a retrospective study including Japanese patients, Uemura et al. found that the baseline sarcopenia in patients with advanced pancreatic adenocarcinoma who received FOLFIRINOX was not associated with OS either [24]. However, these researchers did report the negative impact of an early decrease in skeletal muscle mass on the OS, which may indicate that, more than sarcopenia at diagnosis, maintaining muscle mass throughout treatment is an important factor for improving survival.

Interestingly, the incidence of grade ≥ 3 adverse events was not significantly greater in patients with sarcopenia in our study. Anemia occurred surprisingly more often in patients without sarcopenia, but this should be interpreted with caution as we were unable to identify patients who underwent a blood transfusion or treatment with erythropoietin-stimulating agents. Various studies have reported an association between sarcopenia and chemotherapy toxicity [25–27]. More specifically, sarcopenic obesity has been associated with increased chemotherapy toxicity [27–30]. The administration of cytotoxic agents is usually determined by the body surface area (BSA), calculated from weight and height. It has been hypothesized that patients with obesity and sarcopenia would have a large BSA despite a low lean body mass. Therefore, sarcopenic obese patients would receive a high dose of chemotherapy despite a reduced volume of distribution [9]. We did not evaluate the impact of sarcopenic obesity on FOLFIRINOX tolerability in our study as we included only one obese sarcopenic patient.

Our study has several limitations. First, it is a single-center study, which could have led to patient and treatment strategy selection bias. Second, it is a retrospective study with missing data, especially regarding the toxicity assessment. Finally, as discussed above, one of the major limitations to sarcopenia studies is the lack of consensus on the SMI threshold.

To date, specific cut-offs for sarcopenia in patients with pancreatic cancer have not been reported in large studies or meta-analyses.

5. Conclusions

Sarcopenia at the time of diagnosis does not affect OS, PFS, or chemotherapy toxicity in selected patients receiving FOLFIRINOX for metastatic pancreatic carcinoma. Isolated sarcopenia should not be an exclusion criterion for the triplet chemotherapy regimen in patients deemed eligible by a comprehensive physician assessment. However, our results show a trend toward early death in sarcopenic patients, which should advocate for the early reversion of skeletal muscle loss as part of the global management of patients with metastatic pancreatic carcinoma.

Author Contributions: Conceptualization, L.L., M.B. and R.C., methodology, L.L., M.B. and R.C., validation, L.L., M.B., A.P., J.L., F.C., R.H., A.A., C.B., M.D., P.S. and R.C.; investigation, L.L., M.B. and R.C.; resources, L.L., M.B. and R.C., data curation, L.L. and M.B.; writing—original draft preparation, L.L.; writing—review and editing, L.L. and R.C.; visualization, R.C.; supervision, R.C.; project administration, R.C. All authors have read and agreed to the published version of the manuscript.

Funding: This research received no external funding.

Institutional Review Board Statement: Our study received approval from our local institutional review board, entitled Comité Local des publications, CLEP (AAA-2022-08011).

Informed Consent Statement: No informed consent was necessary.

Data Availability Statement: Data are available.

Conflicts of Interest: R.C has acted as a paid consultant or oral presenter for AAA, Bayer, Servier, Ipsen, Novartis, and Keocyt. C.B has acted as a paid consultant for IPSEN. All other authors have no conflict of interest to declare.

Abbreviations

5-FU: 5-fluorouracil, BMI: body mass index, BSA: body surface area, CI: confidence interval, CSS: cancer-specific survival, CT: computed tomography, CTCAE: Common Terminology Criteria for Adverse Events, ECOG: Eastern Co-operative Oncology Group, HR: hazard ratio, LBM: lean body mass, OS: overall survival, PDAC: pancreatic ductal adenocarcinoma, PFS: progression-free survival, PS: performance status, RECIST: Response Evaluation Criteria In Solid Tumors, SD: standard deviation, SMI: skeletal muscle index.

References

1. Rahib, L.; Smith, B.D.; Aizenberg, R.; Rosenzweig, A.B.; Fleshman, J.M.; Matrisian, L.M. Projecting Cancer Incidence and Deaths to 2030: The Unexpected Burden of Thyroid, Liver, and Pancreas Cancers in the United States. *Cancer Res.* **2014**, *74*, 2913–2921. [CrossRef] [PubMed]
2. Fogel, E.L.; Shahda, S.; Sandrasegaran, K.; DeWitt, J.; Easler, J.J.; Agarwal, D.M.; Eagleson, M.A.B.; Zyromski, N.J.; House, M.G.; Ellsworth, S.; et al. A Multidisciplinary Approach to Pancreas Cancer in 2016: A Review. *Am. J. Gastroenterol.* **2017**, *112*, 537–554. [CrossRef] [PubMed]
3. Burris, H.A.; Moore, M.J.; Andersen, J.; Green, M.R.; Rothenberg, M.L.; Modiano, M.R.; Cripps, M.C.; Portenoy, R.K.; Storniolo, A.M.; Tarassoff, S.; et al. Improvements in survival and clinical benefit with gemcitabine as first-line therapy for patients with advanced pancreas cancer: A randomized trial. *J. Clin. Oncol.* **1997**, *15*, 2403–2413. [CrossRef] [PubMed]
4. Von Hoff, D.D.; Ervin, T.; Arena, F.P.; Chiorean, E.G.; Infante, J.; Moore, M.; Seay, T.; Tjulandin, S.A.; Ma, W.W.; Saleh, M.N.; et al. Increased Survival in Pancreatic Cancer with nab-Paclitaxel plus Gemcitabine. *N. Engl. J. Med.* **2013**, *369*, 1691–1703. [CrossRef] [PubMed]
5. Conroy, T.; Desseigne, F.; Ychou, M.; Bouché, O.; Guimbaud, R.; Bécouarn, Y.; Adenis, A.; Raoul, J.-L.; Gourgou-Bourgade, S.; de la Fouchardière, C.; et al. FOLFIRINOX versus Gemcitabine for Metastatic Pancreatic Cancer. *N. Engl. J. Med.* **2011**, *364*, 1817–1825. [CrossRef] [PubMed]
6. Siegel, R.L.; Miller, K.D.; Jemal, A. Cancer statistics, 2019. *CA Cancer J. Clin.* **2019**, *69*, 7–34. [CrossRef]
7. Fearon, K.; Strasser, F.; Anker, S.D.; Bosaeus, I.; Bruera, E.; Fainsinger, R.L.; Jatoi, A.; Loprinzi, C.; MacDonald, N.; Mantovani, G.; et al. Definition and classification of cancer cachexia: An international consensus. *Lancet Oncol.* **2011**, *12*, 489–495. [CrossRef]

8. Baracos, V.E.; Martin, L.; Korc, M.; Guttridge, D.C.; Fearon, K.C.H. Cancer-associated cachexia. *Nat. Rev. Dis. Prim.* **2018**, *4*, 17105. [CrossRef]
9. Prado, C.M.M.; Lieffers, J.R.; McCargar, L.J.; Reiman, T.; Sawyer, M.B.; Martin, L.; Baracos, V.E. Prevalence and clinical implications of sarcopenic obesity in patients with solid tumours of the respiratory and gastrointestinal tracts: A population-based study. *Lancet Oncol.* **2008**, *9*, 629–635. [CrossRef]
10. Kazemi-Bajestani, S.M.R.; Mazurak, V.C.; Baracos, V. Computed tomography-defined muscle and fat wasting are associated with cancer clinical outcomes. *Semin. Cell Dev. Biol.* **2016**, *54*, 2–10. [CrossRef]
11. Martin, L.; Birdsell, L.; MacDonald, N.; Reiman, T.; Clandinin, M.T.; McCargar, L.J.; Murphy, R.; Ghosh, S.; Sawyer, M.B.; Baracos, V.E. Cancer Cachexia in the Age of Obesity: Skeletal Muscle Depletion Is a Powerful Prognostic Factor, Independent of Body Mass Index. *J. Clin. Oncol.* **2013**, *31*, 1539–1547. [CrossRef] [PubMed]
12. Bozzetti, F. Forcing the vicious circle: Sarcopenia increases toxicity, decreases response to chemotherapy and worsens with chemotherapy. *Ann. Oncol.* **2017**, *28*, 2107–2118. [CrossRef] [PubMed]
13. Shachar, S.S.; Williams, G.R.; Muss, H.B.; Nishijima, T.F. Prognostic value of sarcopenia in adults with solid tumours: A meta-analysis and systematic review. *Eur. J. Cancer* **2016**, *57*, 58–67. [CrossRef]
14. Mintziras, I.; Miligkos, M.; Wächter, S.; Manoharan, J.; Maurer, E.; Bartsch, D.K. Sarcopenia and sarcopenic obesity are significantly associated with poorer overall survival in patients with pancreatic cancer: Systematic review and meta-analysis. *Int. J. Surg.* **2018**, *59*, 19–26. [CrossRef] [PubMed]
15. Bundred, J.; Kamarajah, S.K.; Roberts, K.J. Body composition assessment and sarcopenia in patients with pancreatic cancer: A systematic review and meta-analysis. *HPB* **2019**, *21*, 1603–1612. [CrossRef]
16. Kurita, Y.; Kobayashi, N.; Tokuhisa, M.; Goto, A.; Kubota, K.; Endo, I.; Nakajima, A.; Ichikawa, Y. Sarcopenia is a reliable prognostic factor in patients with advanced pancreatic cancer receiving FOLFIRINOX chemotherapy. *Pancreatology* **2019**, *19*, 127–135. [CrossRef]
17. National Institutes of Health. *Common Terminology Criteria for Adverse Events. Version 4*; US Department of Health and Human Services: Bethesda, MD, USA, 2010.
18. Eisenhauer, E.A.; Therasse, P.; Bogaerts, J.; Schwartz, L.H.; Sargent, D.; Ford, R.; Dancey, J.; Arbuck, S.; Gwyther, S.; Mooney, M.; et al. New response evaluation criteria in solid tumours: Revised RECIST guideline (version 1.1). *Eur. J. Cancer* **2009**, *45*, 228–247. [CrossRef]
19. Barat, M.; Jannot, A.S.; Dohan, A.; Soyer, P. How to report and compare quantitative variables in a radiology article. *Diagn. Interv. Imaging* **2022**, *103*, 571–573. [CrossRef]
20. Chow, R.; Chiu, N.; Bruera, E.; Krishnan, M.; Chiu, L.; Lam, H.; DeAngelis, C.; Pulenzas, N.; Vuong, S.; Chow, E.; et al. Inter-rater reliability in performance status assessment among health care professionals: A systematic review. *Ann. Palliat. Med.* **2016**, *5*, 83–92. [CrossRef]
21. Kelly, C.M.; Shahrokni, A. Moving beyond Karnofsky and ECOG Performance Status Assessments with New Technologies. *J. Oncol.* **2016**, *2016*, 6186543. [CrossRef]
22. Portal, A.; Pernot, S.; Tougeron, D.; Arbaud, C.; Bidault, A.T.; de la Fouchardière, C.; Hammel, P.; Lecomte, T.; Dréanic, J.; Coriat, R.; et al. Nab-paclitaxel plus gemcitabine for metastatic pancreatic adenocarcinoma after Folfirinox failure: An AGEO prospective multicentre cohort. *Br. J. Cancer* **2015**, *113*, 989–995. [CrossRef] [PubMed]
23. Neuzillet, C.; Bouché, O.; Tournigand, C.; Chibaudel, B.; Bouguion, L.; Bengrine-Lefevre, L.; Ataz, D.L.-T.; Mabro, M.; Metges, J.-P.; Péré-Vergé, D.; et al. Adapted physical activity in patients (Pts) with advanced pancreatic cancer (APACaP): Results from a prospective national randomized GERCOR trial. *J. Clin. Oncol.* **2022**, *40*, 4007. [CrossRef]
24. Uemura, S.; Iwashita, T.; Ichikawa, H.; Iwasa, Y.; Mita, N.; Shiraki, M.; Shimizu, M. The impact of sarcopenia and decrease in skeletal muscle mass in patients with advanced pancreatic cancer during FOLFIRINOX therapy. *Br. J. Nutr.* **2021**, *125*, 1140–1147. [CrossRef] [PubMed]
25. Prado, C.M.M.; Baracos, V.E.; McCargar, L.J.; Reiman, T.; Mourtzakis, M.; Tonkin, K.; Mackey, J.R.; Koski, S.; Pituskin, E.; Sawyer, M.B. Sarcopenia as a Determinant of Chemotherapy Toxicity and Time to Tumor Progression in Metastatic Breast Cancer Patients Receiving Capecitabine Treatment. *Clin. Cancer Res.* **2009**, *15*, 2920–2926. [CrossRef] [PubMed]
26. Tan, B.H.L.; Brammer, K.; Randhawa, N.; Welch, N.T.; Parsons, S.L.; James, E.J.; Catton, J. Sarcopenia is associated with toxicity in patients undergoing neo-adjuvant chemotherapy for oesophago-gastric cancer. *Eur. J. Surg. Oncol.* **2015**, *41*, 333–338. [CrossRef]
27. Cousin, S.; Hollebecque, A.; Koscielny, S.; Mir, O.; Varga, A.; Baracos, V.E.; Soria, J.C.; Antoun, S. Low skeletal muscle is associated with toxicity in patients included in phase I trials. *Investig. New Drugs* **2014**, *32*, 382–387. [CrossRef]
28. Anandavadivelan, P.; Brismar, T.B.; Nilsson, M.; Johar, A.M.; Martin, L. Sarcopenic obesity: A probable risk factor for dose limiting toxicity during neo-adjuvant chemotherapy in oesophageal cancer patients. *Clin. Nutr.* **2016**, *35*, 724–730. [CrossRef]
29. Carneiro, I.P.; Mazurak, V.C.; Prado, C.M. Clinical Implications of Sarcopenic Obesity in Cancer. *Curr. Oncol. Rep.* **2016**, *18*, 62. [CrossRef]
30. Baracos, V.E.; Arribas, L. Sarcopenic obesity: Hidden muscle wasting and its impact for survival and complications of cancer therapy. *Ann. Oncol.* **2018**, *29*, ii1–ii9. [CrossRef]

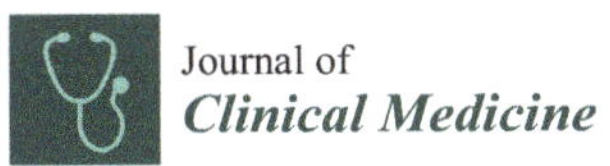

Journal of
Clinical Medicine

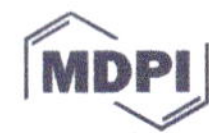

Article

Sarcopenia Is a Prognostic Factor in Patients Undergoing Percutaneous Endoscopic Gastrostomy

Shingo Ono [1,*], Hiroto Furuhashi [1], Shunsuke Kisaki [2], Hideka Horiuchi [1], Hiroaki Matsui [1], Akira Dobashi [1], Hiroya Ojiri [2] and Kazuki Sumiyama [1]

[1] Department of Endoscopy, The Jikei University School of Medicine, 3-25-8 Nishi-Shimbashi, Minato-ku, Tokyo 105-8461, Japan
[2] Department of Radiology, The Jikei University School of Medicine, 3-25-8 Nishi-Shimbashi, Minato-ku, Tokyo 105-8461, Japan
* Correspondence: onoshingo@jikei.ac.jp; Tel.: +81-3-3433-1111; Fax: +81-3-3459-4524

Abstract: (1) Background: Percutaneous endoscopic gastrostomy (PEG) is a widely used long-term enteral nutrition method, but little is known about the associated prognostic factors in patients with PEG. Sarcopenia, a condition characterized by a loss of skeletal muscle mass, increases the risk of developing various gastrointestinal disorders. Yet, the relationship between sarcopenia and the prognosis after PEG remains unclear. (2) Methods: We conducted a retrospective study of patients who underwent PEG consecutively from March 2008 to April 2020. We analyzed preoperative sarcopenia and the prognosis of patients after PEG. We defined sarcopenia as a skeletal muscle index at the level of the third lumbar vertebra of ≤ 29.6 cm^2/m^2 for women and ≤ 36.2 cm^2/m^2 for men. Cross-sectional computed tomography images of skeletal muscle at the level of the third lumbar vertebra were evaluated using DICOM image analysis software (OsiriX). The primary outcome was the difference in overall survival after PEG based on the status of sarcopenia. We also performed a covariate balancing propensity score matching analysis. (3) Results: Of 127 patients (99 men, 28 women), 71 (56%) were diagnosed with sarcopenia, and 64 patients died during the observation period. The median follow-up period did not differ between patients with and without sarcopenia ($p = 0.5$). The median survival time after PEG was 273 days in patients with sarcopenia and 1133 days in those without ($p < 0.001$). Cox proportional hazard model analyses identified three factors that were significantly associated with overall survival: sarcopenia (adjusted hazard ratio [HR]: 2.9, 95% confidence interval [CI]: 1.6–5.4, $p < 0.001$), serum albumin level (adjusted HR: 0.34, 95% CI: 0.21–0.55, $p < 0.001$) and male sex (adjusted HR: 2.0, 95% CI: 1.1–3.7, $p = 0.03$). Propensity score-matched analysis ($n = 37$ vs. 37) showed that the survival rate was lower in the sarcopenia group than in the non-sarcopenia group (at 90 days: 77% (95% CI, 59–88) vs. 92% (76–97), at 180 days: 56% (38–71) vs. 92% (76–97), and at one year: 35% (19–51) vs. 81% (63–91), $p = 0.0014$). (4) Conclusions: Sarcopenia was associated with poor prognosis in patients having undergone PEG.

Keywords: sarcopenia; L3 skeletal muscle index; percutaneous endoscopic gastrostomy; prognostic factor

Citation: Ono, S.; Furuhashi, H.; Kisaki, S.; Horiuchi, H.; Matsui, H.; Dobashi, A.; Ojiri, H.; Sumiyama, K. Sarcopenia Is a Prognostic Factor in Patients Undergoing Percutaneous Endoscopic Gastrostomy. *J. Clin. Med.* **2023**, *12*, 3360. https://doi.org/10.3390/jcm12103360

Academic Editor: Hidekazu Suzuki

Received: 14 February 2023
Revised: 1 May 2023
Accepted: 1 May 2023
Published: 9 May 2023

1. Introduction

Percutaneous endoscopic gastrostomy (PEG), which was first described in 1980 [1], has been widely used as a long-term enteral nutrition method for patients with malnutrition due to dysphagia and maintained functional gut. PEG has fewer complications and lower associated mortality than surgical gastrostomy and is a minimally invasive and safe procedure that can be applied even in elderly and debilitated patients [2].

Although the severe complication rate of PEG is low, the procedure is sometimes associated with early mortality. Risk factors associated with post-PEG prognosis may include hypoalbuminemia, a history of aspiration pneumonia, and elevated C-reactive protein levels [3–5]. Despite the high number of procedures performed, there is insufficient evidence to identify clear risk factors for poor prognosis in patients undergoing PEG. Knowing these factors at baseline is key to reducing medical procedures and their associated expenses.

Sarcopenia was recognized as an independent condition with an International Classification of Diseases-10 code in 2016 [6]. The prevalence of sarcopenia has increased, and it has become a serious global public health concern for an aging society [7]. Sarcopenia is a syndrome characterized by progressive and generalized loss of skeletal muscle mass and strength with a risk of adverse outcomes such as physical disability, poor quality of life, and poor prognosis. Recently, CT-defined sarcopenia, such as skeletal mass index at the L3 level (L3-SMI), psoas muscle mass index at the L3 level (L3-PMI), and skeletal muscle radiation attenuation at the L3 level (L3-MRA), became known as a prognostic factor in patients with liver diseases and patients after surgery [8–14]. However, the relationship between sarcopenia and prognosis in PEG patients is still unknown.

In this study, we evaluated whether the existence of sarcopenia at the time of undergoing PEG affects overall survival. We also investigated which of the sarcopenia indices, including L3-SMI, L3-PMI, and L3-MRA, would be the most useful factor for demonstrating the association with poor prognosis.

2. Materials and Methods

2.1. Study Design

We conducted a retrospective study of patients who consecutively underwent PEG from March 2008 to April 2020 at the Jikei University Hospital (Tokyo, Japan). Patients who had baseline cross-sectional abdominal computed tomography (CT) scans within one month before or two weeks after PEG were included. Exclusion criteria were as follows: (1) advanced pharyngeal, laryngeal, or esophageal cancer; (2) other malignant tumors with palliative therapy; (3) unavailability of cross-sectional CT images at the third lumbar vertebra (L3) level; (4) receiving PEG for a purpose other than nutritional support (i.e., the decompression of the gastrointestinal tract); and (5) lack of clinical data for the analysis (e.g., body height and laboratory data).

2.2. Diagnosis of Sarcopenia

L3-SMI derived from CT scan was used for the diagnosis of sarcopenia. L3-SMI is a surrogate parameter for evaluating sarcopenia in study participants whose grip strength and walking speed could not be measured (e.g., due to dementia and/or gait disturbance) [15,16]. The patients undergoing PEG at our institution routinely receive preoperative CT scans to verify the anatomical relationship between the stomach and adjacent organs. In this study, a single image that included the spinous process of L3 was collected from the preoperative CT image file for each patient. Then, the skeletal muscle area (SMA) (cm^2) was automatically quantified within a Hounsfield unit (HU) range of -30 to 110 [17–20] using OsiriX DICOM viewer (version 12.0.3; Pixmeo SARL, Bernex, Switzerland) after the intra-abdominal organs in that range were manually traced and excluded (Figure 1A). SMA was normalized for body height in meters squared (m^2) to calculate the lumbar skeletal muscle index (SMI) (cm^2/m^2) [21–23]. In addition, L3-PMI (psoas muscle area/body height2 [cm^2/m^2]) (Figure 1B) and L3-MRA (HU) (Figure 1C) were also evaluated. To diagnose sarcopenia, we used L3-SMI cut-off values of 29.6 cm^2/m^2 for women and 36.2 cm^2/m^2 for men [24] and L3-PMI cut-off values of 3.92 cm^2/m^2 for women and 6.36 cm^2/m^2 for men as previously reported [25], whereas the L3-MRA was dichotomized by the median for each gender due to lack of appropriate cut-off values. All measurements were performed by a single trained physician in a blinded manner.

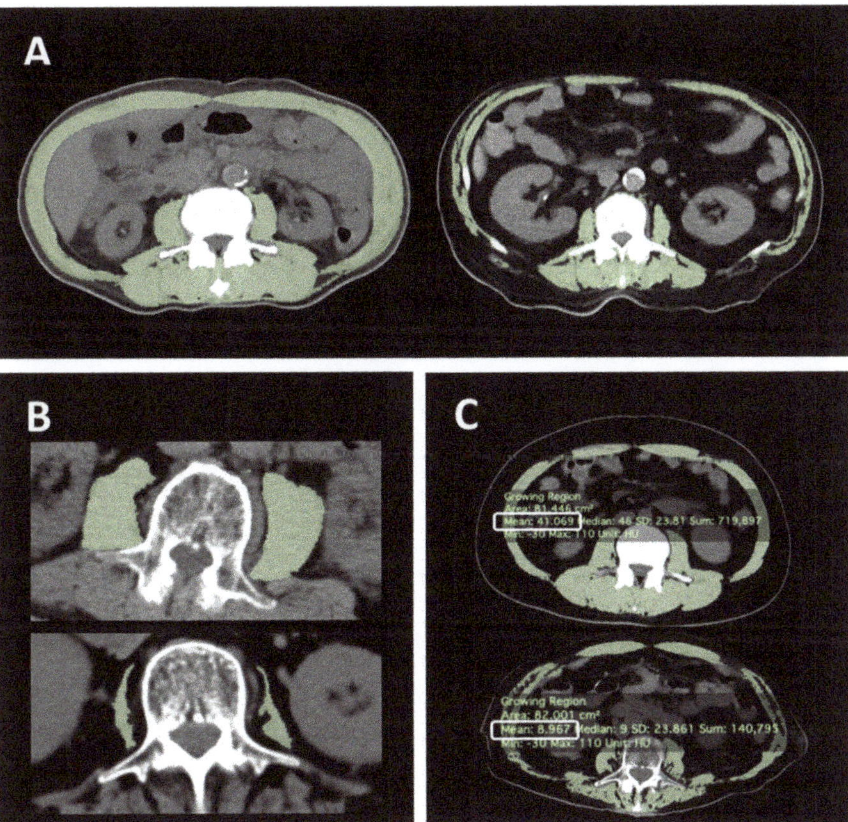

Figure 1. Representative CT images at the level of the third lumbar vertebra. The CT images of patients with (**A**) (**left**) high and (**right**) low L3-SMI and (**B**) (**above**) high and (**below**) low L3-PMI. The areas in green represent the region of skeletal muscle automatically annotated by OsiriX DICOM viewer (version 12.0.3; Pixmeo SARL, Switzerland). (**C**) The images of the skeletal muscles with (**above**) high and (**below**) low values of L3-MRA. The numbers in white squares denote the L3-MRA values that present the average density values (HU) of the skeletal muscle mass at the L3 level. CT, computed tomography; L3-SMI, skeletal muscle mass index at the level of the third lumbar vertebra; L3-PMI, psoas muscle mass index at the level of the third lumbar vertebra; HU, Hounsfield Units; and L3-MRA, muscle radiation attenuation at the level of the third lumbar vertebra.

2.3. Outcomes

The primary outcome was the difference in overall survival between patients with low and high L3-SMI. Secondary outcomes were (1) the difference in overall survival between patients with low and high L3-PMI, (2) the difference in overall survival between patients with low and high L3-MRA, and (3) the difference in overall survival between patients with low and high L3-SMI in a subgroup with the covariate balancing propensity score matching (CBPS). Primary disease warranting PEG was selected from one of the following: (a) Parkinson's disease; (b) amyotrophic lateral sclerosis; (c) multiple system atrophy; (d) other neurological disease; (e) cerebral infarction; (f) cerebral hemorrhage; (g) subarachnoid hemorrhage; (h) other cerebrovascular disease; (i) dementia, and (j) other disease.

2.4. Statistical Analysis

Between-group differences in demographics and clinical data were evaluated using the Chi square test or Fisher exact test for categorical variables and the Student *t*-test and

Mann–Whitney U test for continuous variables. Overall survival was determined using the Kaplan–Meier method. Cox proportional hazards regression model was used to determine the relationship of explanatory variables with overall survival as hazard ratios (HR) and 95% confidence intervals (CI). The cut-off date was set for May 2021. In case of loss to follow-up, the final date the patient was confirmed as alive was censored.

To control for confounding, the following variables were used as the explanatory variables in Cox proportional hazard regression analyses: (1) age (years), (2) sex (male/female), (3) body mass index (BMI) (kg/m^2]), (4) serum albumin level (g/dL), (5) C-reactive protein (mg/dL), (6) total lymphocyte count [26], and (7) previous history of pneumonia (yes/no). Continuous variables were categorized into binary variables: <1.0 and $\geq$1.0 (mg/dL) for C-reactive protein (4) and <1.5 and $\geq$1.5 ($\times10^9$/L) for total lymphocyte count [26]. Bayesian information criterion was used for model selection. CBPS was performed using 'CBPS' package in R using nearest-neighbor matching (1:1 ratio) with a caliper width of 0.2 of the SD of the logit of the score. Matched variables were (1) age (years), (2) sex (male/female), (3) serum albumin level (g/dL), (4) C-reactive protein (mg/dL), (5) total lymphocyte count (TLC) (mg/dL), and (6) previous history of pneumonia (yes/no).

Log-rank test was applied to compare overall survival between groups after matching. Sensitivity analysis was performed for the cut-off values, binarization of variables, the method selecting explanatory variables used for multivariate analysis, and survival analysis when propensity score was used as a covariate instead of matching. Two-tailed tests were used to compare two groups, and $p < 0.05$ was considered significant. All statistical analyses and graphing were carried out using R version 4.0.2 (R Foundation for Statistical Computing, Vienna, Austria) online.3.

3. Results

3.1. Patients Enrollments

Of the 410 patients who underwent PEG during the study period, 283 met at least one of the exclusion criteria, so 127 were selected for analysis. Of these 127 patients, 71 cases (56%) were classified as low L3-SMI, 101 cases (80%) as low L3-PMI, and 63 cases (50%) as low L3-MRA (Figure 2).

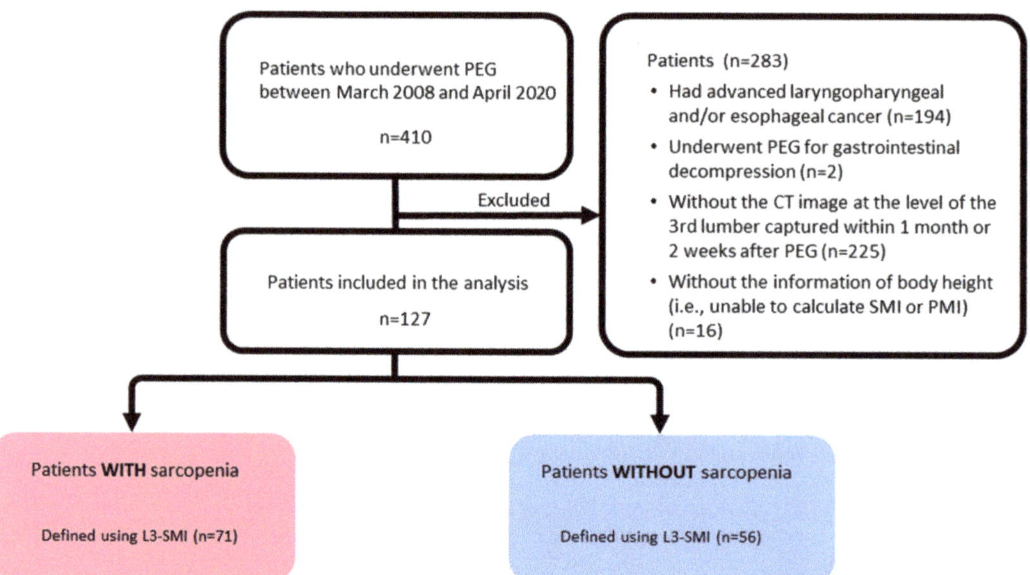

Figure 2. Flow diagram of the study selection process.

PEG, percutaneous endoscopic gastroplasty; CT, computed tomography; L3-SMI, skeletal muscle mass index at the level of the third lumbar vertebra; L3-PMI, psoas muscle mass index at the level of the third lumbar vertebra; and L3-MRA, skeletal muscle radiation attenuation at the level of the third lumbar vertebra.

3.2. Patients Characteristics

Table 1 shows the characteristics of all patients and each group based on the status of L3-SMI, L3-PMI, and L3-MRA. The low L3-SMI group was significantly older ($p = 0.04$) and had lower BMI ($p < 0.001$) compared with the high L3-SMI group. There was no difference in albumin levels between these two groups ($p = 0.2$). Men ($p = 0.001$) were significantly more represented in the low L3-PMI group. The high L3-PMI group had significantly lower albumin levels ($p = 0.03$), cholinesterase ($p = 0.002$), and platelets ($p = 0.002$).

Table 1. Difference in background characteristics of the patients in high and low groups of L3-SMI, L3-PMI, and L3-MRA.

Factor		L3-SMI High		L3-SMI Low		*p* Value	L3-PMI High		L3-PMI Low		*p* Value	L3-MRA High		L3-MRA Low		*p* Value
n		56		71			26		101			63		64		
Sex, *n* (%) Female	Female	20	(35.7)	18	(25.4)	0.2	15	(57.7)	23	(22.8)	0.001	19	(30.1)	18	(28.1)	1
	Male	36	(64.3)	53	(74.6)		11	(42.3)	78	(77.2)		44	(70.0)	46	(71.9)	
Age, mean (SD)	years	70.0	(14.3)	75.4	(14.5)	0.04	71.0	(11.5)	73.5	(15.3)	0.4	71.8	(15.3)	74.2	(13.9)	0.4
Body height, mean (SD)	cm	159.9	(9.3)	161.1	(9.1)	0.5	157.1	(7.6)	161.5	(9.4)	0.03	160.4	(8.4)	161.1	(10.0)	0.7
Body weight, mean (SD)	kg	56.1	(15.2)	49.9	(11.6)	0.01	52.8	(14.1)	52.6	(13.6)	0.9	50.0	(12.2)	55.3	(14.6)	0.03
BMI, mean (SD)	kg/m^2	21.7	(4.3)	19.1	(3.7)	<0.001	21.2	(4.9)	20.0	(3.4)	0.2	19.2	(3.7)	21.2	(4.4)	0.01
Pneumonia, *n* (%)	No	38	(67.9)	34	(47.9)	0.03	18	(69.2)	54	(53.5)	0.2	33	(52.4)	38	(60.3)	0.5
	Yes	18	(32.1)	37	(52.1)		8	(30.8)	47	(46.5)		30	(47.6)	25	(39.7)	
Total protein, mean (SD)	g/dL	6.4	(0.8)	6.3	(0.8)	0.6	6.5	(0.6)	6.3	(0.8)	0.1	6.4	(0.8)	6.2	(0.8)	0.4
Serum albumin, mean (SD)	g/dL	3.0	(0.6)	2.9	(0.6)	0.2	3.2	(0.5)	2.9	(0.6)	0.03	3.0	(0.6)	2.8	(0.6)	0.04
Serum TC, mean (SD)	mg/dL	48.8	(90.6)	64.5	(84.6)	0.5	47.8	(71.8)	60.0	(89.1)	0.7	43.6	(71.3)	80.6	(102.2)	0.09
Serum ChE, mean (SD)	U/L	201	(743.7)	183.1	(80)	0.2	2364	(69)	180.8	(76)	0.002	198	(78)	183.2	(77)	0.3
Serum CRP, mean (SD)	mg/dL	1.2	(2.2)	1.8	(2.4)	0.2	1.1	(1.6)	1.6	(2.4)	0.3	1.1	(1.7)	1.9	(2.7)	0.04
PNI, mean (SD)		36.5	(6.9)	35.7	(7.6)	0.5	38.3	(5.6)	35.5	(7.6)	0.09	36.9	(7.1)	35.1	(7.4)	0.2
Hemoglobin, mean (SD)	g/dL	11.7	(1.8)	11.1	(2.0)	0.08	11.9	(1.7)	11.2	(1.9)	0.1	11.7	(1.9)	11.0	(1.9)	0.03
Platelet, mean (SD)	$\times 10^9$/L	261	(121)	233	(106)	0.2	306	(146)	230.1	(99)	0.002	258	(134)	230.9	(87)	0.2
WBC, mean (SD)	$\times 10^9$/L	6.4	(2.0)	9.4	(21.8)	0.3	6.8	(1.7)	8.4	(18.3)	0.7	6.4	(2.4)	9.7	(23.0)	0.3
TLC, mean (SD)	$\times 10^9$/L	1.3	(0.5)	1.4	(0.7)	0.3	1.4	(0.5)	1.4	(0.7)	0.8	1.3	(0.6)	1.4	(0.7)	0.5

L3-SMI, skeletal muscle mass index at the third lumbar level; L3-PMI, psoas muscle mass index at the third lumbar level; L3-MRA, skeletal muscle radiation attenuation at the third lumbar level; SD, standard deviation; BMI, body mass index; TC, total cholesterol; ChE, Choline esterase; CRP, C-reactive protein; PNI, Onodera's prognostic nutritional index; WBC, white blood cell count; and TLC, total lymphocyte count.

3.3. Overall Follow-Up Period and Events

The median follow-up period was 716 (502–941) days, during which 64 patients (50.4%) died. The median overall survival was 666 (387–992) days. The overall survival rate was 95.2% (89.7–97.8) at 30 days, 90.3% (83.6–94.4) at 60 days, 83.6% (75.7–89.1) at 90 days, and 60.1% (50.3–68.6) at 180 days. The median follow-up period did not differ significantly between the low and high groups in each of the three indices: L3-SMI, 645 (356–945) vs. 811 (411–972) days ($p = 0.5$); L3-PMI, 889 (455–1240) vs. 694 (411–941) days ($p = 0.6$); and 582 (52–NA) vs. 943 (688–1378) days ($p = 0.052$).

Of the 64 deaths, 46 deaths were observed in the low L3-SMI group, and 18 deaths were observed in the high L3-SMI group. Among the 46 deaths in the low L3-SMI group, the cause of death was identified in 38 patients. The most frequent cause of death was pneumonia ($n = 29$), and the other deaths were due to cardiovascular disease ($n = 2$), renal failure ($n = 1$), gastrointestinal necrosis ($n = 1$), superior mesenteric artery embolism ($n = 1$), and death due to primary disease (*n* = 4). Among the 18 deaths in the high L3-SMI group, the cause of death was identified in 13 patients. Six patients died of pneumonia. Other deaths were due to cardiovascular disease (*n* = 2), hepatic failure (*n* = 1), gastrointestinal bleeding (*n* = 1), and death of primary disease (*n* = 3). No PEG-related death was observed in either group. The pneumonia mortality rate tended to be higher in the Low L3-SMI group though the difference was not statistically significant (Low SMI group vs. High SMI group = 76.3% vs. 46.2%; *p* = 0.08).

3.4. Survival Rates and Log-Rank Analyses at 90 and 180 Days and One Year

The median survival was significantly shorter in the low SMI group than in the high SMI group: 273 (95% CI, 163–638) vs. 1133 (666–NA) days; *p* < 0.001 (Figure 3A). The survival rate at 90 days was 75.4% (63.4–83.9) in the low L3-SMI group vs. 94.4% (83.6–98.2) in the high L3-SMI group, 60.1% (47.4–70.7) vs. 92.4% (80.9–97.1) at 180 days and 43.7% (31.3–55.3) vs. 82.8% (68.2–91.1) at one year of follow-up.

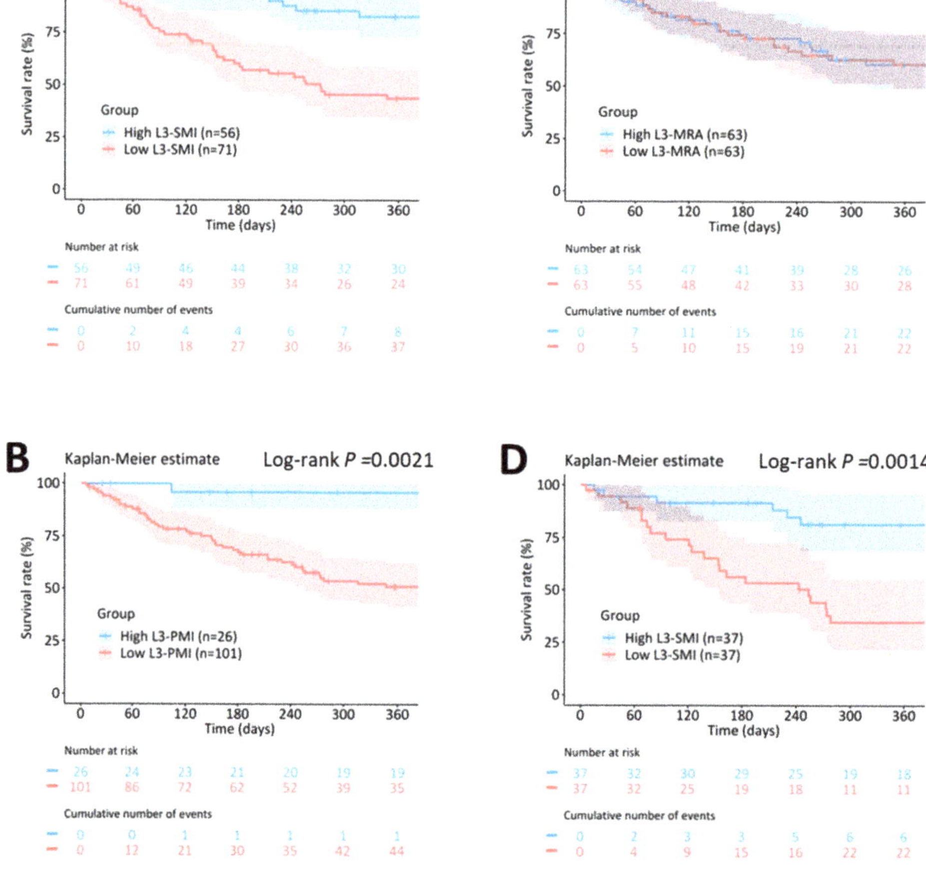

Figure 3. Kaplan–Meier survival curves in patients with and without sarcopenia. Kaplan–Meier survival curves for (**A**) High L3-SMI and Low L3-SMI, (**B**) High L3-PMI and Low L3-PMI, (**C**) High L3-MRA and Low L3-MRA, and (**D**) High L3-SMI and Low L3-SMI after covariate balancing propensity score matching.

The median survival was significantly shorter in the low PMI group than in the high PMI group: 387 (245–863) vs. 1133 (736–NA) days; $p = 0.0021$ (log-rank test) (Figure 3B). The survival rate at 90 days was 79.4% (69.9–86.2) in the low L3-PMI vs. 100% (NA–NA) in the high L3-PMI group, 68.4% (58.0–76.8) vs. 95.8% (73.9–99.4) at 180 days, and 50.9% (39.9–60.9) vs. 95.8% (73.9–99.4) at one year.

The overall survival did not differ significantly between the low and high MRA group (median survival days, 638 (278–867) vs. 1133 (274–NA) days; $p = 0.2$ (log-rank test)) (Figure 3C). We observed no difference between the two groups in the 90-day survival rate (85.0% (73.2–91.9) vs. 83.5% (71.5–90.8)), 180-day survival rate (74.5% (61.3–83.8) vs. 74.7% (61.5–83.9)) or the one-year survival rate (60.6% (46.3–72.2) vs. 60.6% (46.3–72.2)).

Sarcopenia was defined by (A) L3-SMI, (B) L3-PMI, and (C) L3-MRA in all patients ($n = 127$). (D) Subgroup analysis with propensity score matching of known prognostic predictors (high vs. low L3-SMI) ($n = 74$). The color bands represent a 95% confidence interval in each group. L3-SMI, skeletal muscle mass index at the level of the third lumbar vertebra; L3-PMI, psoas muscle mass index at the level of the third lumbar vertebra; and L3-MRA, skeletal muscle radiation attenuation at the level of the third lumbar vertebra.

3.5. Univariate and Multivariate Cox Proportional Hazard Analyses

In univariate analyses, L3-SMI, L3-PMI, and all known risk factors (male sex, age, BMI, hypoalbuminemia, total lymphocyte count $< 1.5 \times 10^9$/L, C-reactive protein ≥ 1.0 mg/dL and underlying pneumonia) emerged as predictive factors related to poor prognosis (Table 2). In multivariate analyses, low L3-SMI, male sex, and hypoalbuminemia were independent risk factors for poor overall survival.

Table 2. Results of univariate and multivariate Cox proportional hazard regression analysis.

Variables	Univariate Cox Proportional Hazard Regression Analysis		Multivariate Cox Proportional Hazard Regression Analysis *	
	HR (95% CI)	*p* Value	Adjusted HR (95% CI)	*p* Value
L3-SMI, low group	2.8 (1.6–4.8)	<0.001	2.9 (1.6–5.4)	<0.001
L3-PMI, low group	3.2 (1.5–7.1)	0.004	(-)	
L3-MRA, low group	1.4 (0.9–2.4)	0.2	(-)	
Sex, male	1.8 (1.0–3.3)	0.046	2.0 (1.1–3.7)	0.03
Age, per year	1.9 (1.2–3.2)	0.01	(-)	
BMI, per kg/mm^2	0.94 (0.89–1.0)	0.049	(-)	
Serum albumin, per g/dL	0.34 (0.21–0.56)	<0.001	0.34 (0.21–0.55)	<0.001
TLC, <1.5 $\times 10^9$/L	1.8 (1.0–3.0)	0.04	(-)	
Serum CRP, $\geq$1.0 mg/dL	2.5 (1.5–4.1)	0.0004	(-)	
Underlying pneumonia, yes	1.9 (1.1–3.2)	0.02	(-)	

* In the multivariate analysis, explanatory variables were selected using Bayesian information criterion. HR, hazard ratio; CI, confidence interval; L3-SMI, skeletal muscle mass index at the third lumber level; L3-PMI, Psoas muscle mass index at the third lumber level; L3-MRA, Muscle radiation attenuation at the third lumber level; BMI, body mass index; CRP, C-reactive protein; PNI, Onodera's prognostic nutritional index; WBC, white blood cell count; and TLC, total lymphocyte count.

3.6. Covariate-Balancing Propensity Score Matching Analyses

Based on the covariate balancing propensity scores, the two groups were matched using the covariates of age, gender, BMI, the coexistence of pneumonia, albumin level, CRP, and lymphocyte count, and 37 patients were selected from each group. Most of the standardized mean differences for the matched factors decreased after matching (Table 3). The log-rank analysis revealed that the overall survival was significantly shorter in the low SMI group (254 (95% CI, 124–538) vs. 1341 (604–NA) days; $p = 0.0014$) (Figure 3D). The survival rate at 90 days was 77.1% (59.3–87.8) in the low L3-SMI group vs. 91.5% (75.8–97.2) in the L3-SMI group, 56.3% (38.3–71.0) vs. 91.5% (75.8–97.2) at 180 days, and 34.7% (19.2–50.6) vs. 81.3% (62.9–91.2) at one year of follow-up.

Table 3. Difference in background characteristics of the patients between low and high L3-SMI group before- and after-covariate balancing propensity score matching.

Factor		Before-Matching					After-Matching				
		High L3-SMI		Low L3-SMI		SMD	High L3-SMI		Low L3-SMI		SMD
n		56		71			37		37		
Matched variables											
Sex, *n* (%)	Female	20	(35.7)	18	(25.4)	0.226	13.0	(35.1)	11.0	(29.7)	0.116
	Male	36	(64.3)	53	(74.6)		24.0	(64.9)	26.0	(70.3)	
Age, mean (SD)	years	70.0	(14.3)	75.4	(14.5)	0.374	73.1	(13.0)	73.2	(17.5)	0.009
BMI, mean (SD)		21.7	(4.3)	19.1	(3.7)	0.644	21.3	(4.7)	20.6	(4.1)	0.15
Pneumonia, *n* (%)	No	38	(67.9)	34	(47.9)	0.413	22.0	(59.5)	24.0	(64.9)	0.112
	Yes	18	(32.1)	37	(52.1)		15.0	(40.5)	13.0	(35.1)	
Albumin, mean (SD)	g/dL	3.0	(0.6)	2.9	(0.6)	0.235	2.9	(0.6)	3.0	(0.7)	0.072
CRP, mean (SD)	mg/dL	1.2	(2.2)	1.8	(2.4)	0.257	1.3	(2.5)	1.4	(2.4)	0.075
TLC, mean (SD)	$\times 10^9$/L	1.3	(0.5)	1.4	(0.7)	0.176	1364.9	(529.8)	1224.3	(530.4)	0.265
Non-matched variables											
Body height, mean (SD)	cm	159.9	(9.3)	161.1	(9.1)	0.134	8.8	(8.8)	161.6	(8.7)	0.341
Body weight, mean (SD)	kg	56.1	(15.2)	49.9	(11.6)	0.462	15.2	(15.2)	54.0	(12.7)	0.005
Total protein, mean (SD)	g/dL	6.4	(0.8)	6.3	(0.8)	0.098	1.0	(0.9)	6.2	(0.7)	0.146
PNI, mean (SD)		36.5	(6.9)	35.7	(7.6)	0.114	6.9	(6.9)	35.6	(7.8)	0.033
ChE, mean (SD)	U/L	201.8	(73.7)	183.1	(79.6)	0.244	64.1	(64.1)	200.1	(88.5)	0.173
WBC, mean (SD)	$\times 10^9$/L	6.4	(2.0)	9.4	(21.8)	0.193	1842.9	(1842.9)	11,329.7	(30,116.8)	0.241
Hemoglobin, mean (SD)	g/dL	11.7	(1.8)	11.1	(2.0)	0.315	1.8	(1.7)	11.0	(2)	0.182
Platelet count, mean (SD)	$\times 10^9$/L	261.7	(121.4)	233.0	(105.8)	0.252	13.7	(13.7)	23.8	(8.1)	0.299

L3-SMI, skeletal muscle mass index at the third lumber level; SMD, standardized mean difference; SD, standard deviation; BMI, body mass index; CRP, C-reactive protein; PNI, Onodera's prognostic nutritional index; WBC, white blood cell count; and TLC, total lymphocyte count.

3.7. Correlation between Sarcopenia-Related Indices and Relationship with Body Mass Index

The correlation coefficient between sarcopenia-related indices and BMI is described in Figure 4. A very strong correlation was observed between L3-SMI and L3-PMI ($r = 0.71$, $p < 0.001$), and each of them showed a moderate correlation with BMI (L3-SMI, $r = 0.48$, $p < 0.001$; L3-PMI, $r = 0.45$, $p < 0.001$; L3-MRA, $r = -0.13$, $p = 0.1$). This trend was observed irrespective of gender. Meanwhile, the relationships between L3-MRA and L3-SMI, L3-PMI, and BMI, respectively, was weak (L3-SMI, $r = 0.28$, $p = 0.002$; L3-PMI, $r = 0.15$, $p = 0.09$; BMI, $r = -0.13$, $p = 0.1$) (Figure 4).

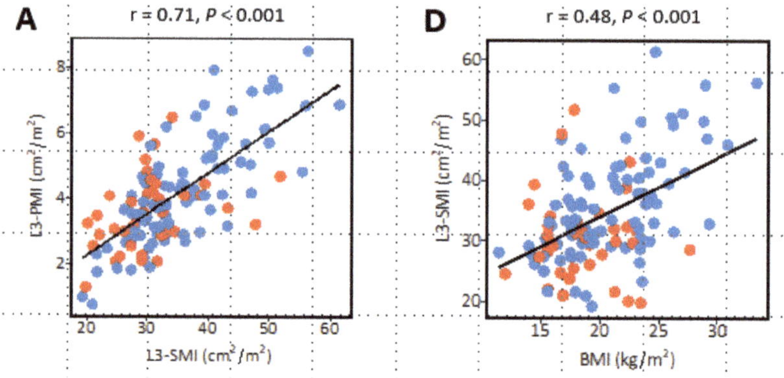

Figure 4. *Cont.*

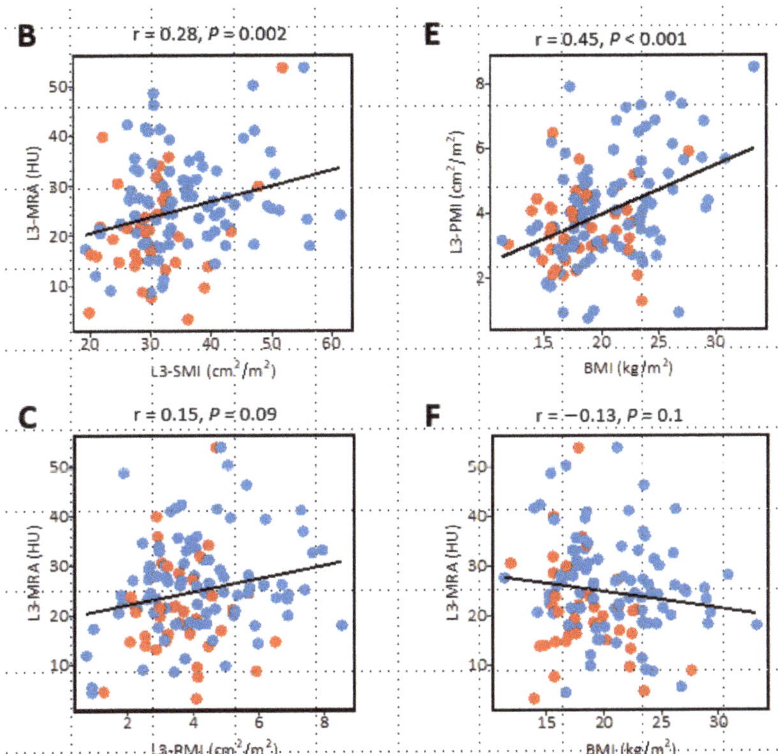

Figure 4. Correlations between each sarcopenia-related indices and between each index and body mass index. Scatterplots for (**A**) L3-SMI and L3-PMI, (**B**) L3-SMI and L3-MRA, and (**C**) L3-PMI and L3-MRA, (**D**) BMI and L3-SMI, (**E**) BMI and L3-PMI, and (**F**) BMI and L3-MRA. Red dots denote female patients, and blue dots show male patients. The black line represents a linear regression line; the region in gray denotes 95% CIs. L3-SMI, skeletal muscle mass index at the level of the third lumbar vertebra. L3-PMI, psoas muscle mass index at the level of the third lumbar vertebra; and L3-MRA, skeletal muscle radiation attenuation at the level of the third lumbar vertebra; and BMI, body mass index.

4. Discussion

To the best of our knowledge, this is the first study to identify preoperative sarcopenia as a prognostic factor for poor survival after PEG in geriatric patients. Hypoalbuminemia was previously established as a prognostic factor associated with PEG, but in this study, sarcopenia emerged as a new prognostic factor associated with PEG independent of hypoalbuminemia.

In the literature, sarcopenia and prognosis have been positively and negatively associated. CT-defined sarcopenia has been known as a prognostic predictor of several hepatic diseases [13,24,27–30], yet sarcopenia does not always worsen survival [31–33]. In our study, sarcopenia negatively affected the prognosis in patients who underwent PEG.

Although there was no significant difference observed in the univariate analysis of L3-SMI with respect to the presence of underlying pneumonia (Supplementary Table S1), pneumonia-related death tended to be more frequent in patients with sarcopenia. Sarcopenia has been identified as a risk factor for pneumonia because of poor chewing and swallowing functions, delayed mobilization, dysphagia, or difficulty in clearing the airway [34]. Sarcopenia is also associated with reduced glutamine production, leading to intestinal dysfunction and infectious complications [35]. These factors may be related to higher mortality related to pneumonia after PEG in patients with sarcopenia.

In this study, among the indicators of sarcopenia, L3-SMI showed significant differences in multivariate analysis. We only diagnosed sarcopenia by skeletal muscle mass in CT images and did not evaluate other factors of sarcopenia. Grip strength and walking speed are commonly used as diagnostic indicators for sarcopenia, but it would be difficult to measure such muscle function in PEG patients because of their severe frailty. However, the correlation between L3-SMI and grip strength has been already reported [36], and L3-SMI has been discerned as an important indicator of sarcopenia. Thus, it was appropriate to use CT images, which are objective and usually taken preoperatively for patients with PEG, for the evaluation of sarcopenia in our study. L3-SMI may be the most suitable factor for predicting prognosis, especially for evaluating sarcopenia in PEG patients.

Median survival did not differ significantly between the low and high L3-MRA groups in this study. A recent study concluded that low L3-MRA, which equally demonstrates sarcopenic obesity, was also associated with higher mortality in patients with hepatocellular carcinoma [24], but we could not confirm that observation. The reason L3-MRA did not affect prognosis in our study may be the limitations of assessing L3-MRA in PEG patients. Since L3-MRA is a method for evaluating tissue components using the CT value of skeletal muscle, it may fluctuate due to the influence of the CT value. In cases with strong edematous changes, as in PEG patients who may have constitutional edema associated with hypoalbuminemia, the CT value in the muscle is expected to decrease due to an increase in water content, and this might affect the L3-MRA level in our study.

In order to minimize the influence of potential confounding variables, we evaluated the prognostic impact of preoperative sarcopenia using CBPS and sensitivity analysis. This analysis provided additional evidence that can support and strengthen the relationship between sarcopenia and poor prognosis and demonstrated that sarcopenia was a robust prognostic factor after PEG compared to other known prognostic factors (Supplementary Table S2).

From our result, assessing sarcopenia in addition to existing independent prognostic factors of PEG may provide important information for patients and their families to discuss the indication of PEG. Evaluating sarcopenia at baseline may lead to the development of tailored preventive strategies, such as early nutritional interventions, physical exercise programs, and individualized care plans for patients with sarcopenia who undergo PEG placement.

This study has limitations. 1. The major population of PEG in the present study was non-malignancy patients with dysphagia (such as Parkinson's disease, amyotrophic lateral sclerosis, multiple system atrophy, and other neurological diseases). We excluded malignancy patients in this study because prognosis can vary depending on cancer stage classification in malignancy patients. Our result may only be limited to non-malignancy patients. 2. Primary and secondary sarcopenia were not distinguished in this study. The results may differ if they were considered separately. Although most of the patients were considered to have secondary sarcopenia associated with malnutrition, low activity, and diseases, it was difficult to distinguish them retrospectively. 3. We excluded patients without pre-procedural CT in this study. It was unclear why procedural CT was not performed in these patients. Although the patients' BMI and survival were similar between patients with and without pre-procedural CT (BMI: 19.7 vs. 19.3, $p = 0.3$, survival days: 384 days vs. 416 days, $p = 0.5$), this exclusion may introduce bias in patient selection. 4. We only included cases with plain CT, as skeletal muscle measurements could be influenced by the use of contrast agent in contrast CT, which may result in selection bias [37]. 5. The cut-off value may not be appropriate in this study. We used the previously reported Asian cut-off value because an association of sarcopenia with PEG patients has not been reported. Since the general condition and nutritional status of patients undergoing PEG tend to be poor, new cut-off values for defining sarcopenia in PEG patients may be considered.

J. Clin. Med. **2023**, *12*, 3360

5. Conclusions

In conclusion, the presence of preoperative sarcopenia was identified as an independent prognostic factor for patients undergoing PEG. Assessing sarcopenia may provide important information for the indication of PEG and may lead to the development of tailored preventive strategies in an increasingly aging society.

Supplementary Materials: The following supporting information can be downloaded at: https://www.mdpi.com/article/10.3390/10.3390/jcm12103360/s1, Table S1: Difference in background characteristics of the patients with or without underlying pneumonia, Table S2: Sensitivity analysis.

Author Contributions: Conceptualization, S.O.; methodology, S.O.; formal analysis, H.F.; resources, S.K. and H.O.; data curation, H.H., H.M. and S.K.; writing—original draft preparation, S.O.; writing—review and editing, H.F. and A.D.; visualization, H.F.; validation H.O.; supervision, K.S. All authors have read and agreed to the published version of the manuscript.

Funding: This research received no external funding.

Institutional Review Board Statement: The study was conducted in accordance with the Declaration of Helsinki and approved by the Ethics Committee of the Jikei University School of Medicine (No. 32-420(10509); 19 April 2021, Tokyo, Japan). The study registration number was UMIN000047005 in the University Hospital Medical Information Network Clinical Trials Registry.

Informed Consent Statement: As this study was retrospective, the documents approved by the ethics committee were posted on the hospital website. We disclosed the information on this study and provided the patients with an opportunity to refuse.

Data Availability Statement: The data that support the findings of this study are available from the corresponding author upon reasonable request.

Acknowledgments: The authors thank Sho Takahashi for advice on statistical analysis.

Conflicts of Interest: The authors declare no conflict of interest.

References

1. Gauderer, M.W.; Ponsky, J.L.; Izant, R.J. Gastrostomy without laparotomy: A percutaneous endoscopic technique. *Nutrition* **1998**, *14*, 736–738. [CrossRef] [PubMed]
2. Rustom, I.K.; Jebreel, A.; Tayyab, M.; England, R.J.A.; Stafford, N.D. Percutaneous endoscopic, radiological and surgical gastrostomy tubes: A comparison study in head and neck cancer patients. *J. Laryngol. Otol.* **2006**, *120*, 463–466. [CrossRef]
3. Suzuki, Y.; Tamez, S.; Murakami, A.; Taira, A.; Mizuhara, A.; Horiuchi, A.; Mihara, C.; Ako, E.; Muramatsu, H.; Okano, H.; et al. Survival of geriatric patients after percutaneous endoscopic gastrostomy in Japan. *World J. Gastroenterol.* **2010**, *16*, 5084–5091. [CrossRef] [PubMed]
4. Blomberg, J.; Lagergren, P.; Martin, L.; Mattsson, F.; Lagergren, J. Albumin and C-reactive protein levels predict short-term mortality after percutaneous endoscopic gastrostomy in a prospective cohort study. *Gastrointest. Endosc.* **2011**, *73*, 29–36. [CrossRef] [PubMed]
5. Tokunaga, T.; Kubo, T.; Ryan, S.; Tomizawa, M.; Yoshida, S.-I.; Takagi, K.; Furui, K.; Gotoh, T. Long-term outcome after placement of a percutaneous endoscopic gastrostomy tube. *Geriatr. Gerontol. Int.* **2008**, *8*, 19–23. [CrossRef] [PubMed]
6. Anker, S.D.; Morley, J.E.; von Haehling, S. Welcome to the ICD-10 code for sarcopenia. *J. Cachexia Sarcopenia Muscle* **2016**, *7*, 512–514. [CrossRef]
7. Shafiee, G.; Keshtkar, A.; Soltani, A.; Ahadi, Z.; Larijani, B.; Heshmat, R. Prevalence of sarcopenia in the world: A systematic review and meta- analysis of general population studies. *J. Diabetes Metab. Disord.* **2017**, *16*, 21. [CrossRef]
8. Kim, G.; Kang, S.H.; Kim, M.Y.; Baik, S.K. Prognostic value of sarcopenia in patients with liver cirrhosis: A systematic review and meta-analysis. *PLoS ONE* **2017**, *12*, e0186990. [CrossRef]
9. Zhang, X.M.; Chen, D.; Xie, X.H.; Zhang, J.E.; Zeng, Y.; Cheng, A.S. Sarcopenia as a predictor of mortality among the critically ill in an intensive care unit: A systematic review and meta-analysis. *BMC Geriatr.* **2021**, *21*, 339. [CrossRef] [PubMed]
10. Ratnayake, C.B.; Loveday, B.P.; Shrikhande, S.V.; Windsor, J.A.; Pandanaboyana, S. Impact of preoperative sarcopenia on postoperative outcomes following pancreatic resection: A systematic review and meta-analysis. *Pancreatology* **2018**, *18*, 996–1004. [CrossRef] [PubMed]
11. Chen, F.; Chi, J.; Liu, Y.; Fan, L.; Hu, K. Impact of preoperative sarcopenia on postoperative complications and prognosis of gastric cancer resection: A meta-analysis of cohort studies. *Arch. Gerontol. Geriatr.* **2022**, *98*, 104534. [CrossRef] [PubMed]
12. Peng, Y.-C.; Wu, C.-H.; Tien, Y.-W.; Lu, T.-P.; Wang, Y.-H.; Chen, B.-B. Preoperative sarcopenia is associated with poor overall survival in pancreatic cancer patients following pancreaticoduodenectomy. *Eur. Radiol.* **2021**, *31*, 2472–2481. [CrossRef] [PubMed]

13. Iritani, S.; Imai, K.; Takai, K.; Hanai, T.; Ideta, T.; Miyazaki, T.; Suetsugu, A.; Shiraki, M.; Shimizu, M.; Moriwaki, H. Skeletal muscle depletion is an independent prognostic factor for hepatocellular carcinoma. *J. Gastroenterol.* **2015**, *50*, 323–332. [CrossRef] [PubMed]

14. Hanai, T.; Shiraki, M.; Nishimura, K.; Ohnishi, S.; Imai, K.; Suetsugu, A.; Takai, K.; Shimizu, M.; Moriwaki, H. Sarcopenia impairs prognosis of patients with liver cirrhosis. *Nutrition* **2015**, *31*, 193–199. [CrossRef] [PubMed]

15. Mourtzakis, M.; Prado, C.M.; Lieffers, J.R.; Reiman, T.; McCargar, L.J.; Baracos, V.E. A practical and precise approach to quantification of body composition in cancer patients using computed tomography images acquired during routine care. *Appl. Physiol. Nutr. Metab.* **2008**, *33*, 997–1006. [CrossRef]

16. Mitsiopoulos, N.; Baumgartner, R.N.; Heymsfield, S.B.; Lyons, W.; Gallagher, D.; Ross, R. Cadaver validation of skeletal muscle measurement by magnetic resonance imaging and computerized tomography. *J. Appl. Physiol.* **1998**, *85*, 115–122. [CrossRef]

17. Mccusker, A.; Khan, M.; Kulvatunyou, N.; Zeeshan, M.; Sakran, J.V.; Hayek, H.; O'Keeffe, T.; Hamidi, M.; Tang, A.; Joseph, B. Sarcopenia defined by a computed tomography estimate of the psoas muscle area does not predict frailty in geriatric trauma patients. *Am. J. Surg.* **2019**, *218*, 261–265. [CrossRef]

18. Dello, S.A.W.G.; Lodewick, T.M.; van Dam, R.M.; Reisinger, K.W.; Broek, M.A.J.V.D.; von Meyenfeldt, M.F.; Bemelmans, M.H.A.; Damink, S.W.M.O.; Dejong, C.H.C. Sarcopenia negatively affects preoperative total functional liver volume in patients undergoing liver resection. *HPB* **2013**, *15*, 165–169. [CrossRef]

19. Tegels, J.J.; van Vugt, J.L.; Reisinger, K.W.; Hulsewé, K.W.; Hoofwijk, A.G.; Derikx, J.P.; Stoot, J.H. Sarcopenia is highly prevalent in patients undergoing surgery for gastric cancer but not associated with worse outcomes. *J. Surg. Oncol.* **2015**, *112*, 403–407. [CrossRef]

20. Reisinger, K.W.; van Vugt, J.L.A.; Tegels, J.J.W.; Snijders, C.; Hulsewé, K.W.E.; Hoofwijk, A.G.M.; Stoot, J.H.; Von Meyenfeldt, M.F.; Beets, G.L.; Derikx, J.P.M.; et al. Functional compromise reflected by sarcopenia, frailty, and nutritional depletion predicts adverse postoperative outcome after colorectal cancer surgery. *Ann. Surg.* **2015**, *261*, 345–352. [CrossRef]

21. Fearon, K.; Strasser, F.; Anker, S.D.; Bosaeus, I.; Bruera, E.; Fainsinger, R.L.; Jatoi, A.; Loprinzi, C.; MacDonald, N.; Mantovani, G.; et al. Definition and classification of cancer cachexia: An international consensus. *Lancet Oncol.* **2011**, *12*, 489–495. [CrossRef]

22. Prado, C.M.; Lieffers, J.R.; McCargar, L.J.; Reiman, T.; Sawyer, M.B.; Martin, L.; Baracos, V.E. Prevalence and clinical implications of sarcopenic obesity in patients with solid tumours of the respiratory and gastrointestinal tracts: A population-based study. *Lancet Oncol.* **2008**, *9*, 629–635. [CrossRef] [PubMed]

23. Martin, L.; Birdsell, L.; MacDonald, N.; Reiman, T.; Clandinin, M.T.; McCargar, L.J.; Murphy, R.; Ghosh, S.; Sawyer, M.B.; Baracos, V.E. Cancer Cachexia in the Age of Obesity: Skeletal Muscle Depletion Is a Powerful Prognostic Factor, Independent of Body Mass Index. *J. Clin. Oncol.* **2013**, *31*, 1539–1547. [CrossRef]

24. Fujiwara, N.; Nakagawa, H.; Kudo, Y.; Tateishi, R.; Taguri, M.; Watadani, T.; Nakagomi, R.; Kondo, M.; Nakatsuka, T.; Minami, T.; et al. Sarcopenia, intramuscular fat deposition, and visceral adiposity independently predict the outcomes of hepatocellular carcinoma. *J. Hepatol.* **2015**, *63*, 131–140. [CrossRef] [PubMed]

25. Hamaguchi, Y.; Kaido, T.; Okumura, S.; Kobayashi, A.; Hammad, A.; Tamai, Y.; Inagaki, N.; Uemoto, S. Proposal for new diagnostic criteria for low skeletal muscle mass based on computed tomography imaging in Asian adults. *Nutrition* **2016**, *32*, 1200–1205. [CrossRef] [PubMed]

26. Cortés-Flores, A.O.; Álvarez-Villaseñor, A.D.S.; Fuentes-Orozco, C.; Ramírez-Campos, K.M.; Ramírez-Arce, A.D.R.; Macías-Amezcua, M.D.; Chavez-Tostado, M.; Hernández-Machuca, J.S.; González-Ojeda, A. Long-term outcome after percutaneous endoscopic gastrostomy in geriatric Mexican patients. *Geriatr. Gerontol. Int.* **2015**, *15*, 19–26. [CrossRef]

27. Okumura, S.; Kaido, T.; Hamaguchi, Y.; Fujimoto, Y.; Masui, T.; Mizumoto, M.; Hammad, A.; Mori, A.; Takaori, K.; Uemoto, S. Impact of preoperative quality as well as quantity of skeletal muscle on survival after resection of pancreatic cancer. *Surgery* **2015**, *157*, 1088–1098. [CrossRef]

28. Zhou, C.-J.; Zhang, F.-M.; Zhang, F.-Y.; Yu, Z.; Chen, X.-L.; Shen, X.; Zhuang, C.-L. Sarcopenia: A new predictor of postoperative complications for elderly gastric cancer patients who underwent radical gastrectomy. *J. Surg. Res.* **2017**, *211*, 137–146. [CrossRef]

29. Miyamoto, Y.; Baba, Y.; Sakamoto, Y.; Ohuchi, M.; Tokunaga, R.; Kurashige, J.; Hiyoshi, Y.; Iwagami, S.; Yoshida, N.; Yoshida, M.; et al. Sarcopenia is a Negative Prognostic Factor After Curative Resection of Colorectal Cancer. *Ann. Surg. Oncol.* **2015**, *22*, 2663–2668. [CrossRef]

30. Harada, K.; Ida, S.; Baba, Y.; Ishimoto, T.; Kosumi, K.; Tokunaga, R.; Izumi, D.; Ohuchi, M.; Nakamura, K.; Kiyozumi, Y.; et al. Prognostic and clinical impact of sarcopenia in esophageal squamous cell carcinoma. *Dis. Esophagus* **2016**, *29*, 627–633. [CrossRef]

31. Benmassaoud, A.; Roccarina, D.; Arico, F.; Leandro, G.; Yu, B.; Cheng, F.; Yu, D.; Patch, D.; Tsochatzis, E. Sarcopenia Does Not Worsen Survival in Patients With Cirrhosis Undergoing Transjugular Intrahepatic Portosystemic Shunt for Refractory Ascites. *Am. J. Gastroenterol.* **2020**, *115*, 1911–1914. [CrossRef] [PubMed]

32. Hayashi, N.; Ando, Y.; Gyawali, B.; Shimokata, T.; Maeda, O.; Fukaya, M.; Goto, H.; Nagino, M.; Kodera, Y. Low skeletal muscle density is associated with poor survival in patients who receive chemotherapy for metastatic gastric cancer. *Oncol. Rep.* **2016**, *35*, "1727–1731. [CrossRef] [PubMed]

33. Grotenhuis, B.A.; Shapiro, J.; Van Adrichem, S.; De Vries, M.; Koek, M.; Wijnhoven, B.P.L.; Van Lanschot, J.J.B. Sarcopenia/Muscle Mass is not a Prognostic Factor for Short- and Long-Term Outcome After Esophagectomy for Cancer. *World J. Surg.* **2016**, *40*, 2698–2704. [CrossRef] [PubMed]

34. Ida, S.; Watanabe, M.; Yoshida, N.; Baba, Y.; Umezaki, N.; Harada, K.; Karashima, R.; Imamura, Y.; Iwagami, S.; Baba, H. Sarcopenia is a Predictor of Postoperative Respiratory Complications in Patients with Esophageal Cancer. *Ann. Surg. Oncol.* **2015**, *22*, 4432–4437. [CrossRef]

35. Biolo, G.; Zorat, F.; Antonione, R.; Ciocchi, B. Muscle glutamine depletion in the intensive care unit. *Int. J. Biochem. Cell. Biol.* **2005**, *37*, 2169–2179. [CrossRef]

36. Cruz-Jentoft, A.J.; Baeyens, J.P.; Bauer, J.M.; Boirie, Y.; Cederholm, T.; Landi, F.; Martin, F.C.; Michel, J.-P.; Rolland, Y.; Schneider, S.M.; et al. Sarcopenia: European consensus on definition and diagnosis. *Age Ageing* **2010**, *39*, 412–423. [CrossRef]

37. Van Der Werf, A.; Dekker, I.M.; Meijerink, M.R.; Wierdsma, N.J.; De Van Der Schueren, M.A.E.; Langius, J.A.E. Skeletal muscle analyses: Agreement between non-contrast and contrast CT scan measurements of skeletal muscle area and mean muscle attenuation. *Clin. Physiol. Funct. Imaging* **2018**, *38*, 366–372. [CrossRef]

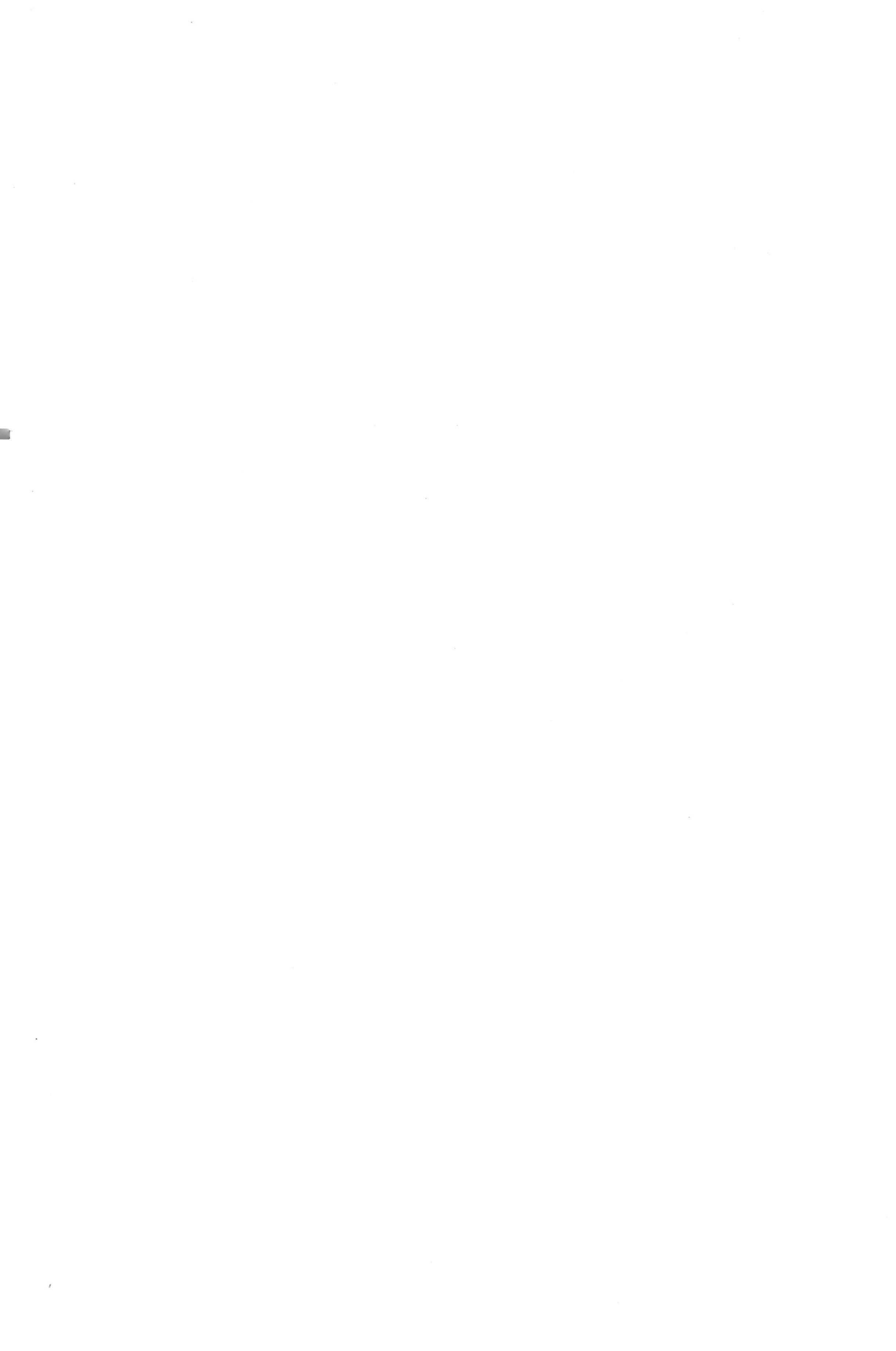

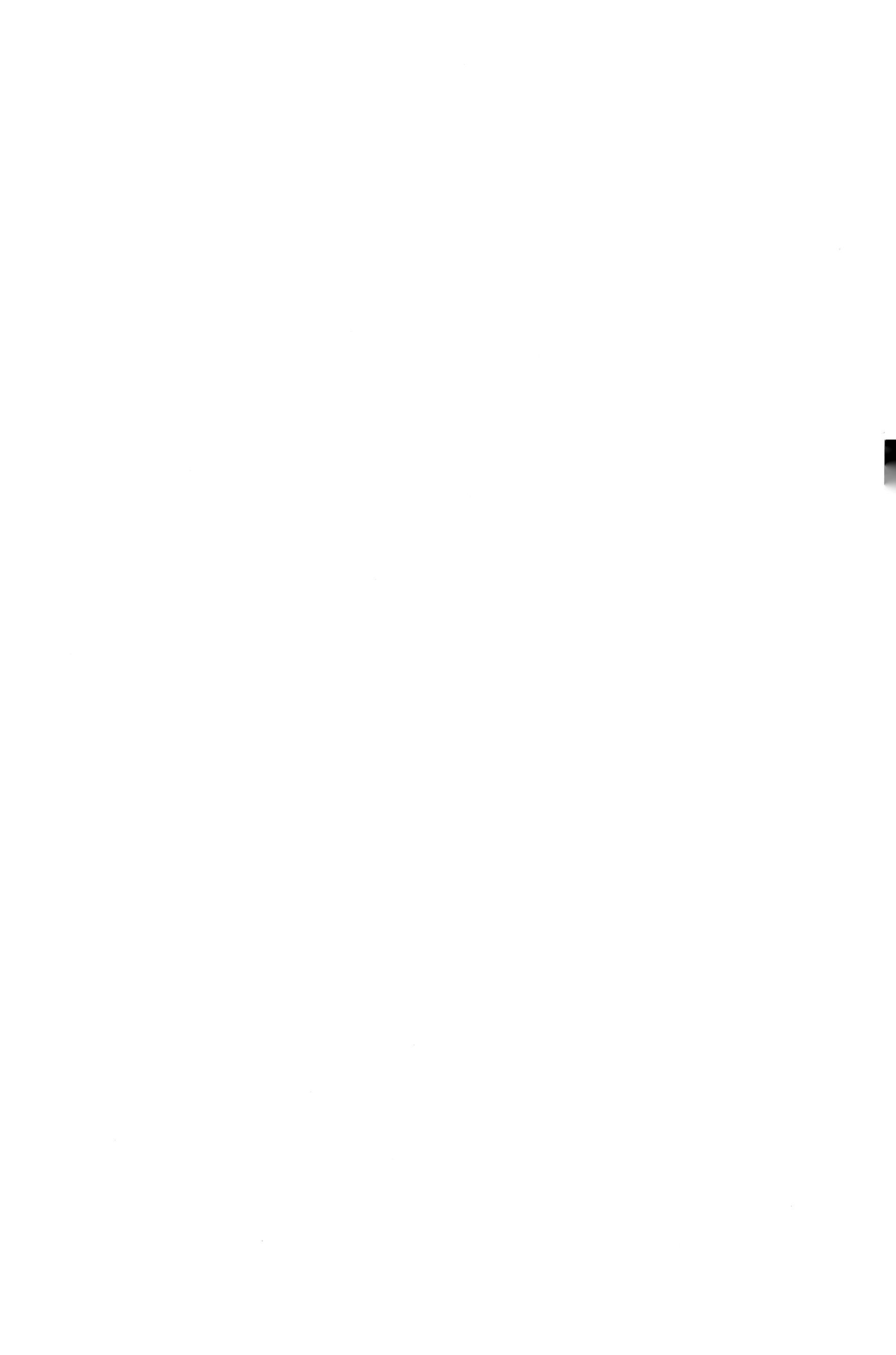

MDPI

St. Alban-Anlage 66

4052 Basel

Switzerland

Tel. +41 61 683 77 34

Fax +41 61 302 89 18

www.mdpi.com

Journal of Clinical Medicine Editorial Office

E-mail: jcm@mdpi.com

www.mdpi.com/journal/jcm

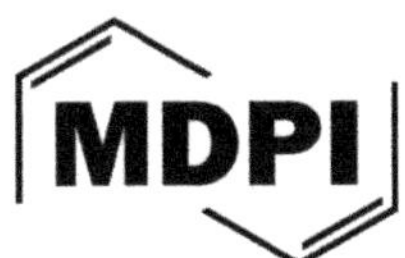

* 9 7 8 3 0 3 6 5 8 3 9 2 1 *